MILD TO MODERATE PSORIASIS

MILD TO MODERATE PSORIASIS

THIRD EDITION

Edited by

John Y. M. Koo, MD
Department of Dermatology, University of California at San Francisco

Ethan C. Levin, MD
Department of Dermatology, University of California at San Francisco

Argentina Leon, MD
Department of Dermatology, University of California at San Francisco

Jashin J. Wu, MD, FAAD
Department of Dermatology, Kaiser Permanente Medical Center, Los Angeles

Mark G. Lebwohl, MD
Department of Dermatology, Mt Sinai School of Medicine, New York

CRC Press
Taylor & Francis Group
Boca Raton London New York

CRC Press is an imprint of the
Taylor & Francis Group, an **informa** business

CRC Press
Taylor & Francis Group
6000 Broken Sound Parkway NW, Suite 300
Boca Raton, FL 33487-2742

Printed on acid-free paper
Version Date: 20140206

International Standard Book Number-13: 978-1-4822-1508-3 (Hardback)

Library of Congress Cataloging-in-Publication Data

Mild to moderate psoriasis / edited by John Y.M. Koo, Ethan C. Levin, Argentina Leon, Jashin J. Wu, Mark G. Lebwohl. -- Third edition.
p. ; cm.
Includes bibliographical references and index.
ISBN 978-1-4822-1508-3 (hardcover : alk. paper)
I. Koo, John Y. M., editor of compilation. II. Levin, Ethan, editor of compilation. III. Leon, Argentina, editor of compilation. IV. Wu, Jashin J. editor of compilation. V. Lebwohl, Mark, editor of compilation.
[DNLM: 1. Psoriasis--therapy. WR 205]

RL321
616.5'26--dc23 2013044937

Visit the Taylor & Francis Web site at
http://www.taylorandfrancis.com

and the CRC Press Web site at
http://www.crcpress.com

CONTENTS

CONTRIBUTORS

April Armstrong
Department of Dermatology
University of Colorado Denver
Anschutz Medical Campus
Denver, Colorado

Daniel C. Butler
University of Arizona College of Medicine
Tucson, Arizona

Maya G. Debbaneh
University of California, Irvine
School of Medicine
Irvine, California

Shannon Famenini
David Geffen School of Medicine at UCLA
Los Angeles, California

Steven R. Feldman
Department of Dermatology
Center for Dermatology Research
Wake Forest School of Medicine
Winston-Salem, North Carolina

Whitney A. Fisk
University of California, Davis
School of Medicine
Sacramento, California

Sarah Fitzmaurice
Department of Dermatology
University of California, Davis
Medical Center
Sacramento, California

Rianne M. J. P. Gerritsen
Department of Dermatology
Radboud University Medical Centre
Nijmegen, The Netherlands

Alice B. Gottlieb
Department of Dermatology
Tufts Medical Center
Boston, Massachusetts

Rishu Gupta
Keck School of Medicine of University of Southern California
Los Angeles, California

Iltefat Hamzavi
Department of Dermatology
Henry Ford Hospital
Detroit, Michigan

Judith Hong
Department of Dermatology
University of California, San Francisco
San Francisco, California

Monica Huynh
Chicago College of Osteopathic Medicine
Chicago, Illinois

Holly A. Kerr
Department of Dermatology
Henry Ford Hospital
Detroit, Michigan

Ashley A. Keyes
Department of Dermatology
Weill Cornell Medical College
New York, New York

Marloes M. Kleinpenning
Department of Dermatology
Radboud University Medical Centre
Nijmegen, The Netherlands

John Y. M. Koo
Department of Dermatology
Psoriasis and Skin Treatment Center
University of California, San Francisco
Medical Center
San Francisco, California

Chrystal A. Landry
Department of Dermatology
Mount Sinai School of Medicine
New York, New York

Mark G. Lebwohl
Department of Dermatology
Mount Sinai School of Medicine
New York, New York

Chai Sue Lee
Kaiser Permanente Medical Group
Milpitas, California

Robert A. Lee
Department of Medicine (Dermatology)
University of California, San Diego
San Diego, California

Argentina Leon
Department of Dermatology
Psoriasis and Skin Treatment Center
University of California, San Francisco
Medical Center
San Francisco, California

Ethan C. Levin
Department of Dermatology
Psoriasis and Skin Treatment Center
University of California, San Francisco
Medical Center
San Francisco, California

Mio Nakamura
Wayne State University School of
Medicine
Detroit, Michigan

Maithily A. Nendedkar-Thomas
Professional Dermatology Care PC
Reston, Virginia

Gabriele B. Poindexter
Department of Dermatology
University of North Carolina
Chapel Hill, North Carolina

Eric Y. Sako
David Geffen School of Medicine at UCLA
Los Angeles, California

Laura F. Sandoval
Department of Dermatology
Center for Dermatology Research
Wake Forest School of Medicine
Winston-Salem, North Carolina

Richard K. Scher
Department of Dermatology
Weill Cornell Medical College
New York, New York

Peter C. M. van de Kerkhof
Department of Dermatology
Radboud University Medical Centre
Nijmegen, The Netherlands

Abby S. Van Voorhees
Department of Dermatology
Hospital of the University of Pennsylvania
Philadelphia, Pennsylvania

Lara Wine-Lee
Department of Dermatology
Hospital of the University of Pennsylvania
Philadelphia, Pennsylvania

Jashin J. Wu
Department of Dermatology
Kaiser Permanente Medical Center
Los Angeles, California

Chapter 1

Introduction

Mark G. Lebwohl

Our knowledge about the pathogenesis of psoriasis and our treatments for psoriasis continue to progress at an extraordinary pace. With the introduction of ustekinumab, the importance of interleukin (IL)-23 in the development of psoriasis was identified which, in turn, lead to the discovery of the importance of the T-helper (Th)-17 cell. Multiple new therapies, including antibodies directed against IL-23, IL-17A, and the IL-17A receptor, have been developed based on this understanding of the pathogenesis of psoriasis.

The importance of new topical therapy for psoriasis is even greater than before. The new systemic therapies in development for psoriasis convert severe disease to mild disease in a majority of patients, a change that is amenable to topical therapy. Many of the systemic therapies work well, but they are slow. Recent studies have shown that patients treated with etanercept and adalimumab respond more quickly when they are concomitantly treated with topical therapies.

Unfortunately, advances in topical therapy lag behind the exciting new developments in systemic treatments. Some new topical therapies are in development and the efficacy of older topical therapies have been enhanced. For example, vehicles have been advanced. Previously, only triamcinolone acetonide was available in spray form. Now, clobetasol and desoximetasone are both available as sprays. The combination of calcipotriene and betamethasone dipropionate has been available in an ointment form for years. Most recently, a suspension has been approved for the scalp and body. Previously, there were only a few topical corticosteroids approved for pediatric use, but in recent years, fluticasone lotion and hydrocortisone butyrate lotion have also been approved for use in pediatrics. There are no new topical calcineurin inhibitors, but much information is available about the safety of calcineurin inhibitors, thereby reducing some of the concerns that emerged when a black box warning was added to the package inserts of tacrolimus ointment and pimecrolimus cream. Both of these agents have been successfully used for psoriasis of the face and intertriginous sites, but neither of them is approved for psoriasis. Numerous topical vitamin D analogs and topical tazarotene are still available for psoriasis. Topical tar preparations and anthralin are still in use. In terms of new agents, topical Janus kinase inhibitors and a combination product consisting of calcipotriene and nicotinamide are in development.

For localized disease that is refractory to topical therapy, targeted ultraviolet B (UVB) phototherapy using the excimer laser has been highly effective. There are now forms of phototherapy that use fine fiber optic cables to deliver narrow band UVB to the scalp, and both narrowband and broadband UVB are still widely used for disease that is refractory to topical therapy.

Although our treatments for mild to moderate psoriasis are better than those in the past, more treatments are still needed. Much of the new information about topical therapies involves their use in combination with the new systemic therapies that have been developed.

In the introduction to the second edition of *Mild to Moderate Psoriasis*, I stated that "we will continue to look for the perfect treatment—a therapy that works for everyone and has no side effects." Although we are still looking for that therapy, we certainly have a lot to offer our patients today.

Chapter 2

General Approach to Psoriasis Treatment

Laura F. Sandoval and Steven R. Feldman

INTRODUCTION

Psoriasis is a complex disease to manage. It may present with wide-ranging severity, affecting vastly the different parts of the body. Very limited areas to very diffuse generalized disease can be present, and the character of the lesions may vary from minimal redness to thick scaly red plaques. The various presentations add to the complexity in choosing the mode of treatment.

Adding to the complexity of the treatment is the availability of a host of different topical, phototherapy, and systemic treatment options. Matching the appropriate treatment with the presentation of the disease is an art. Adding to the complexity of this art is the fact that it is not just lesions that are being treated, but a patient and patients' responses to the lesions vary considerably. Patients also differ in their concern about side effects and the way they tolerate different topical preparations. These variations can be dramatic. In nearly all patients, psoriasis affects the quality of life, including social interactions. The overall impact of psoriasis on quality of life—particularly the effect of psoriasis on social interactions—must be addressed. Management of psoriasis should also include educating patients about certain comorbidities they are at higher risk for so that they can be identified and managed.

Step I: Address Patients' Psychosocial Needs

The first step in managing all patients with psoriasis is to address their psychosocial needs. This approach is fundamental to effective psoriasis treatment. Addressing psychosocial issues helps to establish a strong working relationship between the physician and the patient. By doing so, patients are likely to be more compliant with treatment and should have better health outcomes.

Managing psychosocial needs starts before any physician–patient interaction. Patients should arrive to a practice that presents a caring, competent environment. Parking should be convenient; the check-in window should be open and orderly, with friendly staff; and the waiting room should be clean and well maintained. Initial physician–patient interactions are important in managing psychosocial needs. Physicians should sit within touching distance of the patient. While examining the lesions and talking to the patient, the physician should palpate lesions, with appropriate attention to cultural and patient preferences. While doing so, the physician can remark, "Wow, these lesions are really thick." The purpose of the palpation is not to determine the thickness of the lesions but to communicate to patients that they are touchable. Patients with psoriasis feel isolated from others because of their disease, and by touching the lesions, the physician communicates to the patients that they should not be afraid of having contact with other people. Dr. J. Lamar Calloway, long-time dermatologist at Duke University, would communicate to patients that psoriasis is not an infectious condition; by taking the hand, he would palpate patients psoriasis and rub his own face with it while saying "this is nothing I can catch from you."

While sitting close to the patient, the physician should also proactively ask patients a few questions about their disease. These questions are not likely to change what the physician will prescribe, but they may change how the patient views the doctor, how the patient views the treatment, and ultimately how adherent the patient will be to the treatment recommendations. There are many things about psoriasis that are bothersome to patients, and asking questions about a few of these topics helps communicate to the patient that the dermatologist understands the disease and what the patient is going through. A physician might ask if the itching has been bothersome, if past treatments have been messy or ineffective, or if psychosocial concerns have been an issue. Simply asking a few questions (and listening intently) helps further the bond between the physician and the patient.

Psoriasis affects patients' quality of life and has been associated with a higher risk of depression. Severity or extent of disease does not predict risk of depression in patients with psoriasis [1,2]. Patients are also at increased risk for sleep disturbances, sexual dysfunctions, anxiety, and suicidal ideation [3,4]. Establishing a good physician–patient relationship may enhance open dialog about psychosocial issues and allow physicians to better identify patients experiencing depression and in need of expertise outside the scope of dermatology. Managing psychosocial issues is important not only for the emotional well-being of the patient but also because these stressors can exacerbate psoriasis.

Step II: Educating Patients about Comorbidities

In addition to educating patients about their disease, there are certain comorbidities associated with psoriasis that patients should be aware of. Besides psychosocial issues, an increased risk of cardiovascular disease has been established, including increased risk of myocardial infarction and stroke in mild to severe psoriasis [5,6]. Psoriasis patients also have a higher prevalence of type 2 diabetes mellitus and metabolic syndrome [7–9]. In both conditions, the association is greatest in patients with severe psoriasis.

Although there are no current screening guidelines for these comorbidities in psoriasis patients, it is important to inquire about patients' overall health and encourage health awareness and routine exams with a primary care provider. When appropriate, a discussion about a patient's weight may be warranted, especially because patients with psoriasis have a higher prevalence of obesity, and obesity is a factor in all these comorbidities [10]. A discussion of the risks of these comorbidities benefits the patient while also strengthening the physician–patient relationship by showing that the physician cares about the patient.

No health care provider has enough time to explain to patients everything they would like to know about psoriasis. All of us, however, have the time to encourage patients to join the National Psoriasis Foundation (www.psoriasis.org) or similar organizations in other countries, such as European Psoriasis Organisation (EUROPSO) (www.europso.eu) or International

Federation of Psoriasis Associations (IFPA) (www.ifpa-pso.org). The Psoriasis Foundation and other psoriasis support organizations provide numerous benefits to patients. First, these organizations help patients to feel less isolated. Second, the foundation helps educate patients about available treatment options. Resources on access to health care and financial assistance programs for some treatments are also available. Third, information is provided on comorbidities associated with psoriasis. Fourth, the foundation encourages patients to be compliant with their dermatologists' recommendations. If that were not enough, the foundation also empowers patients to work toward a cure for the disease.

The National Psoriasis Foundation offers a variety of brochures that are very useful for educating patients about specific treatment options. The Psoriasis Foundation periodical for patients entitled *Psoriasis Advance* helps patients answer many of the psychosocial issues that physicians may not feel comfortable addressing, for example, what to do if the lifeguard says you cannot go in the pool, what to do when people point and ask questions, or other social situations. Communication among members is very supportive. Patients can be encouraged to join the Psoriasis Foundation by simply visiting the website at www.psoriasis.org, writing to the foundation (6600 SW 92nd Avenue, Suite 300, Portland, OR 97223, USA), or calling (1-800-723-9166). Anyone can join, even without paying, although there is a recommended donation of US$35 (to cover mailing costs).

Step III: Categorization of Psoriasis

Once psychosocial issues are addressed, further treatment planning is dependent on determining whether patients have relatively localized disease suitable for topical therapy or more extensive disease where phototherapy or systemic treatments will be used. This book focuses on the treatment of people with relatively localized disease. Formerly, the common categorization scheme of mild, moderate, and severe psoriasis was used. However, these three categories do not correspond well to treatment decision making. Typically, one would hear categorizations of mild to moderate versus moderate to severe psoriasis for treatment purposes. Mild to moderate psoriasis tends to refer to patients with relatively localized psoriasis. The moderate to severe category tends to refer to the patient with more generalized disease or disease that is otherwise disabling. Treatment of this latter group has been covered in an excellent textbook entitled *Moderate to Severe Psoriasis* [11]. This chapter and this book focus on the treatment of the patient with mild to moderate, or localized psoriasis.

GENERAL CONSIDERATIONS IN THE TREATMENT OF LOCALIZED PSORIASIS

The treatment of localized psoriasis focuses on local treatments, predominately topical treatments, although certain localized phototherapy and intralesional injection treatments are also used. For topical treatments, multiple agents are available, including tar, anthralin, topical corticosteroids, topical vitamin D and vitamin A analogs, topical immunomodulators (e.g., tacrolimus and pimecrolimus), and keratolytics (e.g., salicylic acid). Whichever of these agents are chosen, a primary consideration determining patients' outcomes will be patients' adherence to the topical treatment regimen.

When patients with psoriasis have been asked about their adherence to topical therapy, approximately 40% reported nonadherence [12,13]. Adherence to topical therapy is lower than with other treatments, including oral therapy, phototherapy, and biologic therapy [14,15]. Patients may not even fill the prescription; one study reported that only about 50% of psoriasis prescriptions were filled [16]. The reasons for poor adherence to treatment are manifold. Frustration with medication efficacy, inconvenience, and fear of side effects are among the most important reasons patients do not use their medication as directed. Other factors affecting patients' use of medication include cost, the medication feeling unpleasant, unclear instructions, and directions that are too complicated [12].

Even when patients have the medicine, they may not use it well. In a clinical trial that assessed adherence using both patient diaries and electronic monitors, psoriasis patients vastly overstated their true use of the treatment [17]. Patients are not always truthful with their doctors about their adherence to topical therapy. Topical therapy is time-consuming and messy. Over time, use of topical therapy decreases. Chronic diseases such as psoriasis are frustrating and wear on people over time. The treatment of these diseases, particularly topical therapy, can be frustrating, too.

Outcomes of localized psoriasis treatment can be improved by encouraging better adherence. There are many practical measures physicians can take to improve a patient's use of his or her medication [18]. First, as discussed above, physicians should establish a strong working relationship with the patient. The patient should also be involved in treatment decision making. Vehicles that the patients do not mind applying should be chosen. Although it was commonly thought that ointments are more effective, less messy vehicles may be able to deliver active drugs just as well as traditional ointments, and better adherence with a nonmessy product may actually lead to greater efficacy than is seen with ointments. There is generally one vehicle that delivers topical therapy better than all the others—the vehicle that a particular patient is willing to use.

Patients are also reluctant to apply topical therapy for long periods before they see improvement. Fast-acting agents should be used, especially initially. The sequential therapy approach addresses this need. Sequential therapy consists of using stronger, faster acting but potentially more risky treatments early in the course of therapy and then transitioning to slower acting but safer treatments for the long-term maintenance of the disease. This approach has the advantage of helping patients see early in the course of therapy that treatments work, thereby improving patients' compliance. The complexity of sequential treatment may make it more difficult for patients to adhere to treatment; giving patients clear, written instructions may help. Other approaches are to use the stronger topical agents such as clobetasol-containing topical corticosteroid products initially and then use them intermittently as needed to control the disease.

Another way to help improve patients' use of medication is to encourage patients to return to the office or at least contact the physician shortly after treatment has begun, for example, in one to two weeks. Patients' adherence to medication improves around the time of follow-up visits, a pattern referred to as "white coat compliance" [17]. A long interval before a return visit may lead to poor compliance if the patient feels that it will be impossible to be adherent for that length of time. By seeing patients back in just a week, patients are more likely to use their medication over that week, thereby seeing the potential benefits the treatment offers. Once patients have seen that the treatment actually works, they will use the treatment intermittently knowing that it will be effective for them. A very short interval between initiation of treatment and the first return visit may be especially important for patients with scalp psoriasis, because use of topical scalp treatment regimens is exceedingly time consuming and difficult.

Some patients have disease that is poorly responsive to all attempts at management with self-administered treatments. Such resistance may not be due to defective steroid receptors but may be due to exceedingly poor adherence to treatment. In these instances, the use of physician-administered treatments may be appropriate. Adherence can be ensured with intralesional injection treatment. Office-based localized phototherapy, or office-based application of topical agents, may be helpful alternatives.

CONCLUSIONS

Treating mild to moderate psoriasis (relatively localized psoriasis) can be frustrating for both the patient and the physician. Much of this frustration can be alleviated by addressing patients' psychosocial concerns upfront. All patients with psoriasis should be encouraged to join the National Psoriasis Foundation or similar patient advocacy groups. These organizations help reduce patients' isolation and increase their knowledge about treatments, ultimately resulting in improved adherence to the physician-recommended treatment regimen.

Topical treatments are safe and effective for most patients with mild to moderate psoriasis. Getting patients to actually use the treatment is a critical component in maximizing topical treatment efficacy. Patients should be encouraged to participate in the treatment planning process, choosing vehicles, and other treatment characteristics (e.g., dosing) that fit the patients' lifestyles. Using rapidly acting agents initially and encouraging patients to come in for an early follow-up visit may help improve the compliance. The resulting improvement should help reduce the frustration of psoriasis on both the patient and the physician.

ACKNOWLEDGMENTS

Center for Dermatology Research is funded by an unrestricted educational grant from Galderma Laboratories, LP. Dr. Feldman has also received support from Abbott, Amgen, Anacor Pharmaceuticals, Astellas, Caremark, Causa Research, Celgene, Centocor Ortho Biotech, Coria Laboratories, Dermatology Foundation, Doak, Gerson Lehrman Group, Hanall Pharmaceutical, Informa Healthcare, Kikaku, Leo Pharma, Medical Pharmaceutical, Medicis, Medscape, Merck, Merz, Novan, Novartis, Peplin, Pfizer, Pharmaderm, Photomedex, Reader's Digest, Sanofi-Aventis, SkinMedica, Steifel/GSK, Taro, U.S. Department of Justice, and Xlibris.

REFERENCES

1. Kimball AB, Jacobson C, Weiss S, et al. The psychosocial burden of psoriasis. *Am J Clin Dermatol* 2005; 6: 383–392.
2. Finzi A, Colombo D, Caputo A, et al. Psychological distress and coping strategies in patients with psoriasis: the PSYCHAE Study. *J Eur Acad Dermatol Venereol* 2007; 21: 1161–1169.

3. Rieder E, Tausk F. Psoriasis, a model of dermatologic psychosomatic disease: psychiatric implications and treatments. *Int J Dermatol* 2012; 51: 12–26.
4. Shutty BG, West C, Huang KE, et al. Sleep disturbances in psoriasis. *Dermatol Online J* 2013; 19: 1.
5. Mehta NN, Yu Y, Pinnelas R, et al. Attributable risk estimate of severe psoriasis on major cardiovascular events. *Am J Med* 2011; 124: 775.
6. Armstrong EJ, Harskamp CT, Armstrong AW. Psoriasis and major adverse cardiovascular events: a systematic review and meta-analysis of observational studies. *J Am Heart Assoc* 2013; 2: e000062.
7. Armstrong AW, Harskamp CT, Armstrong EJ. Psoriasis and the risk of diabetes mellitus: a systematic review and meta-analysis. *JAMA Dermatol* 2013; 149: 84–91.
8. Armstrong AW, Harskamp CT, Armstrong EJ. Psoriasis and metabolic syndrome: a systematic review and meta-analysis of observational studies. *J Am Acad Dermatol* 2013; 68: 654–662.
9. Gelfand JM, Yeung H. Metabolic syndrome in patients with psoriatic disease. *J Rheumatol Suppl* 2012; 89: 24–28.
10. Herron MD, Hinckley M, Hoffman MS, et al. Impact of obesity and smoking on psoriasis presentation and management. *Arch Dermatol* 2005; 141: 1527–1534.
11. Koo J, Lee CS, Lebwohl MG, et al. *Moderate to Severe Psoriasis*. 3rd edn. New York, NY: Informa Health Care; 2009.
12. Brown KK, Rehmus WE, Kimball AB. Determining the relative importance of patient motivations for nonadherence to topical corticosteroid therapy in psoriasis. *J Am Acad Dermatol* 2006; 55: 607–613.
13. Richards HL, Fortune DG, O'Sullivan TM, et al. Patients with psoriasis and their compliance with medication. *J Am Acad Dermatol* 1999; 41: 581–583.
14. Bewley A, Burrage DM, Ersser SJ, et al. Identifying individual psychosocial and adherence support needs in patients with psoriasis: a multinational two-stage qualitative and quantitative study. *J Eur Acad Dermatol Venereol* 2013.
15. Chan SA, Hussain F, Lawson LG, et al. Factors affecting adherence to treatment of psoriasis: comparing biologic therapy to other modalities. *J Dermatolog Treat* 2013; 24: 64–69.
16. Storm A, Andersen SE, Benfeldt E, et al. One in 3 prescriptions are never redeemed: primary nonadherence in an outpatient clinic. *J Am Acad Dermatol* 2008; 59: 27–33.
17. Carroll CL, Feldman SR, Camacho FT, et al. Adherence to topical therapy decreases during the course of an 8-week psoriasis clinical trial: commonly used methods of measuring adherence to topical therapy overestimate actual use. *J Am Acad Dermatol* 2004; 51: 212–216.
18. Feldman SR. *Practical Ways to Improve Patients' Treatment Outcomes*. Winston-Salem, NC: Medical Quality Enhancement Corporation; 2008.

Chapter 3

General Guidelines for Administration of Topical Agents

Shannon Famenini, Eric Y. Sako, and Jashin J. Wu

INTRODUCTION

Psoriasis is a chronic, immune-mediated skin disease that affects 2%–4% of the world population [1]. In a survey of dermatologists who belong to the American Academy of Dermatology, approximately 70% of psoriasis patients were treated with topical therapies and 30% with phototherapy and systemic therapy [2]. However, according to a systematic analysis in 2011, almost two-thirds of topical prescriptions were written without sufficient information for patients to manage their psoriasis correctly [3]. Another questionnaire that evaluated adherence to topical regimens highlighted the importance of giving patient information in enhancing the efficacy of topical therapies [4]. In fact, patients' needs can be better met by providing more information on the side effects, proper use, and efficacy of topical treatments [5].

Topical therapies are usually used as first-line treatments; they are safe and effective, easy to administer, and cost-effective. However, topical treatments may not result in complete clearance of psoriatic lesions [6]. In the past 35 years, new advances in the development of systemic therapy and phototherapy have allowed for partial to complete clearance in some psoriatic patients.

In this chapter, we discuss the various factors to be considered when choosing whether to use topical agents or systemic therapies. We then discuss different issues to be considered before prescribing topical agents for psoriasis. We hope these general guidelines for the use of topical therapies will help physicians choose the optimal topical therapy for their patients.

ASPECTS OF PSORIASIS

Body Surface Area

Patients can be classified as having mild, moderate, or severe psoriasis based on their body surface area (BSA); the BSA value can then be used to determine a treatment regimen. The patient's palms, including the fingers and the thumb (i.e., from the wrist to the tip of the fingers), constitute approximately 1% of the total BSA as measured in clinical trials. According to the National Psoriasis Foundation, 0%–3% BSA is mild disease, 3%–10% BSA is moderate disease, and >10% BSA is severe disease. Patients with mild disease can generally be managed with topical treatments. For patients with severe psoriasis, the application of topical agents would be too time consuming, impractical, and expensive. Furthermore, it would be difficult to apply a sufficient quantity to all affected areas. Also, some topical medications, such as topical corticosteroids, calcipotriene, and calcitriol, have safety limitations that reduce the amount of drug applied. Moderate and severe psoriasis are usually treated with systemic treatments or phototherapy in addition to topical agents. It is important to note that BSA does not take into account body location or the emotional impact on the patient, factors that may warrant more aggressive therapy.

Psoriasis Area Severity Index

The Psoriasis Area and Severity Index (PASI) is a quantitative measurement of psoriasis severity that combines BSA with the degree of erythema, scaling, and thickness (induration). However, the PASI is generally too cumbersome to be used in the general practice setting and is mostly used by clinical trials as required by the Food and Drug Administration (FDA). In fact, a systematic review of randomized clinical trials showed a high degree of correlation between the PASI and the Physician's Global Assessment (PGA) score, although the PASI score is more detailed [7]. Please see previously published work [8–11] for details on using the PASI. Recent use of PASI training videos is an effective tool in improving accuracy of PASI scoring among dermatologists [12].

A PASI score of 72.0 correlates to 100% BSA with a score of 4 for erythema, scaling, and thickness. It has been suggested that PASI < 7.0 should correspond to mild plaque psoriasis, PASI of 7.0–12.0 to moderate psoriasis, and PASI > 12.0 to severe psoriasis [13].

PASI is also used to measure relative clinical changes that are often endpoints used in clinical trials. A PASI50 improvement indicates 50% improvement in the PASI score compared with the same patient's baseline PASI score. PASI75 and PASI50 at a future time point are commonly measured endpoints for efficacy [14], and PASI75 at week 12 is often required by the FDA to demonstrate efficacy. A systematic review of 13 randomized controlled trials demonstrated that PASI75 also translates to significant quality-of-life improvements as measured by the Dermatology Life Quality Index (DLQI) [15].

Location on Body and Types of Psoriasis

Location of psoriasis as well as the ease of therapeutic response can also affect psoriasis therapy. Because the face is often the most noticeable region of the body, more aggressive treatments may be applied. Also, a person who is concerned about public exposure of their psoriasis may wish to have these areas more aggressively treated. However, topical corticosteroids should be used carefully and sparingly on the face because the skin is relatively thin and side effects such as acne or rosacea may result. The eyelids are another region where topical corticosteroids should be applied with care.

Inverse psoriasis affects intertriginous areas, where natural occlusion of skin planes increases the potency of topical corticosteroids 10–100 times [16]. Potent topical corticosteroids should be avoided because the risk of skin atrophy is greatly increased. For short-term treatment, low-to-mid potency topical corticosteroids are recommended. For long-term treatment, calcipotriene, calcitriol, tacrolimus, or pimecrolimus is recommended [17].

In palmar–plantar psoriasis, the thickness of the skin on the palms and soles decreases the penetration of topical steroids into the skin. Thus, although these areas may represent a small BSA, systemic therapy or phototherapy in addition to topical agents may be necessary.

Response to Therapy

When patients with mild psoriasis fail to improve with topical therapies, the use of phototherapy, systemic treatments, or a combination is warranted. Sometimes, the psoriasis can be emotionally and socially disabling, thereby necessitating more aggressive therapy. Furthermore, as mentioned, treatment with systemic therapies in adjunct to topical steroids can greatly enhance quality of life in patients experiencing involvement of more sensitive regions such as the face.

Presence or Absence of Psoriatic Arthritis

According to the National Psoriasis Foundation, 10%–30% of people with psoriasis also develop psoriatic arthritis [18]. Although psoriasis affecting the skin can be cleared without any residual manifestations, psoriatic arthritis causes irreversible bone changes. Topical therapies have not been shown to have any efficacy in improving the symptoms of pain or slowing down of joint destruction in psoriatic arthritis. Biologic therapy, including adalimumab, etanercept, and infliximab, reduces signs and symptoms, improves physical function and inhibits progression of structural damage in patients with psoriatic arthritis [19,20]. In September 2013, the U.S. Food and Drug Administration approved ustekinumab for the treatment of adult patients with active psoriatic arthritis.

Methotrexate is also effective in improving the clinical features of the disease. Although the coadministration of methotrexate with tumor necrosis factor (TNF) inhibitors resulted in similar responses in a longitudinal observational study, methotrexate was shown to increase TNF inhibitor drug survival, defined as duration and rate of adherence to TNF inhibitor treatment [21]. Thus, if a patient has mild psoriasis but is also suffering from debilitating psoriatic arthritis, he or she should be considered for treatment with systemic therapies, such as adalimumab, etanercept, infliximab, or methotrexate.

MEDICATIONS

Several topical therapies are available (Table 3.1), and a brief overview is presented here. When choosing a topical agent, it is best to take into consideration the side effect profile, efficacy, and appropriate patient selection. The main topical therapies available are topical steroids, calcipotriene, calcitriol, tacrolimus, pimecrolimus, tar-based products, and tazarotene, each of which has quantitative data on efficacy.

Tacrolimus and pimecrolimus are topical immunomodulators that have been tested particularly for inverse psoriasis. They are now occasionally used off-label for moderate psoriasis but are only moderately effective. Recent in vivo and in vitro studies have suggested that tacrolimus-loaded liquid crystalline nanoparticles may be a possible method to increase the effectiveness of this treatment compared with tacrolimus dissolved in propylene glycol [22]. Anthralin and coal tar preparations are older therapies that are less frequently used today because they are messy. Keratolytics such as lactic acid, salicylic acid, and the numerous nonmedicated moisturizers are complementary therapies that help to improve quality-of-life symptoms and are useful for thick scaling areas such as the palms and soles.

TABLE 3.1 Major Topical Therapies Used to Treat Psoriasis

Topical steroids
Calcipotriene/calcitriol
Tazarotene
Anthralin
Crude coal tar
Lactic acid
Salicylic acid
Pimecrolimus
Tacrolimus
Nonmedicated moisturizers

Moisturizers (lotions, creams, and ointments) in general are helpful for dry scaly skin and in dry climates. Lotion preparations are more useful for scalp and intertriginous areas, whereas thick creams and ointments are suited for trunk and extremities. Fissured psoriatic lesions that appear on palms and soles may benefit from thick ointments or petroleum, whereas alcohol-based solutions would cause burning. Patients with psoriasis should be encouraged to use a moisturizer regularly as part of dry skin care.

Algorithm of Which Topical Agent to Select

The selection of which topical medication to use initially is a matter of choice, experience, cost, and prior patient responses to these therapies. A prescribing algorithm is presented here.

First-Line Topical Therapies

1. Topical corticosteroids: choice of potency depends on severity and location of disease.
    - Range of potencies from weak (class 7) to moderate to potent to superpotent (class 1) (seven classes of potency).
    - It is the authors' suggestion that physicians new to the use of topical corticosteroids select one steroid from one of the weak, moderate, and potent classes to learn what formulations are available (e.g., lotion, cream, ointment), packaging sizes (30 g [1 oz], 60 g, 120-g tubes), and generic/brand names. This approach will facilitate writing prescriptions and providing an adequate amount of medication for the extent of BSA that is to be treated.
    - Weak potencies for children.
    - Weak-to-moderate potencies for face to minimize risks of skin atrophy.
    - Potent-to-superpotent strength for trunk/extremities.
    - Lotion, foam, solution, or gel formulation is usually preferred for scalp.
    - Lotion or cream is usually preferred for intertriginous areas.
    - For treatment of nail psoriasis, 8% clobetasol nail lacquer can be considered [23].
    - Clobetasol propionate 0.05% spray for up to four weeks is effective and well tolerated in scalp psoriasis [24].
    - All classes of topical steroids have generic preparations to decrease cost.

- If used correctly, side effect profile for steroids is minimal.
  One of the disappointing aspects of using topical steroids is its relatively limited duration of effectiveness, known as tachyphylaxis. Tachyphylaxis refers to the development of resistance or loss of efficacy over a period of two to four months. However, some studies suggest that tachyphylaxis may be due to loss of compliance over time instead of to a reduction in efficacy [25].

2. Calcipotriene and calcitriol
   - Cream and solution preparations used twice daily (BID).
   - Slow effectiveness—approximately two months for best effect.
   - Maintains effectiveness without tachyphylaxis in contrast to topical steroids.
   - Minimal side effect profile.
   - Expensive, proportional to amount of use and BID application.
   - A synergistic response occurs when used in combination with topical steroids.
3. Tazarotene
   - Tazarotene is a unique retinoid available as a gel or cream in 0.05% and 0.1% concentrations.
   - It is applied once daily.
   - Irritation is the main side effect.
   - It has a longer remission time compared with topical steroids.
4. Combination topical therapies
   - Medium-to-potent topical corticosteroids when used in combination with either calcipotriene/calcitriol [26–30] or tazarotene [31] preparations will produce a higher response level, approximating 70%–90% in some clinical trials.
   - These combinations may be most useful in patients with difficult but limited lesions of psoriasis.
   - Once-daily application of the two-compound formulation of calcipotriol and betamethasone has shown significant improvements in treatment of scalp psoriasis and has been demonstrated to be more effective than either of its individual components [27,29].

Amount to Dispense

The amount of topical therapy that should be used is directly proportional to the BSA involvement. Generally, approximately 2 g covers the face or hands, 3 g covers one arm or the anterior or posterior trunk, 4 g covers one leg, and 30 g (1 oz) covers the entire body. Thus, if a patient's arms were affected, for 30 days the patient would require 180 g (6 oz) of medication in one prescription. Unfortunately, the prescribed amount of topical agents is frequently too little.

Type of Vehicle

Topical therapies are available as creams, foams, gels, liquid solutions, lotions, ointments, and drug-impregnated tapes. The appropriate vehicle depends on the location of the lesions, the patient's symptoms, and the patient's preference. Patient's preference often takes precedence as long as there are no safety concerns. In fact, it has been suggested that taking into account the patient's preference in choosing a delivery system improves patient adherence [32,33]. Thus, choosing a method that patients are more likely to follow is important in successful disease management.

Thicker (ointment) vehicles, such as a petroleum jelly base, are more moisturizing based on a quasi-occlusive effect produced by the ointments. Thus, based on the same active ingredients, ointments were thought to be stronger than creams, and creams were considered stronger than lotions. Creams spread across the skin easily and quickly, are more quickly absorbed than ointments, and do not produce a greasy effect on clothes. Thus, creams may be more suitable for in the morning when application of the medication may stain clothes, and ointments may be more appropriate for in the evening when patients have more time to apply the medication and are less concerned about staining their clothes. Thus, it is reasonable to prescribe both a cream and an ointment of the same therapy. Recent analyses have challenged the conventional thought that ointments are more effective [34]. In fact, a systematic review of the different formulations for clobetasol propionate showed similar efficacies, again demonstrating how patient preference and compliance are important determinants in selecting the appropriate vehicle for delivery [35].

The symptoms may also guide the vehicle choice. Dry or itchy skin may benefit from an ointment or cream because they are more moisturizing. Thick ointment and petroleum are more beneficial for fissured psoriatic lesions on the palms and soles. The drying effect of gels and foams renders them more suitable for people with oily skin or those who dislike the greasiness of ointments and creams. An alcohol-based vehicle, such as liquid solution or foam, will be painful for those with fissures or cracked lesions.

The location of the psoriasis also affects which vehicle to use. The scalp is especially difficult to treat because the hair blocks direct application to the lesions and prevents patients from using cosmetically unsuitable vehicles such as ointments and creams. Gels, foams, liquid solutions, and lotions are typically the best vehicle for the scalp. However, some African American patients with scalp psoriasis may prefer ointments. In the intertriginous areas of the body, such as axillae, groin, and inframammary folds, a lotion or cream will be more comfortable than an ointment.

Weather or environmental conditions may suggest the appropriate type of vehicle/medication. For example, in a warm and moist climate, lotions and creams will be better tolerated than ointments. The opposite would be true for dry or cold climates.

Patients should be instructed on the correct use of these agents. Most therapies can be applied either on a damp scalp after towel drying or on a dry scalp. It is imperative to instruct the patient on appropriate application so that the agent reaches the scalp lesions and not just the hair. Demonstrating the application in the office may help with compliance. Patients should also be taught that these medicines must be left on the scalp and thus used after a shampoo rather than before. Active medications to the scalp are often applied at night and shampooed out in the morning with standard hair preparations and conditioners as desired. One must also consider that "active" medications in shampoo preparations may be self-defeating because they would be rapidly removed by completing of the shampooing process.

Patients should be instructed for the quantity of topical medications applied to the skin. Basically, one should be rubbing in a thin film to the skin without leaving a thick or visible coating on the surface, which is wasteful and expensive because the excessive medication will be rubbed off by the clothes. Keep in mind that in optimal conditions, only about 1% of the active ingredient, for example, corticosteroid, applied to the skin actually penetrates into the skin. Indeed, topical therapy is not an ideal way to get a drug into the skin. However, it does have the obvious advantage of limiting the drug to only affected areas of the skin in contrast to taking a drug orally. There are vasoconstriction assays with topical steroids that show penetration into the stratum corneum "reservoir." Plastic film occlusion several days after steroid application will still produce vasoconstriction, demonstrating a reservoir effect.

New delivery methods of topical medications have become available for use. Calcitriol is available as an ointment. Calcipotriene is available as an ointment, solution, cream, and as a combination ointment with betamethasone dipropionate. Calcipotriene 0.005% has recently been developed as foam and provides a new therapeutic option for psoriasis patients [36]. Furthermore, a two-compound calcipotriol/betamethasone suspension has been developed to provide an alternative approach for patients who dislike ointments. Clinical trials have shown this formulation to be effective, with few adverse events and rapid onset of action [37].

Some topical agents are most effective when applied twice a day, for example, topical corticosteroids and calcipotriene/calcitriol. The patient who is not happy with a particular vehicle for practical reasons is much less likely to use the agent as directed and may report that the therapy is ineffective when it actually would be effective if used correctly. This behavior may limit the doctor's therapeutic options and force the use of stronger medications. It is best to encourage the patients to use the therapies as directed and to ask their opinion and feedback about the prescribed medicine. Maintaining a good physician–patient relationship, individualized treatment strategy, and adequate return visits are important in ensuring patient compliance and treatment efficacy.

Strength of the Agent

In choosing a topical steroid, it is important to take into account the patient's age. Due to their thinner skin, pediatric and elderly patients are more prone to the side effects of topical corticosteroids. Therefore, it is reasonable to choose a less potent topical corticosteroid in the treatment of these populations.

Techniques to Enhance Topical Therapy

Special tape that is impregnated with steroids (flurandrenolide tape) and produces an occlusive effect can be used when patients have a small number of lesions and are willing to take the time to cut the tape to fit each plaque. Lesions on the extremities may be good candidates for this treatment because they are thick, usually resistant to traditional treatment, and are less likely to develop skin atrophy from the constant contact with corticosteroids.

Occlusion is another technique that is used to enhance topical therapy (corticosteroids in particular). For example, for the patient can apply a low-to medium-class topical steroid and wrap the affected areas with plastic wrap, place gloves over the hands or a shower cap over the feet. One can use a sock or thin cotton glove to keep the plastic in place. Application of corticosteroid under occlusion is only done for a few hours or in the evening. Occlusion produces a greater penetration of the steroid into the skin lesion. Recent study showed that an occlusive hydrogel dressing after the application of calcipotriene/betamethasone dipropionate ointment can result in substantial decreases in PASI compared with application without occlusion. Thus, hydrogel dressings are an effective and safe occlusive option to augment the effects of topical therapy [38].

Extensive use of corticosteroid under occlusion can produce side effects such as atrophy of the skin leading to fragility of the skin and purpura. In past years for severe psoriasis, steroids and occlusion were used extensively or even to the entire body, leading to risks of systemic steroid effects such as damage involving the hypothalamus–pituitary–adrenal (HPA) axis, or the eventual development of pustular psoriasis in some patients. Fortunately, with the advent of many more treatments for moderate to severe psoriasis, extensive steroid/occlusion is rarely used today.

For patients with small, 2.54–10.16-cm (1–4-in.) lesions on the trunk and extremities, a quasi-topical approach would be an intralesional technique using the injection of small doses of corticosteroids, mainly triamcinolone, in an aqueous formulation. The most typical injection formulation is in a vial with a concentration of 10 mg/mL. Using dilutions with normal saline, a concentration of 2.5 mg/mL is prepared in the vial or syringe and injected into the epidermis and upper dermis. As concentrations are increased to 5 or 10 mg/mL, the risk of atrophy in the injection site is increased. The injection approach is often very effective for small, scattered lesions such as on the elbows and knees and can produce a beneficial effect that will last several months.

COMBINATION, ROTATIONAL, AND SEQUENTIAL THERAPY

Patients with more resistant psoriasis may benefit from combination, rotational, or sequential therapy. These techniques are detailed in subsequent chapters, but we present here the general rationale behind each technique. Combination therapy works on the premise of using two medications with different mechanisms of action to maximize efficacy and minimize the side effects of each individual agent. For example, a medication with a rapid onset of action but unfavorable side effect profile can be combined with a slower-acting agent but more favorable side effect profile.

Combination therapy, however, tends to be expensive. Combinations of corticosteroids with calcipotriol are the most extensively studied and offer a safe and effective treatment option [39]. In fact, a meta-analysis comparing the efficacy of vitamin D analogs in combination with topical steroids versus the use of vitamin D analogs alone showed that the combination is more effective and has a better cost per success profile [28]. A combination of calcipotriol/betamethasone dipropionate ointment has been shown to be safe and effective in patients with psoriasis vulgaris [40]. The combination of the two-compound formulation has proven to be especially effective in the treatment of scalp psoriasis [29,31]. Topical therapies have also been used in combination with immunomodulators and phototherapy [41,42].

Rotational therapy decreases cumulative toxicity by switching between medications with differing toxicity profiles. This technique is also commonly used with systemic therapy [43].

Sequential therapy is when medications are used in a set sequence to maximize the initial speed of improvement while minimizing long-term toxicity. The three phases of this technique are the clearing phase, the transitional phase, and the maintenance phase. Although the classic example is halobetasol propionate and calcipotriene, sequential therapy can be performed with any combination of a rapid-acting therapy and a maintenance medication that is safe for the long-term use. The Yin-Yang strategy also proposes a new effective sequential topical therapy with treatment by clobetasol spray for one month followed by calcitriol ointment for the next month [44].

REFERENCES

1. Parisi R, Symmons DP, Griffiths CE, et al. Global epidemiology of psoriasis: a systematic review of incidence and prevalence. *J Invest Dermatol* 2013;133:377–85.
2. Peckham PE, Weinstein GD, McCullough JL. The treatment of severe psoriasis. A national survey. *Arch Dermatol* 1987;123:1303–7.
3. Pouplard C, Gourraud PA, Meyer N, et al. Are we giving patients enough information on how to use topical treatments? Analysis of 767 prescriptions in psoriasis. *Br J Dermatol* 2011;165:1332–6.
4. Puig L, Carrascosa JM, Belinchón I, et al. Adherence and patient satisfaction with topical treatment in psoriasis, and the use, and organoleptic properties of such treatments: a Delphi study with an expert panel and members of the Psoriasis Group of the Spanish Academy of Dermatology and Venereology. *Actas Dermosifiliogr* 2013;104:488–96.
5. Martin SL, McGoey ST, Bebo BF, Jr, et al. Patients' educational needs about topical treatments for psoriasis. *J Am Acad Dermatol* 2012;68:e163–8.
6. Horn EJ, Fox KM, Patel V, et al. Are patients with psoriasis undertreated? Results of National Psoriasis Foundation survey. *J Am Acad Dermatol* 2007;57:957–62.
7. Robinson A, Kardos M, Kimball AB. Physician Global Assessment (PGA) and Psoriasis Area and Severity Index (PASI): why do both? A systematic analysis of randomized controlled trials of biologic agents for moderate to severe plaque psoriasis. *J Am Acad Dermatol* 2012;66:369–75.
8. Fleischer AB, Jr, Rapp SR, Reboussin DM, et al. Patient measurement of psoriasis disease severity with a structured instrument. *J Invest Dermatol* 1994;102:967–9.
9. Langley RG, Ellis CN. Evaluating psoriasis with Psoriasis Area and Severity Index, psoriasis global assessment, and lattice system physician's global assessment. *J Am Acad Dermatol* 2004;51:563–9.
10. Jacobson CC, Kimball AB. Rethinking the Psoriasis Area and Severity Index: the impact of area should be increased. *Br J Dermatol* 2004;151:381–7.
11. Feldman SR, Fleischer AB, Jr, Reboussin DM, et al. The self-administered Psoriasis Area and Severity Index is valid and reliable. *J Invest Dermatol* 1996;106:183–6.
12. Armstrong AW, Parsi K, Schupp CW, et al. Standardizing training for psoriasis measures: effectiveness of an online training video on Psoriasis Area and Severity Index assessment by physician and patient raters. *JAMA Dermatol* 2013;149:577–82.
13. Schmitt J, Wozel G. The Psoriasis Area and Severity Index is the adequate criterion to define severity in chronic plaque-type psoriasis. *Dermatology* 2005;210:194–9.
14. Carlin CS, Feldman SR, Krueger JG, et al. A 50% reduction in the Psoriasis Area and Severity Index (PASI 50) is a clinically significant endpoint in the assessment of psoriasis. *J Am Acad Dermatol* 2004;50:859–66.
15. Mattei PL, Corey KC, Kimball AB. Psoriasis Area Severity Index (PASI) and the Dermatology Life Quality Index (DLQI): the correlation between disease severity and psychological burden in patients treated with biological therapies. *J Eur Acad Dermatol Venereol* 2013.
16. Koo J, Kochavi G, Kwan JC. Topical medications for psoriasis. In: Koo J, Kochavi G, Kwan JC, eds. *Contemporary Diagnosis and Management of Psoriasis*. 1st edn. Newtown, PA: Handbooks in Health Care; 2004, pp. 18–38.

17. Samarasekera EJ, Sawyer L, Wonderling D, et al. Topical therapies for the treatment of plaque psoriasis: systematic review and network meta-analyses. *Br J Dermatol* 2013;168:954–67.
18. Kalb RE, Bagel J, Korman NJ, et al. Treatment of intertriginous psoriasis: from the Medical Board of the National Psoriasis Foundation. *J Am Acad Dermatol* 2009;60:120–4.
19. Cuchacovich R, Perez-Alamino R, Garcia Valladares I, et al. Steps in the management of psoriatic arthritis: a guide for clinicians. *Ther Adv Chronic Dis* 2012;3:259–69.
20. Esposito M, Giunta A, Mazzotta A, et al. Efficacy and safety of subcutaneous anti-tumor necrosis factor-alpha agents, etanercept and adalimumab, in elderly patients affected by psoriasis and psoriatic arthritis: an observational long-term study. *Dermatology* 2012;225:312–19.
21. Fagerli KM, Lie E, van der Heijde D, et al. The role of methotrexate co-medication in TNF-inhibitor treatment in patients with psoriatic arthritis: results from 440 patients included in the NOR-DMARD study. *Ann Rheum Dis* 2013.
22. Thapa RK, Yoo BK. Evaluation of the effect of tacrolimus-loaded liquid crystalline nanoparticles on psoriasis-like skin inflammation. *J Dermatolog Treat* 2013.
23. Nakamura RC, Abreu Ld, Duque-Estrada B, et al. Comparison of nail lacquer clobetasol efficacy at 0.05%, 1% and 8% in nail psoriasis treatment: prospective, controlled and randomized pilot study. *An Bras Dermatol* 2012;87:203–11.
24. Sofen H, Hudson CP, Cook-Bolden FE, et al. Clobetasol propionate 0.05% spray for the management of moderate to severe plaque psoriasis of the scalp: results from a randomized controlled trial. *J Drugs Dermatol* 2011;10:885–92.
25. Miller JJ, Roling D, Margolis D, et al. Failure to demonstrate therapeutic tachyphylaxis to topically applied steroids in patients with psoriasis. *J Am Acad Dermatol* 1999;41:546–9.
26. Devaux S, Castela A, Archier E, et al. Topical vitamin D analogues alone or in association with topical steroids for psoriasis: a systematic review. *J Eur Acad Dermatol Venereol.* 2012;26(Suppl 3):52–60.
27. Mrowietz U, Macheleidt O, Eicke C. Effective treatment and improvement of quality of life in patients with scalp psoriasis by topical use of calcipotriol/betamethasone (Xamiol®-gel): results. *J Dtsch Dermatol Ges* 2011;9:825–31.
28. van der Velden HM, Pasch MC, van Erp PE, et al. Treatment of plaque psoriasis with the two-compound product calcipotriol/betamethasone dipropionate versus both monotherapies: an immunohistochemical study. *J Dermatolog Treat* 2010;21:13–22.
29. van de Kerkhof PC, Hoffmann V, Anstey A, et al. A new scalp formulation of calcipotriol plus betamethasone dipropionate compared with each of its active ingredients in the same vehicle for the treatment of scalp psoriasis: a randomized, double-blind, controlled trial. *Br J Dermatol* 2009;160:170–6.
30. Tyring S, Mendoza N, Appell M, et al. A calcipotriene/betamethasone dipropionate two-compound scalp formulation in the treatment of scalp psoriasis in Hispanic/Latino and Black/African American patients: results of the randomized, 8-week, double-blind phase of a clinical trial. *Int J Dermatol* 2010;49:1328–33.
31. Talpur R, Cox K, Duvic M. Efficacy and safety of topical tazarotene: a review. *Expert Opin Drug Metab Toxicol* 2009;5:195–210.
32. Tan X, Feldman SR, Chang J, et al. Topical drug delivery systems in dermatology: a review of patient adherence issues. *Expert Opin Drug Deliv* 2012;9:1263–71.
33. Feldman SR. Approaching psoriasis differently: patient-physician relationships, patient education and choosing the right topical vehicle. *J Drugs Dermatol* 2010;9:908–11.
34. Zivkovich AH, Feldman SR. Are ointments better than other vehicles for corticosteroid treatment of psoriasis? *J Drugs Dermatol* 2009;8:570–2.
35. Feldman SR, Yentzer BA. Topical clobetasol propionate in the treatment of psoriasis: a review of newer formulations. *Am J Clin Dermatol* 2009;10:397–406.
36. Feldman SR, Matheson R, Bruce S, et al. Efficacy and safety of calcipotriene 0.005% foam for the treatment of plaque-type psoriasis: results of two multicenter, randomized, double-blind, vehicle-controlled, phase III clinical trials. *Am J Clin Dermatol* 2012;13:261–71.
37. Reich K, Bewley A. What is new in topical therapy for psoriasis? *J Eur Acad Dermatol Venereol* 2011;25(Suppl 4):15–20.
38. Patel T, Bhutani T, Busse KL, et al. Evaluating the efficacy and safety of calcipotriene/betamethasone ointment occluded with a hydrogel patch: a 6-week bilaterally controlled, investigator-blinded trial. *Cutis* 2011;88:149–54.

39. Hendriks AG, Keijsers RR, de Jong EM, et al. Efficacy and safety of combinations of first-line topical treatments in chronic plaque psoriasis: a systematic literature review. *J Eur Acad Dermatol Venereol* 2013;27:931–51.
40. Menter A, Gold LS, Bukhalo M, et al. Calcipotriene plus betamethasone dipropionate topical suspension for the treatment of mild to moderate psoriasis vulgaris on the body: a randomized, double-blind, vehicle-controlled trial. *J Drugs Dermatol* 2013;12:92–8.
41. Koo J, Kochavi G, Kwan JC. Combination, rotational, and sequential therapy. In: Koo J, Kochavi G, Kwan JC, eds. *Contemporary Diagnosis and Management of Psoriasis.* 1st edn. Newtown, PA: Handbooks in Health Care; 2004, pp. 59–66.
42. van de Kerkhof PC. Therapeutic strategies: rotational therapy and combinations. *Clin Exp Dermatol* 2001;26:356–61.
43. Weinstein GD, White GM. An approach to the treatment of moderate to severe psoriasis with rotational therapy. *J Am Acad Dermatol* 1993;28:454–9.
44. Bhutani T, Zitelli KB, Koo J. Yin-yang strategy: proposing a new, effective, repeatable, sequential therapy for psoriasis. *J Drugs Dermatol* 2011;10:831–4.

Chapter 4

Topical Corticosteroids

Laura F. Sandoval and Steven R. Feldman

INTRODUCTION

Although psoriasis can be very extensive, the majority of affected individuals suffer from limited disease, with lesions that encompass a relatively small portion of their total body surface area [1,2]. Thus, most people with psoriasis can be treated with topical medications alone. For patients who do have more extensive disease, topical treatments are often used for the worst spots to complement phototherapy or systemic treatments. A topical corticosteroid, either exclusively or in combination with other treatments, is the primary treatment for psoriasis in the United States. At least three out of four psoriasis patients are treated with topical corticosteroids, most commonly with clobetasol propionate [1].

Topical corticosteroids are a cornerstone of treatment for many inflammatory skin conditions. There is a plethora of topical corticosteroid agents available that may be categorized by potency; formulations, such as creams, ointments, lotions, sprays, foams, shampoos, gels, solutions, oils, and tapes; or a combination. Understanding the nuances of topical corticosteroid vehicles and potency is a critical aspect of dermatologic care in general, and psoriasis treatment in particular. Each formulation has advantages and disadvantages, and the many available formulations provide the clinician with great flexibility when prescribing these medications. This chapter addresses many aspects of topical corticosteroid use, challenging older paradigms and offering suggested approaches to optimize topical corticosteroid treatment.

RATIONALE FOR PSORIASIS THERAPY

Psoriasis is a complex immune-mediated disease where inflammation and hyperproliferation are key features. Activation of both innate and adaptive immune systems has been implicated in the pathogenesis. In psoriasis, T cells are activated—a process that presumably involves presentation of an unknown antigen by an antigen presentation cell (APC) to naïve T cells. After complex intercellular signaling and recruitment of memory T-cell subpopulations to the psoriasis lesion, there is extensive inflammation that is propagated by cytokines and growth factors that are necessary for immune response. Specifically, elevated cytokines from CD4+ T-helper (T_H)1 cells, cytokines overexpressed through the interleukin (IL)-23/T_H17 pathway, including IL-17 and IL-22, and T_H22 cells, all play a role in the pathogenesis of psoriasis [3]. Several of these cytokines function both as inflammatory mediators and growth factors and help to explain the clinical characteristics of plaque psoriasis.

Although the immune pathways that govern psoriasis may be extraordinarily complex, with subtleties remaining to be discovered, the common treatment is rather straightforward.

Topical corticosteroids work by modulating the immune system at multiple levels and by limiting vascular permeability that propagate the immune-mediated inflammatory response. A reduction in the local production of cytokines and vasodilatory substances in lesional skin, along with apoptosis of inflammatory cells, explains three essential abilities of topical corticosteroids:

1. Suppression of the local immune response
2. Reduction of inflammation
3. Slowing of hyperproliferation

MECHANISM OF ACTION AND BIOLOGIC POTENCY

The first recorded clinical use of corticosteroids occurred in 1948 when a woman with severe rheumatoid arthritis was successfully treated with an oral corticosteroid preparation. Two years later, in 1950, the Nobel Prize was awarded for the discovery of this new class of anti-inflammatory medication. Sulzberger and Witten's description of "compound F" in 1952 is the first documented account of topical corticosteroid use.

The biologic and pharmacologic activity of the corticosteroid molecule primarily stems from its ability to alter gene transcription and, ultimately, protein expression. For this alteration to occur, the corticosteroid molecule must first pass through the cell membrane where it reversibly binds to a corticosteroid receptor in the cytoplasm. This newly formed corticosteroid–corticosteroid receptor complex has increased DNA-binding capacity and diffuses into the cell nucleus, where it binds to the control sites on the DNA. Once bound to the cell's DNA, the corticosteroid complex modulates the transcription of mRNA [4]. One downstream effect of corticosteroid-modulated transcription is a decrease in the production of inflammatory protein mediators, such as IL-1, IL-2, IL-6, and interferon-α. Corticosteroids exert their vasoconstrictive abilities by decreasing the production of key vasodilatory proteins by using this same mechanism [5]. Although the efficacy of a given topical corticosteroid is determined by several factors, the first key element is the quantitative ability of the active molecule to bind corticosteroid receptors and promote subsequent transcriptional modulation.

Almost immediately after the discovery and first descriptions of hydrocortisone, attempts to increase its potency were initiated. One way to increase potency is halogenation with fluoride or chlorine at the C-6 α or C-9 α structural positions (Figure 4.1). In addition, fluorination in part produces a molecule with superior potency via protection of the steroid ring backbone structure from routine metabolic breakdown [6]. As more potent corticosteroids were developed, side effects of corticosteroid treatment became evident. Historically, more potent corticosteroids were created by fluorination; thus, fluorinated products became associated with higher risk of adverse events. But *it is not fluorination (or halogenation) per se that results in corticosteroid side effects*. The extent to which a drug activates the corticosteroid receptor determines the drug's capacity to produce unwanted side effects. Side effects are not determined by how the molecule is made to be potent; the side effects are determined by the potency. It is an incorrect assumption bordering on myth that nonhalogenated corticosteroids are in any way safer than halogenated corticosteroids; generally, we can expect that corticosteroids of similar potency will have similar side effect profiles.

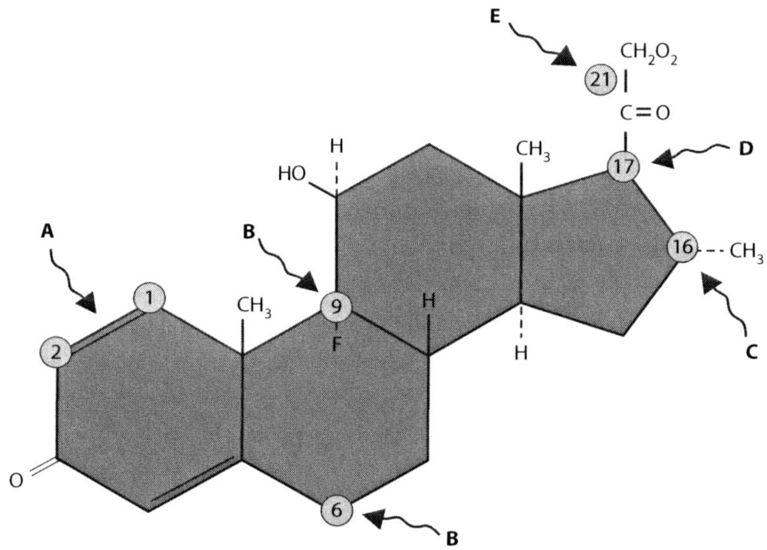

FIGURE 4.1 (See color insert.) Functional effects of changing corticosteroid structural elements. The steroid base contains four rings. Corticosteroids have a dihydroxyacetone side chain attached to the carbon atom at position 17. The addition of a double bond between the C-1 and C-2 atoms of the cholesterol backbone (A) increases potency by increasing the lipophilicity of the molecule. Halogenation (with fluoride or chlorine) at the C-6 or C-9 structural positions (B) increases corticosteroid potency through interactions with the corticosteroid receptor. Reduced polarity of the molecule, and therefore greater lipophilicity, can also be achieved by removal of the C-16 α-hydroxyl group (C) or the C-17 dihydroxyacetone side chain (D), or by masking hydrophilic side groups via esterification of the C-17 or C-21 positions (E).

DELIVERY AND PHYSIOLOGIC POTENCY

As with systemic corticosteroid therapy, topical corticosteroid therapy and efficacy rely on activation of the cytoplasmic corticosteroid receptor. However, unlike systemic corticosteroids that are ingested or injected intramuscularly, topical corticosteroids must reach their target cells by first diffusing across the stratum corneum. Therefore, topical corticosteroid potency is a function of not only the agent's physiologic potency to activate its cellular receptor but also the ability of that agent to penetrate the skin barrier. Thus, the ability of the topical drug vehicle to deliver the active drug molecule plays a key role in determining topical corticosteroid potency.

The ability of a given corticosteroid compound to traverse the stratum corneum involves complex physical chemistry. Furthermore, the ability of a formulation to deliver a corticosteroid cannot be predicted; it must be assessed clinically. The potency of a formulation depends on the ability of the active agent to separate from the vehicle and diffuse across the stratum corneum. We can envision this process as a two-phase system in which the vehicle and the stratum corneum resemble the water and oil phase in a balsamic vinegar and oil salad dressing. The amount of drug that penetrates the skin is determined in large part by how the drug partitions between the vehicle and stratum corneum phases. This partitioning determines how much of the drug enters the skin, thereby affecting the potency of the corticosteroid product.

Vehicles that drive the corticosteroid into the skin because of good partitioning—whether they be ointments, creams, gels, solutions, foams, lotions, or other vehicles—tend to be potent agents.

Alterations of the corticosteroid, its vehicle, or the stratum corneum may affect partitioning. For instance, polar, hydrophilic molecules move poorly through the stratum corneum, whereas lipophilic, nonpolar molecules diffuse through this barrier wall [7–9]. There are several methods by which the lipophilicity, and thus the diffusion capacity, of the active corticosteroid may be enhanced. These methods include the removal of the C-17 dihydroxyacetone side chain or the C-16 α-hydroxyl group and the addition of a double bond between the C-1 and C-2 atoms of the cholesterol backbone (Figure 4.1). Alternatively, by masking hydrophilic side groups, via esterification of the C-17 or C-21 positions or by the addition of acetonide side groups (Figure 4.1), a more lipophilic molecule is created.

Increasing the concentration of the active drug within the vehicle generally (but not always) tends to increase the delivery of the active drug from the vehicle to the skin. Propylene glycol is often present in topical corticosteroid vehicles. This large molecule binds water and is used to make corticosteroid products more potent by increasing the effective concentration of the active drug, thereby increasing diffusion of the drug into skin. Contrary to what one might think, however, changing the concentration of the corticosteroid compound does not always lead to predictable effects on potency. If the concentration is increased to the point that a drug crystallizes out of solution, the drug may lose potency. A compound's partition coefficient may also be affected by small changes in the composition of the vehicle.

Changing the vehicle or the concentration of a corticosteroid may or may not increase the potency. Indeed, when 0.1% triamcinolone cream is diluted 1:1 with another base, the resulting 0.05% concentration may have similar, higher, or lower potency compared with the original 0.1% cream. The potency effects of changes to a formulation, such as dilution with another vehicle or combined use with other agents, cannot be predicted. The only way to know the resulting potency is to test the actual preparation in a clinical study.

Alteration of the stratum corneum by increasing its permeability generally enhances the delivery of the agent to the targeted skin. Pretreatment with catalytic or fat solvents, removal of scale by chemical or physical modalities, increased hydration, and temperature elevation all tend to result in a more permeable stratum corneum [6,7]. The ability of ointments to hydrate the skin barrier can result in increased drug delivery as well. Dogma therefore suggests that in general ointment vehicles will be more potent. This dogma is not necessarily true, however, if the active drug remains partitioned in the ointment vehicle. Moreover, the dogma is not true if patients do not like, and therefore do not apply, the ointment.

Given the multitude of variables that affect the potency of a given topical corticosteroid, the clinical potency of a particular compound is unpredictable until clinical testing is done. The standard modality of objectively measuring corticosteroid potency is the vasoconstrictor assay introduced by McKenzie and Stoughton in 1962 [10,11]. Topical corticosteroid application results in vasoconstriction of the dermal blood supply via the alteration of gene transcription and subsequent vasoactive mediator production. The vasoconstrictor assay measures the ability of topical corticosteroid products to cause blanching of the skin. Thus, by measuring objective data produced by corticosteroid receptor activation, the vasoconstrictor assay provides information regarding not only the compound's inherent ability to activate its receptors but also the ability of the topical corticosteroid vehicle to deliver the active drug. The vasoconstrictor assay is a good guide to how compounds will perform in clinical practice, although because this assay is performed on normal skin, it may not fully reflect the potency of drugs used on diseased skin. The vasoconstrictor assay is used to place a formulation into one of seven potency classes.

The potency of topical drugs is dependent on the characteristics of the vehicle, but the specifics of which vehicles are more potent are not always predictable. Many clinicians have been taught that ointments, primarily due to their occlusive properties and superior hydration of the stratum corneum, are inherently more potent than creams (as an aside, there are no strict definitions of what is an ointment vs. a cream; these names are applied by manufacturers). Although some ointments may be more potent than creams, lotions, solutions, and other formulations, this concept does not necessarily hold across all topical corticosteroids [12]. Clobetasol propionate foam (Olux, Connetics Corporation) and lotion (Clobex, Galderma Laboratories, LP) preparations are similar in potency to ointment preparations as demonstrated by comparable vasoconstriction scores and by roughly similar efficacy rates in clinical trials [13].

ADHERENCE

Steroid receptor–binding characteristics and the physical chemistry of drug delivery affect the potency of topical corticosteroids. However, another key determinant of efficacy is adherence to treatment, also termed "compliance." A corticosteroid that partitions through the stratum corneum easily and strongly activates corticosteroid receptors may not be very potent if the medication is never applied. Adherence, or compliance, describes the tendency of a patient to apply a medication as prescribed. Nonadherence to topical psoriasis therapy is greater than with oral therapy, phototherapy, or biologic therapy [13,14]. Prescriptions for psoriasis may not even be filled, much less used [15]. Patient compliance is a tremendously complex issue and one that, at best, is only partially understood and appreciated. Numerous factors affect a patient's willingness to adhere to a given prescribed regimen of topical corticosteroids. Among the most prevalent of these factors are frustration with poor efficacy, inconvenience, and fear of side effects [16].

Vehicle preference is also a key characteristic of topical treatment that is thought to affect compliance. Several factors influence a patient's preference with regard to the vehicle used to deliver the corticosteroid agent. Among these factors are product characteristics such as subjective greasiness, messiness, and the degree to which the product stains clothing. As a general rule, patients prefer nonmessy preparations, such as solution, spray, and foam vehicles over other preparations [17]. Nevertheless, individual patient preference with regard to desirable vehicle characteristics may be difficult to predict. For instance, some patients with psoriasis prefer ointment-based agents. This preference is perhaps due in part to the immediate "disappearance" of scale that results from ointment application [18]. We use the word "disappearance" literally. Although the scale is no longer visible, the scale is still present and would be seen histologically. The immediate alteration of the scale's refractive index, and therefore its visibility, may be gratifying to the patient, potentially increasing patient satisfaction and compliance. Another patient may prefer a less messy vehicle on exposed areas. It may not be possible to predict patients' preference for different vehicles. Across a wide array of vehicles, clobetasol propionate products exhibit high-efficacy rates in psoriasis studies [18]. We suggest that clinicians discuss the options with patients and find a vehicle that best meets patients' lifestyles and needs. There is probably one vehicle that works better than all the others; it is the vehicle that the patient is most willing to use.

The astute clinician, in an effort to maximize patient compliance, integrates patient's individual preferences when prescribing a topical corticosteroid regimen. Measuring compliance as it pertains to the "real-world" practice of medicine is difficult, especially in dermatology where often an arbitrary amount of a topical drug is applied to a skin region. Self-reported compliance measures are not to be trusted; electronic monitoring permits a more accurate account of patient compliance. In a trial of 30 patients treated with topical 6% salicylic acid gel twice daily, adherence rates were consistently lower when measured by electronic monitoring caps than when adherence rates were calculated based upon patient medication logs or medication weights—the traditional methods of determining patient compliance. In addition, there was a sudden initial decrease in compliance within five days after the clinical encounter with a continued gradual decrease over subsequent weeks. Compliance rates measured by electronic monitors declined from 85% to 51% over the course of the eight-week trial [19]. This study was done with presumably highly motivated individuals who were paid as part of participating in a clinical trial, who were given the medication, who were told they were being monitored, who were filling out treatment diaries and who had multiple visits as part of the study; it is not unrealistic to predict that compliance rates in clinical practice—where none of these adherence-promoting factors are helping—may be even lower.

An interesting feature of the salicylic acid gel trial was an intermittent increase in compliance at two-week intervals that appeared related to study visits. An increase in compliance shortly before visits should not be unexpected, a phenomenon that has been termed "white-coat compliance," especially by those of us who floss more often before we see the dentist (we therefore like to call this effect the "dental floss phenomenon") [20]. Frequent return visits are common in clinical trials and may explain in part the tendency for clinical trials of a topical agent to show greater efficacy than the same topical agent in clinic populations. Clinicians can use this effect to improve patients' compliance and treatment outcomes by offering a return visit in one to two weeks. Compliance over the first one to two weeks may be improved by this early return visit. In addition, this approach reduces the apparent burden of treatment, because psychologically it is far easier to comply with a request for daily application for one week than for an eight-week or longer period. The early follow-up also encourages patients to fill their prescription and get started on the treatment. Setting such short-term goals may help improve initial treatment outcomes and patients' satisfaction with treatment, thereby fostering better adherence over the long run, improved outcomes, and, ultimately, lower costs.

The concept of tachyphylaxis needs to be reconsidered in light of the data on poor adherence. Tachyphylaxis is classically defined as a "rapidly decreasing response to a drug or physiologically active agent after administration of a few doses" [21]. This form of tachyphylaxis is observed with vasoconstrictor assays. Another phenomenon that is commonly called tachyphylaxis is the tendency for topical corticosteroids to slowly lose efficacy over time; this tachyphylaxis, perhaps better termed "bradyphylaxis," is widely recognized in clinical practice, yet there is little objective data from clinical trials to support the phenomenon. No tachyphylaxis was observed in a 12-week study of psoriasis treated with twice-daily application of betamethasone dipropionate 0.05% ointment [21], and it was suggested that perhaps loss of topical corticosteroid efficacy is observed in clinical practice and not clinical trials because of greater noncompliance in the clinical setting compared with the clinical trial setting. The observation of a steady reduction in the use of the 6% topical salicylic acid gel over an eight-week study also suggests that—with regard to topical corticosteroid treatment—a better definition of the tachyphylaxis seen in clinical practice is probably "a decreased response to topical corticosteroids as the patient gradually stops applying the medication because they are tired of doing it." One goal of dermatology in general and in psoriasis treatment in particular is how to intervene and improve patients' adherence behavior.

LESSONS FROM SKIN CAP

Skin Cap, an over-the-counter spray marketed as a psoriasis treatment, was introduced in North America in 1995 [22]. It was marketed as having zinc pyrithione as its active ingredient. Skin Cap quickly became a popular treatment option; patients, as well as dermatologists, enjoyed the remarkable efficacy the product offered to even the most therapeutically challenging psoriatic patient. The formulation provided for easy and nonmessy application, and no adverse effects were expected for a zinc pyrithione spray. It was so effective that it was suggested that psoriasis patients no longer needed corticosteroid injections, methotrexate, or psoralen + ultraviolet A (PUVA) treatment [23]. "It's a miracle," said some patients. Resistant scalp psoriasis cleared in as little as four days [23].

At the height of the clinical success of Skin Cap spray, however, reports began to surface in Europe that the product contained potent corticosteroids. In 1997, the Food and Drug Administration (FDA) removed Skin Cap from the U.S. market when several independent laboratories discovered that it contained clobetasol propionate. Some clinicians noted, though, that Skin Cap seemed far more effective than topical clobetasol propionate ointment. Some suggested the possibility of a synergistic effect existing between the zinc and the corticosteroid [22]. The corticosteroid receptor contains "zinc fingers," providing a theoretical basis, or at least a notion of a mechanism, for this synergy hypothesis. However, a left–right comparison trial was performed in which clobetasol propionate was applied to all lesions and zinc pyrithione to half the body and zinc pyrithione vehicle to the other half. The zinc-treated side did no better than the control side. Indeed, the side that got zinc did marginally worse—although not statistically significantly worse—than the side that did not get zinc [24].

Three factors probably accounted for the dramatic efficacy of Skin Cap compared with other clobetasol propionate preparations: compliance, compliance, and compliance. As discussed above, ointment vehicles are not inherently more potent than other vehicles and could be less potent if patients do not apply them. For many dermatologists who had been taught that ointments are more potent and who had integrated this idea into their being, the efficacy of Skin Cap may be the best clinical evidence that a drying spray product can be as effective or more effective than an ointment containing the same active ingredient! Because Skin Cap is easily applied, compliance is likely improved. Also, patients are concerned about potential adverse effects with regard to the use of topical corticosteroids; some find the idea of using "a steroid" frightful. When patients are told to apply clobetasol, they are warned about cutaneous and internal risks. When doctors recommended Skin Cap, it was without these warning (and without the many other scary warnings in topical corticosteroid package inserts), also likely enhancing compliance. Finally, because patients paid for Skin Cap themselves, they had probably invested in the product and more likely to use it.

The Skin Cap story provides us important guidance to success with topical corticosteroids for psoriasis. High levels of efficacy can be expected *if we can get patients to use the treatment regimen*. Patients should be involved in the choice of treatment, vehicles and application frequencies should be chosen that fit patients' lifestyles, potential side effects of treatment should not be overstated, written instructions are helpful, and a return visit (or other contact) shortly after starting treatment may improve adherence and treatment outcomes.

EFFICACY

The clinical effectiveness of topical corticosteroids in treating psoriasis and other inflammatory dermatoses has been documented in numerous clinical studies. Several studies using traditional ointment or cream vehicles for class I agents demonstrate rapid improvement in approximately 80% of subjects [25–27]. Newer, less messy formulations of the superpotent corticosteroid clobetasol reveal similar efficacy rates [18,28]. The speed at which topical clobetasol clears psoriasis is as great or greater than even our most potent systemic treatments.

Less potent topical corticosteroids may also be effective in treating psoriasis and tend to be used in situations for which use of class I agents is to be avoided or minimized. For relatively thin plaque psoriasis, a mid-potency corticosteroid is often appropriate. Areas of the body where the stratum corneum is relatively thin—such as the face, intertriginous areas, and genitals—are areas where a relatively low-strength topical corticosteroid may be all that is needed; there are also several noncorticosteroid topical anti-inflammatory agents now available. Prudent use of lower potency topical corticosteroids and noncorticosteroid agents helps to ensure that adverse events are minimized.

The use of niche vehicles such as oils, gels, tapes, and injectable preparations may be of value in specific situations. Flurandrenolide-impregnated tape (Cordran) is an invaluable resource for small-to-medium or stubborn plaques; the application of the tape one to three times weekly helps to avoid problems with poor compliance. It is difficult to classify flurandrenolide tape in the traditional class system. Flurandrenolide is a class V corticosteroid, but when used in the occlusive tape, it is expected that the bioavailability below the dermis and epidermis is enhanced; therefore, monitoring for adverse events is important. The efficacy of many corticosteroids may be enhanced when combined with certain noncorticosteroid topical agents, a practice that is commonplace in dermatology. The use of a single product that contains more than one active drug may have adherence benefits over the use of separate products.

SAFETY

Fear of adverse effects from the use of topical corticosteroids are widespread among patients and physicians alike and may represent a significant barrier to effective treatment of inflammatory skin diseases such as psoriasis. Nearly 75% of patients prescribed topical corticosteroids have some degree of concern regarding the potential adverse effects related to their use; the greatest concerns are skin atrophy, or thinning, and the fear of absorption [29].

Adverse events from corticosteroid use are best grouped into local, or cutaneous, and systemic. Numerous studies have been reported regarding local skin atrophy and striae formation at the site of topical corticosteroid application [30,31]. Improved ultrasound techniques have provided objective evidence of skin thinning by potent and very potent topical corticosteroids within six weeks of treatment onset [16,32–35]. However, the precise degree of skin thinning required for clinical significance is yet to be determined. Other cutaneous and systemic side effects are summarized in Table 4.1.

Perhaps the most worrisome aspect of therapy with topical corticosteroids is the potential for systemic absorption and subsequent metabolic derangements. Disturbance of the hypothalamic–pituitary axis, iatrogenic Cushing syndrome, adrenal insufficiency, and necrosis of the femoral head are a few reported examples of systemic effects from topical corticosteroids [36–39]. Several reports have failed to demonstrate evidence of cortisol suppression with the use of low-, mid-, or high-potency topical corticosteroids [16,40–45].

TABLE 4.1 Potential Side Effects from Topical Corticosteroid Use

Cutaneous effects
Allergic and contact dermatitis
Irritation
Atrophy
Striae
Telangiectasia
Ecchymoses and purpura
Hypopigmentation
Steroid rosacea
Perioral dermatitis
Folliculitis
Rebound and pustular flares
Systemic effects
Hypothalamus–pituitary axis suppression
Iatrogenic Cushing syndrome
Iatrogenic adrenal suppression
Avascular necrosis of the femoral head

Other evidence supports mild, transient cortisol suppression with high-potency topical corticosteroid use [16,46–48]. Although there is evidence for these systemic events, the frequency of clinically significant events is low. The possibility should be considered that poor adherence to treatment may be one of the factors that limits the risk. Patients who have extensive psoriasis are at the highest risk for systemic effects, although the amount required to create systemic side effects is not well described. A reasonable rule is no more than 50 g of a class I agent or 100 g of a class II agent each week used in appropriate regions.

SAFER TOPICAL CORTICOSTEROIDS: ARE THEY POSSIBLE?

Since Sulzberger and Witten's description of compound F in 1952, there have been great strides in the development and formulation of topical corticosteroids. The potency of today's topical corticosteroids has reached a level capable of effectively treating challenging and recalcitrant inflammatory dermatoses. With greater potency comes a greater potential for adverse events. Research and development has attempted to dissociate potency from adverse events to create safer potent topical corticosteroids.

Improving the safety profile of topical corticosteroids while maintaining potency has proven elusive. Creating nonfluorinated potent corticosteroids is not the solution; it is the strength of the corticosteroid, not the fluorine atom covalently bound in the molecule, that contributes to adverse events. There is no reason whatsoever to expect that potent nonfluorinated corticosteroids will have fewer or less severe side effects than fluorinated corticosteroids of equal potency. Mometasone furoate uses chlorination rather than fluorination to achieve potency. Some studies claim a reduced risk of adverse effects with mometasone furoate [32,49]. These studies, however, were not adequately designed to demonstrate comparable potency while decreasing adverse event rates. For example, one study comparing mometasone to hydrocortisone found greater potency with mometasone but not significantly greater adverse events; this study was powered to find differences in efficacy but was not powered to identify the likely real differences in adverse event profiles [50]. Studies of the nonfluorinated prednicarbate have also claimed a dissociation between benefit and risk. Although both a reduction in adverse effect rate and equal potency have been demonstrated independently [34,35,51,52], studies have not shown the occurrence of both outcomes simultaneously under identical conditions. Therefore, we conclude that the existence of safer topical corticosteroids with equal potency is yet to be demonstrated.

One adverse effect that is directly related to the specific structure of the corticosteroid molecule is allergic or contact dermatitis [53,54]. An allergy to topical corticosteroids is important to consider in a patient that fails therapy, and identifying such allergy may prevent further exacerbating the problem by avoiding prescription of more potent corticosteroids with potentially greater side effects.

COST CONSIDERATIONS

Very recently, there has been increasing attention given to the economics of psoriasis care. Annual U.S. cost estimates of treating psoriasis range from $650 million to $2 billion [55]. Topical corticosteroids are the most common class of medications used to treat psoriasis, and there are economic considerations for their use as adjunctive or primary therapy. The first and most obvious consideration is the ability of the patient (and potential third-party payers) to pay for a certain medication. In today's complex setting of copays and insurance caps, a patient's ability to afford a medication should be addressed. There is tremendous variation seen not only among classes of topical steroids but also within them [56] (Figure 4.1); there are generic alternatives in all potency classes. Some large retailers have $4 drug list that may include select generic topical corticosteroids, and it may be a benefit for providers to be familiar with such programs. Also, on a macro scale, the effect of corticosteroids on the cost of caring for psoriasis patients needs to be considered. A recent analysis demonstrated that the use of topical corticosteroids is a primary driver for reduced health care costs in psoriasis management [57]. This study highlights the concept of topical corticosteroids as controller medications that reduce cost and improve well-being.

PRACTICAL USE OF TOPICAL CORTICOSTEROIDS

The in vitro potency and vasoconstrictor assay–assessed efficacy of a given topical corticosteroid is meaningless if the patient does not apply the product as instructed. Therefore, maximization of patient compliance is crucial to the practical use of topical corticosteroids and to all topical and oral medications. There are numerous factors that influence an individual patient's medication adherence, including patient, physician, and vehicle factors. Although it may not be practical to change genetic factors that affect patients' compliance, physicians can work to increase compliance in several practical ways. First, physicians should establish a close, empathetic relationship with psoriasis patients. Greater compliance can be expected when clinicians touch the psoriasis and ask questions about the patient's disease and how it affects his or her life. Second, physicians should encourage patients to join the National Psoriasis Foundation and make use of the foundation's educational resources. The foundation encourages patients to adhere to their dermatologists' treatment recommendations. Through increasing patients' understanding of psoriasis, the National Psoriasis Foundation also empowers patients to take control of their disease and its treatments; such an approach likely leads to greater adherence and better treatment outcomes.

Next, physicians should involve the patient in treatment planning and choose treatment options that the patient finds acceptable. If less messy vehicles are preferred, solution, foam, or lotion vehicles may be offered. For patients who prefer ointments, ointments should be used. Setting realistic expectations is important; 35% of psoriasis patients feel their physicians do not tell them what to expect from treatment and 69% expect a cure when trying a new psoriasis treatment [13]. Finally, physicians should consider several psychologic factors known to influence patient compliance. Duration of treatment affects compliance rates for those patients on chronic medication regimens, as is often the case with psoriasis patients. Compliance decreases as treatment duration lengthens in patients requiring chronic, oral calcium channel–blocker therapy [58]. One early return office visit may be all it takes to improve initial adherence, initial efficacy, and patients' satisfaction with treatment. Patient compliance increases during the period surrounding a clinical encounter with a physician or other health care provider. Compliance rates of 88% and 86% to epilepsy medications were observed five days before and after a clinical visit, respectively; however, compliance rates fell to approximately 73% when measured for one month after the patient's clinical visit [59]. Similarly, a clinical study of 30 patients on stable antiepileptic drug regimens demonstrated a 33% increase in drug levels simply by decreasing average clinical visit intervals from three months to one month [60]. This phenomenon has been referred to in the medical literature as the "toothbrush effect", white coat effect [61], and, most recently, the dental floss phenomenon. Irrespective of the terminology, the phenomenon is well established and should be exploited by the practitioner in an effort to maximize patient compliance. A return visit, or some other expected contact with the patient, one or two weeks after initiating topical treatment may be a strong incentive to adhere to the treatment.

STEROID ALTERNATIVES: COMPLEMENTARY, NOT REALLY ALTERNATIVES

The perceived and actual potential for adverse effects associated with long-term, high-potency topical corticosteroid use propels a search for even safer topical therapies. Topical calcipotriene (Dovonex) obtained FDA approval in December 1993. It is a synthetic vitamin D_3 derivative indicated for the topical treatment of psoriasis. Topical calcipotriene quickly replaced anthralin and tars as the primary noncorticosteroid treatment for psoriasis, and by 1996, it accounted for 71% of the noncorticosteroid medications used at psoriasis visits [62]. Although approved for monotherapy in the topical treatment of psoriasis, dermatologists swiftly realized the drug's limitations and the need to use it as an adjunct to topical corticosteroids rather than as a substitute for corticosteroids. In 1994, the drug's inaugural year of FDA approval, it was used as monotherapy in 44% of the patients to whom it was prescribed. By 1996, this number had fallen to only 16%. Conversely, cases in which the drug was used as an adjunct to topical corticosteroids increased from 17% to 84% between these same years [62]. Central to calcipotriene's decline as a monotherapy agent are the extended treatment period before clinical response and the agent's principal adverse effect, skin irritation. Fortunately, both of these factors are lessened by combined use with a topical corticosteroid agent [63–65].

Another topical vitamin D product, topical calcitriol, is available with lower risk of irritation. These topical vitamin D products are commonly used as a topical corticosteroid adjunct rather than as an alternative. A combination topical product with calcipotriene and betamethasone dipropionate (Taclonex, Leo Pharma Inc.) is also available. By reducing the complexity of treatment and offering once a day application, this combination product may improve adherence and treatment outcomes [66].

A second topical agent heralded as a corticosteroid alternative in the treatment of psoriasis, topical tacrolimus (Protopic), is an immunosuppressant agent produced by *Streptomyces tsukubaensis*. When topical tacrolimus is combined with salicylic acid, a penetration-enhancing agent, it is modestly efficacious for common plaque psoriasis [67]. Topical tacrolimus 0.1% is effective in the treatment of facial and inverse psoriasis, with 81% of patients demonstrating complete clearing [68]. The efficacy of topical tacrolimus in the treatment of facial and inverse psoriasis is likely a result of the greater penetration of topical agents typically observed in these regions. Topical tacrolimus may be a good alternative to topical corticosteroids in the treatment of facial and inverse psoriasis, or it may be used in combination with topical corticosteroids as has been done with topical calcipotriene.

POTENTIAL PITFALLS

The greatest potential pitfall in the use of topical corticosteroids for psoriasis is poor compliance. In both clinical trials and actual clinical practice, superpotent topical corticosteroids can be highly effective [18,69,70]. When psoriasis does not respond to a topical corticosteroid as anticipated, poor adherence to treatment should be considered. It may be tempting to complicate the treatment regimen by using penetration enhancers, other combinations of medications, or sequential treatment regimens. However, simplifying the regimen, choosing a less messy vehicle, and using other measures to enhance adherence may be more logical and effective.

SUMMARY

Psoriasis is a common, chronic inflammatory skin condition requiring long-term medical management. The majority of psoriasis patients have mild to moderate disease that can be managed with topical corticosteroids. The chronicity of the disease and its treatment are major hurdles for patients and their dermatologists. Chronic adherence to the use of any medication is problematic, and chronic applications of time-consuming, messy topical preparations are particularly difficult.

Selection of the appropriate agent for a given patient is critical to maximize compliance; no agent, regardless of biologic or physiologic potency, can be effective if it is not applied. For the prescriber, this compliance means considering patients' preferences in the choice of topical corticosteroids. Characteristics such as ease and frequency of application, messiness, cost, and duration of therapy influence patient compliance. Unrealistic expectations from treatment and then disappointment when treatment does not meet these expectations may lead to poor adherence. Concerns regarding adverse effects are common among patients prescribed topical corticosteroids and are a frequent source of noncompliance. To maximize the benefits of topical corticosteroids, physicians should seek to identify and minimize these barriers.

When used well, how effective are topical corticosteroids for psoriasis? Clinical studies and clinical experience with Skin Cap demonstrate the high level of efficacy that can be achieved with topical corticosteroids when patients actually apply them. By paying attention to the factors that influence patients' adherence to topical agents, topical corticosteroids can be among our most potent psoriasis treatment options.

REFERENCES

1. Pearce DJ, Stealey KH, Balkrishnan R, et al. Psoriasis treatment in the United States at the end of the 20th century. *Int J Dermatol* 2006; 45(4): 370–374.
2. Koo J. Population-based epidemiologic study of psoriasis with emphasis on quality of life assessment. *Dermatol Clin* 1996; 14(3): 485–496.
3. Kagami S, Rizzo HL, Lee JJ, et al. Circulating Th17, Th22, and Th1 cells are increased in psoriasis. *J Invest Dermatol* 2010; 130: 1371–1383.
4. Kragballe K. Topical corticosteroids: mechanisms of action. *Acta Derm Venereol Suppl (Stockh)* 1989; 151: 7–10.

5. Van De Kerkhof PC, Vissers WH. The topical treatment of psoriasis. *Skin Pharmacol Appl Skin Physiol* 2003; 16(2): 69–83.
6. Murray JR. The history of corticosteroids. *Acta Derm Venereol Suppl (Stockh)* 1989; 151: 4–6.
7. Fritz KA, Weston WL. Topical glucocorticosteroids. *Ann Allergy* 1983; 50(2): 68–76.
8. Lee SS. Topical steroids. *Int J Dermatol* 1981; 20(10): 632–641.
9. Katz M, Shaikh ZI. Percutaneous corticosteroid absorption correlated to partition co-efficient. *J Pharm Sci* 1965; 54(4): 591–594.
10. Hepburn DJ, Aeling JL, Weston WL. A reappraisal of topical steroid potency. *Pediatr Dermatol* 1996; 13(3): 239–245.
11. Mckenzie AW, Stoughton RB. Method for comparing percutaneous absorption of steroids. *Arch Dermatol* 1962; 86: 608–610.
12. Gao HY, Li Wan PA. Topical formulations of fluocinolone acetonide. Are creams, gels and ointments bioequivalent and does dilution affect activity? *Eur J Clin Pharmacol* 1995; 46(1): 71–75.
13. Bewley A, Burrage DM, Ersser SJ, et al. Identifying individual psychosocial and adherence support needs in patients with psoriasis: a multinational two-stage qualitative and quantitative study. *J Eur Acad Dermatol Venereol* 2013.
14. Chan SA, Hussain F, Lawson LG, et al. Factors affecting adherence to treatment of psoriasis: comparing biologic therapy to other modalities. *J Dermatolog Treat* 2013; 24: 64–69.
15. Storm A, Andersen SE, Benfeldt E, et al. One in 3 prescriptions are never redeemed: primary nonadherence in an outpatient clinic. *J Am Acad Dermatol* 2008; 59: 27–33.
16. Brown KK, Rehmus WE, Kimball AB. Determining the relative importance of patient motivations for nonadherence to topical corticosteroid therapy in psoriasis. *J Am Acad Dermatol* 2006; 55(4): 607–613.
17. Feldman S, Housman T. Patients' vehicle preference for corticosteroid treatments of psoriasis. *Am J Clin Dermatol* 2003; 4(4): 221–224.
18. Warino L, Balkrishnan R, Feldman SR. Clobetasol propionate for psoriasis: are ointments really more potent? *J Drugs Dermatol* 2006; 5(6): 527–532.
19. Carroll CL, Feldman SR, Camacho FT, et al. Adherence to topical therapy decreases during the course of an 8-week psoriasis clinical trial: commonly used methods of measuring adherence to topical therapy overestimate actual use. *J Am Acad Dermatol* 2004; 51(2): 212–216.
20. Feldman SR, Camacho FT, Krejci-Manwaring J, et al. Adherence to topical therapy increases around the time of office visits. *J Am Acad Dermatol* 2007; 57(1): 81–83.
21. Miller JJ, Roling D, Margolis D, et al. Failure to demonstrate therapeutic tachyphylaxis to topically applied steroids in patients with psoriasis. *J Am Acad Dermatol* 1999; 41(4): 546–549.
22. Smith K. Skin Cap: what have we learned, and when did we learn it? [Editorial]. *Dermatol Online J* 1997; 3(2): 11c.
23. Shelley WB, Shelley ED. A dermatologic diary. Portrait of a practice. *Cutis* 1997; 59(4): 181–182.
24. Housman TS, Keil KA, Mellen BG, et al. The use of 0.25% zinc pyrithione spray does not enhance the efficacy of clobetasol propionate 0.05% foam in the treatment of psoriasis. *J Am Acad Dermatol* 2003; 49(1): 79–82.
25. Goldberg B, Hartdegen R, Presbury D, et al. A double-blind, multicenter comparison of 0.05% halobetasol propionate ointment and 0.05% clobetasol propionate ointment in patients with chronic, localized plaque psoriasis. *J Am Acad Dermatol* 1991; 25(6 Pt 2): 1145–1148.
26. Blum G, Yawalkar S. A comparative, multicenter, double blind trial of 0.05% halobetasol propionate ointment and 0.1% betamethasone valerate ointment in the treatment of patients with chronic, localized plaque psoriasis. *J Am Acad Dermatol* 1991; 25(6 Pt 2): 1153–1156.
27. Katz HI, Gross E, Buxman M, et al. A double-blind, vehicle-controlled paired comparison of halobetasol propionate cream on patients with plaque psoriasis. *J Am Acad Dermatol* 1991; 25(6 Pt 2): 1175–1178.
28. Gottlieb AB, Ford RO, Spellman MC. The efficacy and tolerability of clobetasol propionate foam 0.05% in the treatment of mild to moderate plaque-type psoriasis of nonscalp regions. *J Cutan Med Surg* 2003; 7: 185–192.
29. Charman CR, Morris AD, Williams HC. Topical corticosteroid phobia in patients with atopic eczema. *Br J Dermatol* 2000; 142(5): 931–936.
30. Goa KL. Clinical pharmacology and pharmacokinetic properties of topically applied corticosteroids. A review. *Drugs* 1988; 36(Suppl 5): 51–61.
31. Jones EW. Steroid atrophy—a histological appraisal. *Dermatologica* 1976; 152 (Suppl 1): 107–115.

32. Kerscher MJ, Hart H, Korting HC, et al. In vivo assessment of the atrophogenic potency of mometasone furoate, a newly developed chlorinated potent topical glucocorticoid as compared to other topical glucocorticoids old and new. *Int J Clin Pharmacol Ther* 1995; 33(4): 187–189.
33. Kerscher MJ, Korting HC. Comparative atrophogenicity potential of medium and highly potent topical glucocorticoids in cream and ointment according to ultrasound analysis. *Skin Pharmacol* 1992; 5(2): 77–80.
34. Kerscher MJ, Korting HC. Topical glucocorticoids of the non-fluorinated double-ester type. Lack of atrophogenicity in normal skin as assessed by high-frequency ultrasound. *Acta Derm Venereol* 1992; 72(3): 214–216.
35. Korting HC, Vieluf D, Kerscher M. 0.25% Prednicarbate cream and the corresponding vehicle induce less skin atrophy than 0.1% betamethasone-17-valerate cream and 0.05% clobetasol-17-propionate cream. *Eur J Clin Pharmacol* 1992; 42(2): 159–161.
36. Levin C, Maibach HI. Topical corticosteroid-induced adrenocortical insufficiency: clinical implications. *Am J Clin Dermatol* 2002; 3(3): 141–147.
37. Nathan AW, Rose GL. Fatal iatrogenic Cushing's syndrome. *Lancet* 1979; 1(8109): 207.
38. Kubo T, Kojima A, Yamazoe S, et al. Osteonecrosis of the femoral head that developed after long-term topical steroid application. *J Orthop Sci* 2001; 6(1): 92–94.
39. Katz HI, Hien NT, Prawer SE, et al. Superpotent topical steroid treatment of psoriasis vulgaris—Clinical efficacy and adrenal function. *J Am Acad Dermatol* 1987; 16: 804–811.
40. Munro DD. The effect of percutaneously absorbed steroids on hypothalamic–pituitary–adrenal function after intensive use in in-patients. *Br J Dermatol* 1976; 94(Suppl 12): 67–76.
41. Crespi HG. Topical corticosteroid therapy for children: alclometasone dipropionate cream 0.05%. *Clin Ther* 1986; 8(2): 203–210.
42. Lucky AW, Grote GD, Williams JL, et al. Effect of desonide ointment, 0.05%, on the hypothalamic-pituitary-adrenal axis of children with atopic dermatitis. *Cutis* 1997; 59(3): 151–153.
43. Rasmussen JE. Percutaneous absorption of topically applied triamcinolone in children. *Arch Dermatol* 1978; 114(8): 1165–1167.
44. Van Der Meer JB, Glazenburg EJ, Mulder PG, et al. The management of moderate to severe atopic dermatitis in adults with topical fluticasone propionate. The Netherlands Adult Atopic Dermatitis Study Group. *Br J Dermatol* 1999; 140(6): 1114–1121.
45. Vernon HJ, Lane AT, Weston W. Comparison of mometasone furoate 0.1% cream and hydrocortisone 1.0% cream in the treatment of childhood atopic dermatitis. *J Am Acad Dermatol* 1991; 24(4): 603–607.
46. Weston WL, Sams WM, Jr, Morris HG, et al. Morning plasma cortisol levels in infants treated with topical fluorinated glucocorticosteroids. *Pediatrics* 1980; 65(1): 103–106.
47. Queille C, Pommarede R, Saurat JH. Efficacy versus systemic effects of six topical steroids in the treatment of atopic dermatitis of childhood. *Pediatr Dermatol* 1984; 1(3): 246–253.
48. Juhlin L. Comparison of fluticasone propionate cream, 0.05%, and hydrocortisone-17-butyrate cream, 0.1%, in the treatment of eczema. *Cutis* 1996; 57(2 Suppl): 51–56.
49. Kelly JW, Cains GD, Rallings M, et al. Safety and efficacy of mometasone furoate cream in the treatment of steroid responsive dermatoses. *Australas J Dermatol* 1991; 32(2): 85–91.
50. Bhardwaj SS, Camacho F, Derrow A, et al. Statistical significance and clinical relevance: the importance of power in clinical trials in dermatology. *Arch Dermatol* 2004; 140(12): 1520–1523.
51. Korting HC, Unholzer A, Schafer-Korting M, et al. Different skin thinning potential of equipotent medium-strength glucocorticoids. *Skin Pharmacol Appl Skin Physiol* 2002; 15(2): 85–91.
52. Schafer-Korting M, Korting HC, Kerscher MJ, et al. Prednicarbate activity and benefit/risk ratio in relation to other topical glucocorticoids. *Clin Pharmacol Ther* 1993; 54(4): 448–456.
53. Davis MD, el-Azhary RA, Farmer SA. Results of patch testing to a corticosteroid series: a retrospective review of 1188 patients during 6 years at Mayo Clinic. *J Am Acad Dermatol* 2007; 56(6): 921–927.
54. Baeck M, Chemelle JA, Rasse C, et al. C(16)-methylated corticosteroids are less allergenic than the non-methylated molecules. *Contact Dermatitis* 2011; 64(6): 305–312.
55. Javitz HS, Ward MM, Farber E, et al. The direct cost of care for psoriasis and psoriatic arthritis in the United States. *J Am Acad Dermatol* 2002; 46(6): 850–860.
56. Pearce DJ, Thomas CG, Fleischer AB, Jr, et al. The cost of psoriasis therapies: considerations for therapy selection. *Dermatol Nurs* 2004; 16(5): 421–428, 432.
57. Kulkarni AS, Balkrishnan R, Richmond D, et al. Medication-related factors affecting health care outcomes and costs for patients with psoriasis in the United States. *J Am Acad Dermatol* 2005; 52(1): 27–31.

58. Farmer KC, Jacobs EW, Phillips CR. Long-term patient compliance with prescribed regimens of calcium channel blockers. *Clin Ther* 1994; 16(2): 316–326.
59. Cramer JA, Scheyer RD, Mattson RH. Compliance declines between clinic visits. *Arch Intern Med* 1990; 150(7): 1509–1510.
60. Wannamaker BB, Morton WA, Jr, Gross AJ, et al. Improvement in antiepileptic drug levels following reduction of intervals between clinic visits. *Epilepsia* 1980; 21(2): 155–162.
61. Feinstein AR. On white-coat effects and the electronic monitoring of compliance. *Arch Intern Med* 1990; 150(7): 1377–1378.
62. Feldman SR, Fleischer AB, Cooper JZ. New topical treatments change the pattern of treatment of psoriasis: dermatologists remain the primary providers of this care. *Int J Dermatol* 2000; 39(1): 41–44.
63. Ruzicka T, Lorenz B. Comparison of calcipotriol monotherapy and a combination of calcipotriol and betamethasone valerate after 2 weeks' treatment with calcipotriol in the topical therapy of psoriasis vulgaris: a multicentre, double-blind, randomized study. *Br J Dermatol* 1998; 138(2): 254–258.
64. Lebwohl M, Siskin SB, Epinette W, et al. A multicenter trial of calcipotriene ointment and halobetasol ointment compared with either agent alone for the treatment of psoriasis. *J Am Acad Dermatol* 1996; 35(2 Pt 1): 268–269.
65. Lebwohl M, Yoles A, Lombardi K, et al. Calcipotriene ointment and halobetasol ointment in the long-term treatment of psoriasis: effects on the duration of improvement. *J Am Acad Dermatol* 1998; 39: 447–450.
66. Zaghloul SS, Goodfield MJ. Objective assessment of compliance with psoriasis treatment. *Arch Dermatol* 2004; 140(4): 408–414.
67. Carroll CL, Clarke J, Camacho F, et al. Topical tacrolimus ointment combined with 6% salicylic acid gel for plaque psoriasis treatment. *Arch Dermatol* 2005; 141(1): 43–46.
68. Freeman AK, Linowski GJ, Brady C, et al. Tacrolimus ointment for the treatment of psoriasis on the face and intertriginous areas. *J Am Acad Dermatol* 2003; 48(4): 564–568.
69. Feldman SR. Effectiveness of clobetasol propionate spray 0.05% added to other stable treatments: add-on therapy in the cobra trial. *Cutis* 2007; 80(5 Suppl): 20–28.
70. Menter A. Topical monotherapy with clobetasol propionate spray 0.05% in the cobra trial. *Cutis* 2007; 80(5 Suppl): 12–19.

Chapter 5

Vitamin D_3 Analogs

Argentina Leon, Chai Sue Lee, and John Y. M. Koo

Calcipotriene (Dovonex®/Divonex®), known as calcipotriol outside of the United States, and calcitriol (Vectical®/Silkis®) are topical vitamin D_3 analogs approved for the treatment of plaque psoriasis. The U.S. Food and Drug Administration (FDA) approved calcipotriene in 1993. At that time, it was the first elegant nonsteroidal topical medication for the treatment of psoriasis. Today, calcipotriene is available in three formulations: ointment, cream, and scalp solution. Calcitriol was approved in the United States in 2009 and is currently available in an ointment formulation. Other topical vitamin D_3 analogs are available outside of the United States, such as tacalcitol (Bonalfa®) and maxacalcitol (Oxarol®).

CHEMISTRY AND MECHANISM OF ACTION

Calcitriol (1,25-dihydroxyvitamin D_3) is a natural occurring, active form of vitamin D_3. Calcipotriene is a synthetic analog of calcitriol. Figure 5.1 shows the chemical structures of calcitriol, calcipotriene, and other vitamin D_3 analogs.

At the molecular level, these agents can regulate gene transcription by binding the intracellular vitamin D receptor [4]. Through this receptor, vitamin D analogs can induce differentiation of keratinocytes and inhibit proliferation of T cells, keratinocytes, and fibroblasts [5–6].

After using topical vitamin D analogs, the psoriatic plaques can have a decrease in the number of basal keratinocytes, normalization of epidermal structure, and a decrease in the number of epidermal T-cell and polymorphonuclear leukocytes in the psoriatic skin [7–9].

Efficacy of Calcipotriene

Multiple clinical trials have confirmed the efficacy of all formulations (ointment, cream, and solution) of calcipotriene in the treatment of psoriasis in adults [5,6,10]. In addition, long-term studies have shown that the benefits of calcipotriene therapy were maintained for up to one year [11–15]. In a non comparative study, 40 patients receiving twice daily calcipotriene ointment had a mean time to healing of 53.5 day. With a mean time to relapse of 43.3 days [16].

Calcipotriene versus Other Vitamin D Analogs

In a large study involving 250 subjects, ointment and calcitriol ointment were found to have similar efficacy [17]. Comparing the two medications, calcitriol ointment was better tolerated

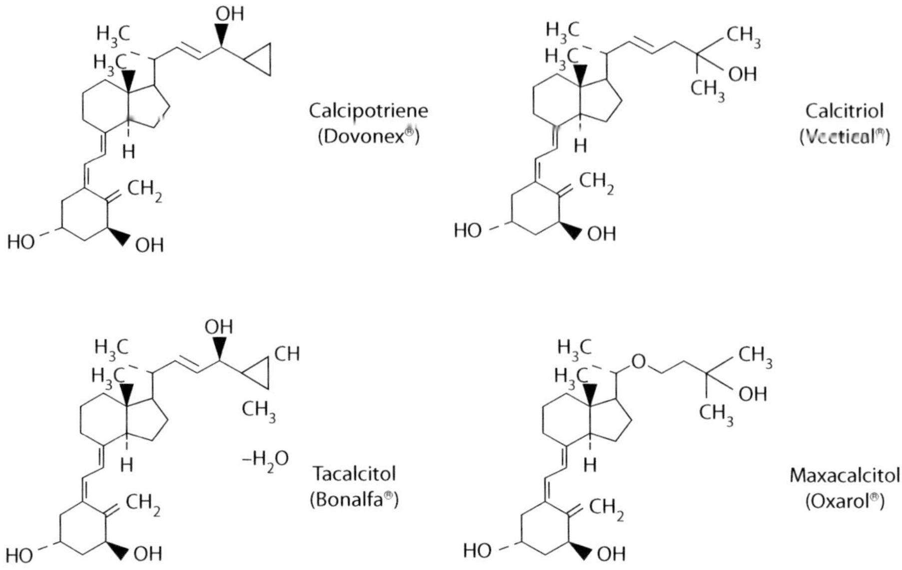

FIGURE 5.1 Chemical structures of vitamin D_3 analogs.

and induced less treatment-related adverse events [17]. Calcipotriene was found to be more effective than tacalcitol [18]. Calcipotriene ointment once daily and maxacalcitol ointment once daily were shown to have similar efficacy [19].

Calcipotriene versus Other Topical Agents

Calcipotriene ointment was shown to have similar or superior efficacy compared with topical corticosteroids, including betamethasone valerate ointment [20–22], betamethasone dipropionate plus salicylic acid (dosages not reported) [23], and fluocinonide ointment [24].

Calcipotriene ointment twice daily (BID) was significantly more effective than twice-daily 5% coal tar plus 2% allantoin (keratolytic) and 0.5% hydrocortisone [25]. In addition, twice-daily calcipotriene ointment provided similar or superior efficacy to once-daily short-contact 0.1%–3% dithranol [26–27]. Calcipotriene ointment also had a significantly greater cosmetic acceptability than short-contact dithranol cream [26].

A comparison of tazarotene 0.1% gel once daily plus mometasone furoate 0.1% cream once daily versus calcipotriene ointment twice daily found similar efficacy after eight weeks of treatment [28]. At the end of eight weeks, 59% of patients in the calcipotriene group versus 60% in the tazarotene plus mometasone group achieved a marked or ≥75% improvement in severity of psoriasis based on investigator assessment. In addition, there were no differences in plaque elevation or scaling scores between the two treatment groups, although erythema scores were significantly better in the tazarotene plus mometasone group. Calcipotriene was better tolerated than tazarotene plus mometasone. Fewer patients in the calcipotriene group experienced burning (8% vs. 42%), pruritus (13% vs. 32%), skin irritation (12% vs. 28%), or erythema (7% vs. 25%).

Efficacy of Calcitriol Clinical trials have demonstrated the efficacy of calcitriol when used as monotherapy, sequential therapy, or in combination with other agents. Two randomized studies compared the efficacy of calcitriol with placebo [29]. In both studies, more patients in the calcitriol groups improved than in the placebo groups ($p \leq .005$ for comparison with placebo in both studies). Patients in the calcitriol groups also achieved greater reduction in pruritus ($p < .001$) compared with the placebo group.

Calcitriol versus Other Topical Agents

In a study that compared calcitriol ointment twice daily versus anthralin cream once daily for eight weeks, Psoriasis Area Severity Index (PASI) improvement from baseline was not different (64% vs. 57%) [30]. However, the calcitriol group experienced higher quality of life during the eight-week study period as measured by the psoriasis disability index (PDI) questionnaire.

In comparison to high-potency topical corticosteroid, calcitriol is less efficacious. A randomized multicenter trial compared the efficacy between calcitriol 3 μg/g ointment BID and betamethasone dipropionate ointment BID after six weeks of treatment [31]. Subjects in the betamethasone dipropionate group achieved better global improvement and global severity scores ($p < .05$). Interestingly, subjects who responded to treatment had a higher remission rate in the calcitriol group (48%) versus betamethasone group (25%) during the eight-week follow-up period. A possible explanation for this observation could be related to the topical steroid rebound effect.

COMBINATION THERAPY

Combination therapy can result in increased efficacy and better medication tolerance. Most dermatologists in the United States use vitamin D_3 analogs in combination with other treatments. For example, when combined with topical steroids, there is reduced incidence of skin irritation from calcipotriene. Furthermore, the vitamin D_3 analogs decrease the risk of skin atrophy from the use of topical steroid. Calcipotriene is a relatively unstable molecule and is inactivated by acidic pH. It is not compatible and should not be mixed or applied in conjunction with salicylic acid, lactic acid, or ammonium lactate lotion unless application times are separated by at least two hours.

Calcipotriene and Topical Steroids

In one study, calcipotriene ointment in the morning combined with halobetasol ointment in the evening was more effective than either agent as twice-daily monotherapy [32]. If both calcipotriene and halobetasol are applied twice daily as combination therapy, efficacy may be further enhanced, provided that the two agents are mixed fresh each time in the palm of the patient just before application. This protocol is to prevent the agents from inactivating each other [33].

In another study, pulse therapy with betamethasone dipropionate once daily (weeks 1 and 3) and calcipotriene ointment twice daily (weeks 2 and 4) was compared with betamethasone dipropionate once daily for four weeks [34]. More patients treated with pulse therapy had "marked improvement" or "complete clearance" than those treated with monotherapy as measured by both the investigators (96% vs. 41%) and subjects (96% vs. 37%).

Another study compared maintenance therapy with halobetasol ointment twice daily on weekends combined with calcipotriene ointment twice daily on weekdays versus halobetasol ointment monotherapy on weekends [35]. Remission was defined as 75% improvement or a physician's global assessment of ≤2. More patients in the combination therapy maintained remission throughout the six-month study period than patients receiving halobetasol ointment weekend therapy (76% vs. 40%).

Calcipotriene and Tazarotene

Calcipotriene combined with tazarotene may have similar efficacy to superpotent topical steroids [36]. In an open-label, bilateral comparison study, the efficacy of calcipotriene ointment twice daily combined with tazarotene 0.1% gel once daily was not different from that of clobetasol ointment twice daily [36]. The study consisted of 15 patients who underwent a two-week treatment course, followed by a four-week posttreatment observation. At the end of the two weeks, lesions treated with calcipotriene and tazarotene had the same improvement in overall lesion severity—reduction in plaque elevation and scaling—as the clobetasol-treated lesions. Not surprisingly, erythema improved more in the clobetasol-treated lesions. Adverse events were more frequent in calcipotriene- and tazarotene-treated lesions than in those treated with clobetasol. The most common adverse effects related to treatment with calcipotriene and tazarotene were asymptomatic erythema and mild peeling. However, no patient had to withdraw or interrupt treatment because of adverse events. The results of this study suggest that calcipotriene ointment and tazarotene gel may be used simultaneously without major concern for inactivation of either compound.

Calcipotriene and Phototherapy

The standard of care for ultraviolet B (UVB) phototherapy is three times weekly treatments to achieve the optimal therapeutic response. Twice weekly UVB phototherapy is often inadequate. However, when combined with calcipotriene cream, twice weekly UVB phototherapy may be as effective as UVB phototherapy three times per week [37]. One of the barriers to phototherapy is the inconvenience associated with three visits per week. Thus, decreasing the visit frequency to two times per week can improve compliance.

In another study, calcipotriene plus narrowband UVB phototherapy (NBUVB) was shown to have a UVB-sparing effect compared with NBUVB alone [38]. In contrast, Brands et al. [39] did not find significant improvement with combination calcipotriene and NBUVB versus NBUVB alone. They suggest that differences in the comparisons with UVB phototherapy may reflect differences in UVB phototherapy techniques, patient noncompliance in applying calcipotriene ointment, or a UVB-blocking action of calcipotriene ointment.

Frappaz and Thivolet [40] showed that the combination of twice-daily calcipotriene ointment and three times a week PUVA phototherapy was more effective than PUVA alone.

In contrast to another study, calcipotriene ointment plus twice weekly PUVA phototherapy provided similar reductions in overall disease severity scores to PUVA monotherapy [41]. Both studies, however, showed a significant decrease in the duration of PUVA therapy, in the cumulative UVA dose, and number of UVA irradiations when PUVA was used in combination with calcipotriene compared with PUVA monotherapy [40,41]. For example, in the larger study, the duration of PUVA therapy was reduced from 34 to 22 days, the cumulative UVA dose reduced from 57 to 30 J/cm^2, and the number of UVA irradiations administered reduced from 15 to 10 [40].

When combined with phototherapy, calcipotriene should be applied a minimum of two hours before light treatment to prevent inactivation by UVA and possible burning sensations from UVB.

Calcipotriene and Systemic Agents

In 1998, van de Kerkhof et al. [42] reported that the addition of calcipotriene ointment twice daily to systemic treatment with acitretin was significantly more effective than acitretin plus placebo ointment. All patients were treated with a starting dose of 20 mg acitretin/day. The dose was increased every two weeks in increments of 10 mg/day until a maximum dose of 70 mg/day was reached, clearance was achieved, or patients developed unacceptable side effects to acitretin. After 12 weeks, 67% of the patients in the calcipotriene and acitretin group achieved clearance or marked improvement compared with 41% of the patients in the acitretin plus placebo ointment group [42]. Furthermore, the median total dose of acitretin required to reach clearing or marked improvement was significantly reduced in the combination therapy group compared with acitretin alone (1680 vs. 2100 mg). In a more recent study with a longer duration of treatment, the duration of treatment and total dose of retinoid required to achieve clearance were not different [43]. After 52 weeks, 60% of patients in the calcipotriene and acitretin combination therapy group and 40% in the acitretin monotherapy group achieved complete clearance. The addition of calcipotriene did not significantly reduce the total duration of treatment (82.8 vs. 92.8 days) and cumulative dose of acitretin required to reach clearance state (1613 vs. 2205 mg).

Combination therapy with calcipotriene ointment twice daily and oral cyclosporine 2 mg/kg/day significantly improved disease severity compared with cyclosporine 2 mg/kg/day alone [44]. After six weeks, complete clearing or 90% improvement in PASI score occurred in 50% of patients in the calcipotriene and cyclosporine group compared with 12% of the patients in the cyclosporine plus placebo ointment group [44].

De Jong et al. [45] has shown that when methotrexate therapy was discontinued, topical therapy with calcipotriene ointment twice daily results in an extension of the remission time before a relapse of psoriasis occurs compared with maintenance treatment with the vehicle only (113 vs. 35 days). Furthermore, the weekly dose of methotrexate needed to treat psoriasis is lower by combining methotrexate with calcipotriene than by combining methotrexate with vehicle. The mean weekly dose of methotrexate was 6.5 mg/week in the patient group treated with calcipotriene versus 9.9 mg/week in the patient group treated with vehicle [45].

This treatment results in lower cumulative dosage and therefore in a substantial reduction of the risk of short- and long-term side effects of methotrexate.

Calcitriol and Phototherapy

Similar to calcipotriene, calcitriol is often used in combination with treatments to increase efficacy or minimize adverse effects. An eight-week double-blind study compared the efficacy of calcitriol plus UVB phototherapy three times per week versus UVB monotherapy three times per week [46]. The combination therapy resulted in greater PASI score reduction and greater psoriasis clearance than in those receiving phototherapy alone. Furthermore, the combination group had a cumulative UVB exposure that was one-third less than that of the group receiving UVB monotherapy.

Calcitriol and Topical Steroids

A small randomized double-blind study compared the combination of betamethasone valerate 0.1% ointment in the morning and calcitriol 3 μg/g ointment at night ($n = 9$) versus betamethasone valerate ointment twice daily for six weeks ($n = 10$) [47]. There was no difference in efficacy between the two treatment groups. However, this study is limited by its small size.

Sequential Therapy with Calcitriol

Calcitriol is useful in sequential therapy. Calcitriol ointment BID on weekends and clobetasol spray BID on the weekdays is an effective regimen [48]. Another sequential treatment is alternating the use of calcitriol ointment BID with clobetasol spray BID every month, also known as the "ying-yang" method [49]. The rationale behind this strategy is to provide "steroid holiday" between treatment cycles, thus lowering the risk of skin atrophy.

ADVERSE EFFECTS

One of the most important features of vitamin D_3 analogs is their safety profile, making them user-friendly for primary care physicians as well as for dermatologists. Vitamin D_3 analogs are steroid free and thus free from steroid side effects such as skin thinning, striae formation, and adrenal suppression. They are generally well tolerated except that calcipotriene can cause more irritation compared with calcitriol.

Calcipotriene

Cutaneous side effects of calcipotriene include lesional and perilesional irritation that may occur in 12%–20% of patients [20,24,26,50,51]. Irritation from calcipotriene usually presents with a red ring of inflamed skin surrounding the treated lesions (Figure 5.2). Patients usually report a mild stinging, itching, or burning sensation. This reaction is usually transient, and patients quickly become accustomed to it [52].

Irritation from calcipotriene is more frequent on the face and intertriginous areas such as the axillae and groin. It appears to depend largely on the penetration of calcipotriene through the skin. The skin-to-skin occlusion inherent in intertriginous areas enhances penetration of calcipotriene and is thought to account for the increased rate of irritation. Calcipotriene is lipophilic and more readily absorbed by skin containing oily sebaceous glands, such as skin on the face.

Irritation from calcipotriene may resolve withless frequent application (e.g., once a day or every other day, instead of twice a day). Once this regimen is tolerated, the frequency can be increased carefully. Also, calcipotriene cream is often less irritating than the ointment formulation. Diluting calcipotriene with an emollient, such as petroleum jelly, can help to reduce irritation.

In rare patients, calcipotriene may cause excessive peeling and apparent expansion of erythema beyond the original border of the psoriasis (Figure 5.3). If this peeling occurs, and if the sensation is not bothersome, one can reassure the patient and encourage continued use of calcipotriene until the erythema resolves. Otherwise, decreasing the amount or frequency of use as described above can be helpful. Another strategy used by most clinicians during the initiation of therapy is to combine calcipotriene with a class I topical steroid.

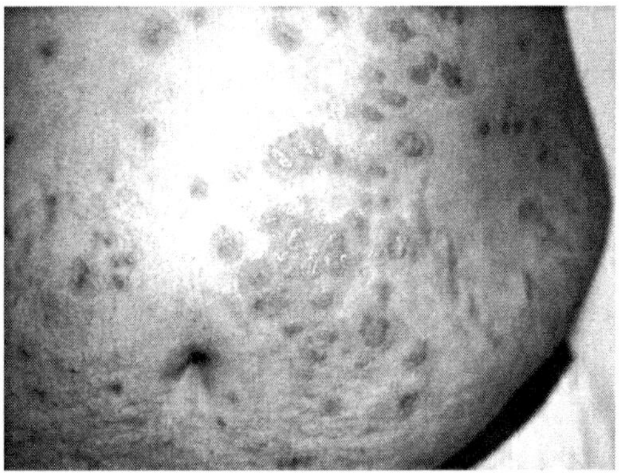

FIGURE 5.2 (See color insert.) Abdominal skin irritation from calcipotriene.

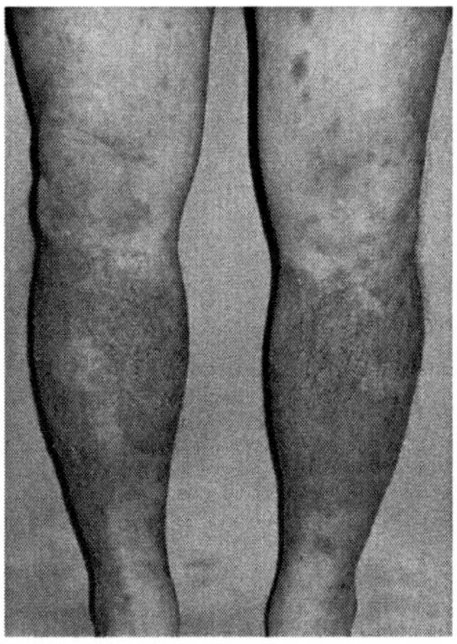

FIGURE 5.3 (See color insert.) Lower extremities skin irritation from calcipotriene.

The risk of developing irritation with calcipotriene is greatly reduced when it is used in conjunction with a topical steroid [32].

Calcitriol

Calcitriol ointment usually has better local tolerability compared with calcipotriene ointment [53]. Cutaneous side effects from calcitriol are usually well tolerated and mild. Similar to calcipotriene, side effects can include local erythema, pruritus, and minor skin irritation. Calcitriol is also more tolerable than calcipotriene when applied to the sensitive areas, such as face, hairline, groin, and flexural areas. A multicenter, randomized study showed that patients with psoriasis in sensitive areas had better local tolerability when treated with calcitriol 3 μg/g ointment than when treated with calcipotriol 50 μg/g ointment ($p < .001$) [53]. The local tolerability parameters included perilesional erythema, perilesional edema, and stinging/burning sensation.

Systemic Side Effects

Calcipotriene

The systemic side effects to be aware of when using calcipotriene are hypercalcemia and hypercalciuria. Although several studies have investigated the effects of calcipotriene twice daily (up to 100 g/week) on serum and urine calcium levels in patients with psoriasis [54–59], only one study showed a small but significant increase in urine calcium levels [55].

In clinical practice, however, there have been isolated case reports of hypercalcemia and hypercalciuria [10]. The majority of cases of hypercalcemia have occurred in patients who exceeded the recommended maximum topical dosage of 100 g/week, although a few occurred in patients using <100 g/week. All reported episodes of hypercalcemia and hypercalciuria have resolved on discontinuation of calcipotriene. A good guideline to follow is to limit total weekly use of calcipotriene in all formulations (ointment, cream, and solution) to 100 g/week to avoid the risk of hypercalcemia.

Calcitriol

Similar to calcipotriene, the most serious concern associated with overuse of calcitriol is hypercalcemia. However, current U.S. labeling indicates that the maximum dose of calcitriol is 200 g/week, twice that of calcipotriene. Calcitriol 3 μg/g ointment twice daily has been used for up to 52 weeks without any clinical effect on calcium homeostasis [60]. Safety regarding use of calcitriol in patients with calcium metabolism disorders or patients with erythrodermic, exfoliative, and pustular psoriasis has not been evaluated [61]. More long-term safety studies are warranted; however, calcitriol appears to have a good safety and side effect profile when used according to FDA labeling.

CONCLUSION

Vitamin D_3 analogs are valuable as first- or second-line therapy for patient with mild to moderate psoriasis and in combination with other antipsoriatic agents for more severe psoriasis. Although vitamin D_3 analogs do not have the same efficacy or speed of action as a superpotent topical corticosteroid, their steroid-sparing effect earns them merits in the realm of psoriasis treatment. Long-term vitamin D_3 analog therapy is not associated with skin atrophy or prominent concerns regarding tachyphylaxis. In addition, vitamin D_3 analog therapy is not associated with the rebound effect observed with several topical steroids whereby psoriasis worsens upon discontinuation of therapy.

Vitamin D_3 analogs are an important adjunct to traditional therapies. When used in combination with a superpotent topical steroid, the two drugs have a synergistic effect. Furthermore, the combination of the two drugs appears to offset the adverse effects of each. The topical steroid helps to decrease the risk of skin irritation from vitamin D_3 analog, and the vitamin D_3 analog helps to prevent skin atrophy by the topical steroid. Vitamin D_3 analogs are also beneficial in combination with UVB or PUVA phototherapy. Therefore, vitamin D_3 analogs may be used as monotherapy, in combination with other agents, or in sequential therapy.

REFERENCES

1. Hansen CM, Mathiasen IS, Binderup L. The anti-proliferative and differentiation-inducing effects of vitamin D analogs are not determined by the binding affinity for the vitamin D receptor alone. *J Invest Dermatol Symp Proc* 1996; 1: 44–48.
2. Berg JP, Liane KM, Bjørhovde SB, et al. Vitamin D receptor binding and biological effects of cholecalciferol analogues in rat thyroid cells. *J Steroid Biochem Mol Biol* 1994; 50: 145–150.
3. Binderup L. Comparison of calcipotriol with selected metabolites and analogues of vitamin D_3: effects on cell growth regulation in vitro and calcium metabolism in vivo. *Pharmacol Toxicol* 1993; 72: 240–244.
4. Binderup L, Bramm E. Effects of a novel vitamin D analogue MC 903 on cell proliferation and differentiation in vitro and on calcium metabolism in vivo. *Biochem Pharmacol* 1988; 37: 889–895.
5. Murdoch D, Clissold SP. Calcipotriol: a review of its pharmacological properties and therapeutic use in psoriasis vulgaris. *Drugs* 1992; 43: 415–429.
6. Lea AP, Goa KL. Calcipotriol: a review of its pharmacological properties and therapeutic efficacy in the management of psoriasis. *Clin Immunother* 1996; 5: 230–248.
7. Glade CP, Van Erp PE, Van Hooijdonk CA, et al. Topical treatment of psoriatic plaques with 1-a24 dihydroxyvitamin D_3: a multiparameter flow cytometrical analysis of epidermal growth, differentiation and inflammation. *Acta Derm Venereol* 1995; 75: 381–385.
8. Van Der Vleuten CJM, De Jong E, Van de Kerkhof PCM. Epidermal differentiation characteristics of the psoriatic plaque during treatment with calcipotriol. *Arch Dermatol Res* 1996; 288: 366–372.
9. Cavicchini S, Brezzi A, Gasparini G, et al. Skin ultrastructure after calcipotriol treatment: a transmission electron microscopic and freeze-fracture study on psoriatic patients. *Acta Derm Venereol* 1996; 76: 186–189.
10. Scott LJ, Dunn CJ, Goa KL. Calcipotriol ointment: a review of its use in the management of psoriasis. *Am J Clin Dermatol* 2001; 2: 95–120.
11. Cullen SI, Calcipotriene Study Group. Long-term effectiveness and safety of topical calcipotriene for psoriasis. Calcipotriene Study Group. *South Med J* 1996; 89: 1053–1056.
12. Ellis JP, Griffiths WAD, Klaber MR. Long-term treatment of chronic plaque psoriasis with calcipotriol ointment in patients unresponsive to short-contact dithranol. *Eur J Clin Res* 1995; 7: 247–257.
13. Ohgawara A, Kobayashi H, Tangami H, et al. Long-term treatment with MC903 (calcipotriol) ointment in patients with psoriasis vulgaris: an open clinical trial [in Japanese]. *Rinsho Iyaku* 1995; 11: 2589–2607.
14. Poyner T, Hughes IW, Dass BK, et al. Long-term treatment of chronic plaque psoriasis with calcipotriol. *J Dermatol Treat* 1993; 4: 173–177.
15. Ramsay CA, Berth-Jones J, Brundin G, et al. Long-term use of topical calcipotriol in chronic plaque psoriasis. *Dermatology* 1994; 189: 260–264.

16. Giannotti B, Carli P, Varotti C, et al. Treatment of psoriasis with calcipotriol: time of onset and healing relapses. *Eur J Dermatol* 1997; 7: 275–278.
17. Zhu X, Wang B, Zhao G, et al. An investigator-masked comparison of the efficacy and safety of twice daily applications of calcitriol 3 μg/g ointment vs. calcipotriol 50 μg/g ointment in subjects with mild to moderate chronic plaque type psoriasis. *J Eur Acad Dermatol Venereol* 2007; 21: 466–472.
18. Veien NK, Bjerke JR, Rossmann-Ringdahl I, et al. Once daily treatment of psoriasis with tacalcitol compared with twice daily treatment with calcipotriol. A double-blind trial. *Br J Dermatol* 1997; 137: 581–586.
19. Barker JN, Ashton RE, Marks R, et al. Topical maxacalcitol for the treatment of psoriasis vulgaris: a placebo-controlled, double-blind, dose-finding study with active comparator. *Br J Dermatol* 1999; 141: 274–278.
20. Cunliffe WJ, Berth-Jones J, Caudy A, et al. Comparative study of calcipotriol (MC 903) ointment and betamethasone 17-valerate ointment in patients with psoriasis vulgaris. *J Am Acad Dermatol* 1992; 26(5 Pt 1): 736–743.
21. Kragballe K, Gjertsen BT, De Hoop D, et al. Double-blind, right/left comparison of calcipotriol and betamethasone valerate in treatment of psoriasis vulgaris [published erratum appears in Lancet 1991; 337: 988]. *Lancet* 1991; 337: 193–196.
22. Ohgawara A, Kobayashi H, Iizuka H, et al. Clinical evaluation of MC903 (calcipotriol) ointment in patients with psoriasis vulgaris: a right to left comparative study against betamethasone valerate ointment (phase III study) [in Japanese]. *Rinsho Iyaku* 1995; 11: 2573–2587.
23. Crosti C, Finzi AB, Mian E, et al. Calcipotriol in psoriasis vulgaris: a controlled trial comparing betamethasone dipropiante + salicylic acid. *Int J Dermatol* 1997; 36: 537–541.
24. Bruce S, Epinette WW, Funicella T, et al. Comparative study of calcipotriene (MC 903) ointment and fluocinonide ointment in the treatment of psoriasis. *J Am Acad Dermatol* 1994; 31(5 Pt 1): 755–759.
25. Pinheiro N. Comparative effects of calcipotriol ointment (50 micrograms/g) and 5% coal tar/2% allantoin/0.5% hydrocortisone cream in treating plaque psoriasis. *Br J Clin Pract* 1997; 51: 16–19.
26. Berth-Jones J, Chu AC, Dodd WA, et al. A multicentre, parallel-group comparison of calcipotriol ointment and short-contact dithranol therapy in chronic plaque psoriasis. *Br J Dermatol* 1992; 127: 266–271.
27. Christensen OB, Mørk NJ, Ashton R, et al. Comparison of a treatment phase and a follow-up phase of short-contact dithranol and calcipotriol in outpatients with chronic plaque psoriasis. *J Dermatol Treat* 1999; 10: 261–265.
28. Guenther LC, Poulin YP, Pariser DM. A comparison of tazarotene 0.1% gel once daily plus mometasone furoate 0.1% cream once daily versus calcipotriene 0.005% ointment twice daily in the treatment of plaque psoriasis. *Clin Ther* 2000; 22: 1225–1238.
29. Lebwohl M, Menter A, Weiss J, et al. Calcitriol 3 microg/g ointment in the management of mild to moderate plaque type psoriasis: results from 2 placebo-controlled, multicenter, randomized double-blind, clinical studies. *J Drugs Dermatol* 2007; 66: 428–435.
30. Hutchingson PE, Marks R, White J. The efficacy, safety and tolerance of topical calcitriol 3 μg/g ointment in the treatment of plaque psoriasis: a comparison with short-contact dithranol. *Dermatology* 2000; 201: 139–145.
31. Camarasa JM, Ortonne JP, Dubertret L. Calcitriol shows greater persistence of treatment effect than betamethasone diproprionate in topical psoriasis therapy. *Dermatolog Treat* 2003; 14: 8–13.
32. Lebwohl M, Siskin SB, Epinette W, et al. A multicenter trial of calcipotriene ointment and halobetasol ointment compared with either agent alone for the treatment of psoriasis. *J Am Acad Dermatol* 1996; 35: 268–269.
33. Koo J, Lebwohl MG, Menter A, et al. Topical psoriasis update: today's topical treatment strategies to optimize patient response and quality of life. *Dermatol Times* 2004; 1–15.
34. Singh S, Reddy DC, Pandey SS. Topical therapy for psoriasis with the use of augmented betamethasone and calcipotriene on alternate weeks. *J Am Acad Dermatol* 2000; 43(1 Pt 1): 61–65.
35. Lebwohl M, Yoles A, Lombardi K, et al. Calcipotriene ointment and halobetasol ointment in the long-term treatment of psoriasis: effects on the duration of improvement. *J Am Acad Dermatol* 1998; 39: 447–450.

36. Bowman PH, Maloney JE, Koo JY. Combination of calcipotriene (Dovonex) ointment and tazarotene (Tazorac) gel versus clobetasol ointment in the treatment of plaque psoriasis: a pilot study. *J Am Acad Dermatol* 2002; 46: 907–913.
37. Ramsay CA, Schwartz BE, Lowson D, et al. Calcipotriol cream combined with twice weekly broad-band UVB phototherapy: a safe, effective and UVB-sparing antipsoriatic combination treatment. *Dermatology* 2000; 200: 17–24.
38. Woo WK, McKenna KE. Combination TL01 ultraviolet B phototherapy and topical calcipotriol for psoriasis: a prospective randomized placebo-controlled clinical trial. *Br J Dermatol* 2003; 149: 146–150.
39. Brands S, Brakman M, Bos JD, et al. No additional effect of calcipotriol ointment on low-dose narrow band UVB phototherapy in psoriasis. *J Am Acad Dermatol* 1999; 41: 991–995.
40. Frappaz A, Thivolet J. Calcipotriol in combination with PUVA: a randomized double blind placebo study in severe psoriasis. *Eur J Dermatol* 1993; 3: 351–354.
41. Youn JL, Park BS, Park SB, et al. Comparison of calcipotriol-PUVA with conventional PUVA in the treatment of psoriasis. *J Dermatol Treat* 2000; 11: 125–130.
42. Van De Kerkhof PC, Cambazard F, Hutchinson PE, et al. The effect of addition of calcipotriol ointment (50 micrograms/g) to acitretin therapy in psoriasis. *Br J Dermatol* 1998; 138: 84–89.
43. Rim JH, Park JY, Choe YB, et al. The efficacy of calcipotriol + acitretin combination therapy for psoriasis: comparison with acitretin monotherapy. *Am J Clin Dermatol* 2003; 4: 507–510.
44. Grossman RM, Thivolet J, Claudy A, et al. A novel therapeutic approach to psoriasis with combination calcipotriol ointment and very low-dose cyclosporine: results of a multicenter placebo-controlled study. *J Am Acad Dermatol* 1994; 31: 68–74.
45. De Jong EM, Mork NJ, Seijger MM. The combination of calcipotriol and methotrexate compared with methotrexate and vehicle in psoriasis: results of a multicentre placebo-controlled randomized trial. *Br J Dermatol* 2003; 148: 318–325.
46. Ring J, Kowalzick L, Christopher E, et al. Topical calcitriol (1,25-dihydroxyvitamin D_3) in the treatment of plaques psoriasis. *J Eur Acad Dermatol Venerol* 2000; 14: S259–S260.
47. Galderma Laboratories. A prospective randomized double-blind, parallel group study of once daily betamethasone valerate 0.1% ointment (BV) in the morning and once daily calcitriol 3.0 μg/g in the evening versus twice daily (BV) in the treatment of patients suffering from chronic plaque psoriasis. Study Report No. 6, H141 901/MC. Lausanne, Switzerland: Galderma Laboratories; 1993.
48. Hudson CP, Kempers S, Menter A, et al. An open-label, multicenter study of the efficacy and safety of a weekday/weekend treatment regimen with calcitriol ointment 3 microg/g and clobetasol propionate spray 0.05% in the management of plaque psoriasis. *Cutis* 2011; 88: 201–207.
49. Bhutani T, Zitelli KB, Koo J. Ying-yang strategy: proposing a new, effective, repeatable, sequential therapy of psoriasis. *J Drugs Dermatol* 2011; 10: 831–834.
50. Highton A, Quell J. Calcipotriene ointment 0.005% for psoriasis: a safety and efficacy study. Calcipotriene Study Group. *J Am Acad Dermatol* 1992; 32: 67–72.
51. Katz HI. Combined topical calcipotriene ointment 0.005% and various systemic therapies in the treatment of plaque-type psoriasis vulgaris: review of the literature and results of a survey sent to 100 dermatologists. *J Am Acad Dermatol* 1997; 37(3 Pt 2): S62–S68.
52. Koo J, Kochavi G, Kwan JC. Topical medications for psoriasis. In: *Contemporary Diagnosis and Management of Psoriasis*. 1st edn. Newtown, PA: Handbooks in Health Care; 2004. pp. 18–38.
53. Ortonne JP, Humbet P, Nicolas JF, et al. Intra-individual comparison of the cutaneous safety and efficacy of calcitriol 3 microg g(-1) ointment and calcipotriol 50 microg g(-1) ointment on chronic plaque psoriasis localized in facial, hairline, retroauricular or flexural areas. *Br J Dermatol* 2003; 148: 326–333.
54. Mortensen L, Kragballe K, Wegmann E, et al. Treatment of psoriasis vulgaris with topical calcipotriol has no short-term effect on calcium or bone metabolism: a randomized, double-blind, placebo-controlled study. *Acta Derm Venereol* 1993; 73: 300–304.
55. Berth-Jones J, Bourke JF, Iqbal SJ, et al. Urine calcium excretion during treatment of psoriasis with topical calcipotriol. *Br J Dermatol* 1993; 129: 411–414.
56. Gumowski-Sunek D, Rizzoli R, Saurat JH. Effects of topical calcipotriol on calcium metabolism in psoriatic patients: comparison with oral calcitriol. *Dermatologica* 1991; 183: 275–279.
57. Berth-Jones J, Bourke JF, Elouzi H, et al. Immediate and long term effects of topical calcipotriol on calcium homeostasis during treatment of psoriasis. *Br J Dermatol* 1992; 127(Suppl 40): 17–18.

58. Saurat JH, Gumowski-Sunek D, Rizzoli R. Topical calcipotriol and hypercalcaemia [letter]. *Lancet* 1991; 337: 1287.
59. Gumowski-Sunek D, Rizzoli R, Saurat JH. Calcium tolerance test in patients with extended body surface psoriasis and treated with calcipotriol. *Dermatology* 1992; 185: 229–230.
60. Lebwohl M, Ortonne JP, Andres P, et al. Calcitriol ointment 3 microg/g is safe and effective over 52 weeks for the treatment of mild to moderate plaque psoriasis. *Cutis* 2009; 83: 205–212.
61. Calcitriol [package insert]. Galderma Laboratories, L.P. Fort Worth, TX 76177, USA.

Chapter 6

Fixed-Dose Corticosteroid and Calcipotriene Combination Therapy

Ethan C. Levin and John Y. M. Koo

The majority of patients with mild to moderate psoriasis are managed with topical therapy [1]. The two most widely prescribed topical medications are corticosteroids and vitamin D_3 analogs. In a survey of 650 patients from an academic dermatology practice in the United States, 79% of patients were prescribed topical corticosteroids [2]. In Europe, the most widely prescribed topical therapy is reported to be the vitamin D_3 analog calcipotriene (known as calcipotriol outside the United States) [3].

Despite their widespread use and demonstrated efficacy, the chronic use of topical corticosteroids or vitamin D_3 analogs is associated with safety and efficacy concerns. Potential side effects from topical corticosteroids include cutaneous atrophy, striae, and suppression of the hypothalamic–pituitary–adrenal axis. The efficacy of long-term topical corticosteroid therapy may be compromised by tachyphylaxis [4]. Although this issue is unresolved, potential explanations include inability of topical corticosteroid monotherapy to completely clear lesions, exacerbation unrelated to the topical corticosteroid, and impaired compliance.

The most common side effect of topical vitamin D_3 analogs is irritation of the lesions, the surrounding skin, or both [5]. In addition, topical calcipotriene in excess of 100 g/week has been associated with hypercalcemia [6].

COMBINATION CORTICOSTEROID AND CALCIPOTRIENE THERAPY

To maximize the benefits of topical therapy, topical corticosteroids are often administered in combination with a second topical agent, such as calcipotriene. Potential benefits of combination therapy include improved disease control and decreased adverse events. Benefits of combination therapy are derived from differing mechanisms of action and less overall exposure to the individual components. For example, the combination of a topical corticosteroid plus topical calcipotriene is reported to be particularly effective at clearing psoriatic lesions without significant risk of skin atrophy from the corticosteroid or cutaneous irritation from calcipotriene. In fact, combination therapy with calcipotriene in the morning and corticosteroid in the evening is more effective than either agent used alone [7–9]. Unfortunately, combination therapy has its own disadvantages. For example, stacking or combining different agents may inactivate one or both products or require complicated dosing schedules that may decrease compliance. Furthermore, relying on the patient to self-administer potentially complicated combination regimens can be challenging. There is a lot of variability in how patients apply combination therapy even if told how much of each agent to use, when to mix them together, and how to apply them. Thus, a fixed-dose combination agent that combines topical corticosteroid with a topical vitamin D_3 analog can eliminate much of the user-dependent error, thereby enhancing efficacy. In addition, the convenience of a single application may increase compliance.

Fixed-Dose Calcipotriene 0.005% and Betamethasone Dipropionate 0.064%

Fixed-dose calcipotriene 0.005% and betamethasone dipropionate 0.064% (Taclonex®) is approved by the U.S. Food and Drug Administration (FDA) for the treatment of plaque psoriasis in adults ≥18 years old in both ointment and suspension formulations (known as "gel" outside of the United States). The ointment formulation has been available in the United States since January 2006 [10] for once-daily application up to four weeks. The suspension formulation was first approved for scalp psoriasis in 2006 and the indication was expanded to include other parts of the body in October 2012 [11] for once-daily application up to eight weeks. As per label, the maximum recommended weekly dose of both the ointment and suspension is 100 g. Outside of the United States, the ointment formulation is called Dovobet® or Daivobet®, and the suspension formulation may be referred to as gel or Xiamiol®.

In the ointment formulation, the two active agents are mixed in an anhydrous vehicle. The atrophogenic potential and bioavailability of betamethasone dipropionate in this formulation appears equal to that of betamethasone dipropionate (Diprosone®) ointment, a class II high-potency topical corticosteroid [12,13]. Calcipotriene, the other component in the combination ointment, has the same biologic activity as in its monotherapy formulation (Dovonex®, Daivonex®) [14].

CLINICAL TRIALS AND ANALYSES OF FIXED-COMBINATION FORMULATIONS OF BETAMETHASONE DIPROPIONATE/CALCIPOTRIENE

Topical fixed-dose betamethasone dipropionate/calcipotriene ointment has been evaluated in seven large international trials of >7000 patients with psoriasis involving 10%–30% of total body surface area. In all trials, psoriasis severity was assessed at baseline, during the treatment, and at the end of treatment using the Psoriasis Area and Severity Index (PASI). All seven trials demonstrated consistent reduction in PASI of approximately 40% after one week and 70% after four weeks of betamethasone dipropionate/calcipotriene therapy [15].

FIXED-DOSE COMBINATION THERAPY MORE EFFECTIVE THAN CORTICOSTEROID OR CALCIPOTRIENE ALONE

Studies with Ointment Formulation

Three double-blind studies investigated the efficacy and safety of fixed-dose combination therapy compared with monotherapy for the treatment of moderate psoriasis. In two studies, the treatment groups included calcipotriene/betamethasone dipropionate ointment (combination therapy), calcipotriene ointment alone, or betamethasone dipropionate ointment alone [15,16]. One of these studies included a vehicle-only control group [16]. More than 2000 patients with an average PASI of 11 were treated twice daily for four weeks. In both studies, patients treated with fixed-dose combination had a greater reduction in PASI score after four weeks than those treated with single agent therapy ($p < .001$ for each comparison). In addition, fixed-dose combination therapy had a rapid onset of action, with a significantly greater reduction in PASI scores after just one week compared with monotherapy or placebo in both studies ($p < 0.001$ for each comparison).

A third study comparing once-daily fixed-dose combination therapy to twice-daily calcipotriene reported similar results [17]. After eight weeks, 41% of patients treated with the once-daily fixed-dose combination therapy reached PASI-75, a greater percentage of patients than in any of the other three treatment groups ($p \leq .004$ for all comparisons) (Figure 6.1) [21].

Fixed-dose combination therapy was well tolerated by patients. In all three studies, more patients treated with calcipotriene monotherapy experienced lesional/perilesional adverse reactions than those treated with the fixed-dose combination therapy (12% vs. 8%, 17% vs. 10%, and 22% vs. 11%) [15–17].

Studies with the Suspension/Gel Formulation

There were three studies that examined the safety and efficacy of the suspension formulation for once-daily treatment of plaque psoriasis on the body [18–20]. The largest study was a double-blind, placebo-controlled study of calcipotriene/betamethasone dipropionate suspension in treating mild to moderate plaque psoriasis [20]. More than 1100 subjects with an average PASI of 7.9 were randomized to one of four treatment groups: (1) calcipotriene/betamethasone dipropionate suspension, (2) betamethasone dipropionate suspension, (3) calcipotriene suspension, or (4) suspension vehicle alone. Patients were treated with once-daily topical suspension for up to eight weeks. After eight weeks, 41% of patients treated with the once-daily fixed-dose combination therapy reached PASI-75 (Figure 6.1) [21]. This value was a greater percentage than any of the other three treatment groups ($p \leq .004$ for all comparisons). The greatest reduction in PASI scores was seen in the combination therapy group at both four and eight weeks ($p \leq .001$ for all comparisons) (Figure 6.2) [21]. Although these data only reflect eight weeks of daily use, the reduction appears comparable to that of some oral or injectable agents.

As in the ointment studies, the fixed-dose topical suspension was well tolerated by the patients. The overall incidence of adverse events was similar in all four treatment groups, and most were not related to the study treatment.

In conclusion, both the ointment and suspension formulations of fixed-dose calcipotriene/betamethasone dipropionate appear to be faster acting and more effective for the treatment of mild to moderate plaque psoriasis compared with calcipotriene monotherapy or betamethasone monotherapy. Furthermore, combination therapy with the ointment or suspension is less irritating than calcipotriene monotherapy.

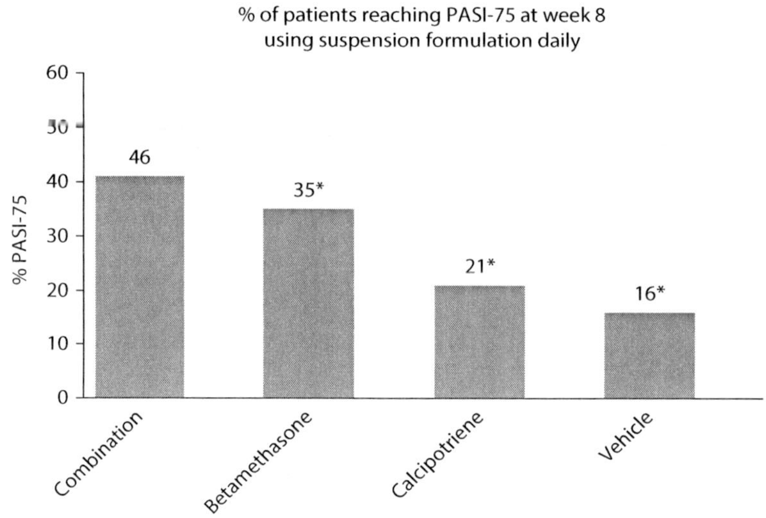

FIGURE 6.1 (See color insert.) All patients treated with once-daily topical suspension. Combination = calcipotriene/betamethasone dipropionate ointment. $^{*}p < .001$ for comparison with combination therapy. (Data from Kragballe K and Noerrelund KL, *J Eur Acad Dermatol Venereol* 16, 276, 2002.)

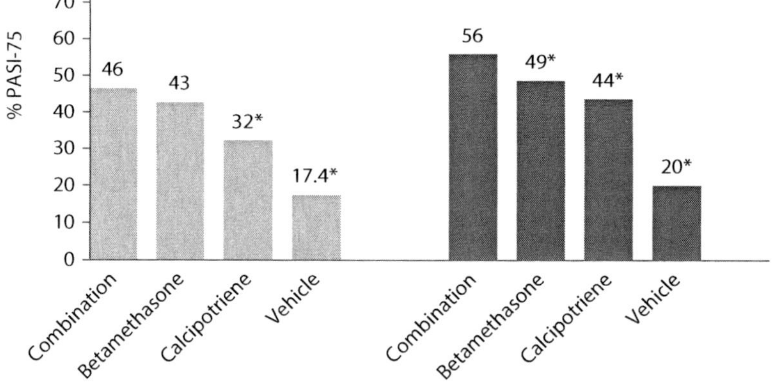

FIGURE 6.2 (See color insert.) All patients treated with once-daily topical suspension. Combination = calcipotriene/betamethasone dipropionate suspension. $^{*}p \leq .004$ for comparison with combination therapy. (Data from Kragballe K and Noerrelund KL, *J Eur Acad Dermatol Venereol* 16, 276, 2002.)

ONCE-DAILY FIXED-DOSE COMBINATION IS AS SAFE AND EFFECTIVE AS TWICE-DAILY THERAPY

A four-week study addressed the efficacy of once-daily versus twice-daily therapy of the ointment formulation [21]. In this study, 828 patients were randomized to four groups: (1) once-daily betamethasone dipropionate/calcipotriene ointment and once-daily vehicle; (2) twice-daily betamethasone dipropionate/calcipotriene ointment; (3) twice-daily calcipotriene ointment; and (4) twice-daily vehicle. The mean PASI at entry was 10.5. After one and four weeks, patients treated with the once- or twice-daily combination therapy had lower average PASI scores than those treated with twice-daily calcipotriene or twice-daily vehicle ($p < .001$ for all comparisons). Furthermore, there was no difference in average PASI scores between the once-daily and twice-daily combination group at one and four weeks ($p = .3$ and $p = .052$) (Figure 6.3).

Lesional/perilesional adverse events were reported more frequently in the calcipotriene group (20%) than in either the once-daily or twice-daily combination group (10% and 11%, respectively) ($p < .01$).

In conclusion, once- and twice-daily topical calcipotriene/betamethasone dipropionate ointment for mild to moderate psoriasis appears to have similar efficacy. In addition, this combination therapy is both more effective and better tolerated than twice-daily calcipotriene ointment.

ONCE-DAILY FIXED-DOSE THERAPY IS EFFECTIVE FOR PATIENTS WITH MILD, MODERATE, AND SEVERE PSORIASIS

Menter et al. [22] reported the results of a pooled analysis of six randomized, double-blind, vehicle-controlled studies, active-controlled studies, or both using the fixed-dose

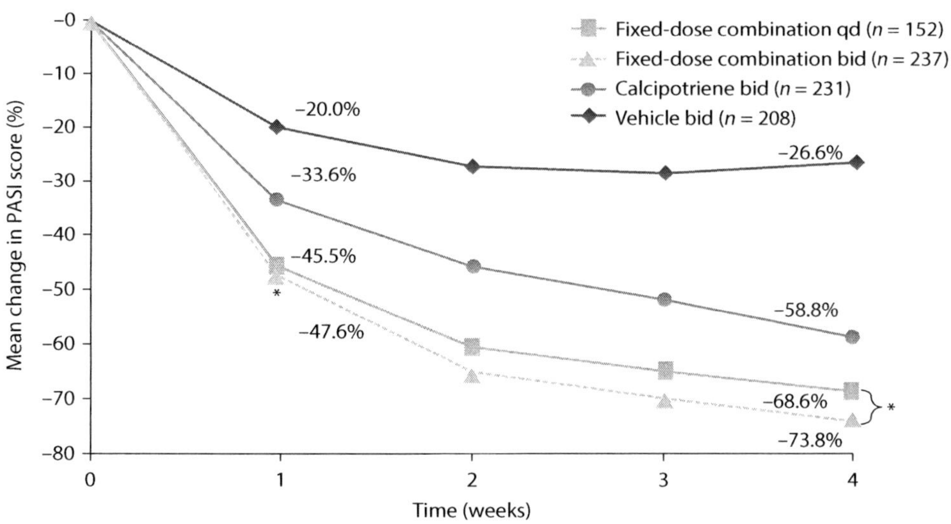

FIGURE 6.3 Once-daily versus twice-daily fixed-dose combination therapy. There was no statistical difference in Psoriasis Area and Severity Index between once-daily and twice-daily combination groups after one and four weeks of treatment (*$p > 0.05$ for both comparisons).

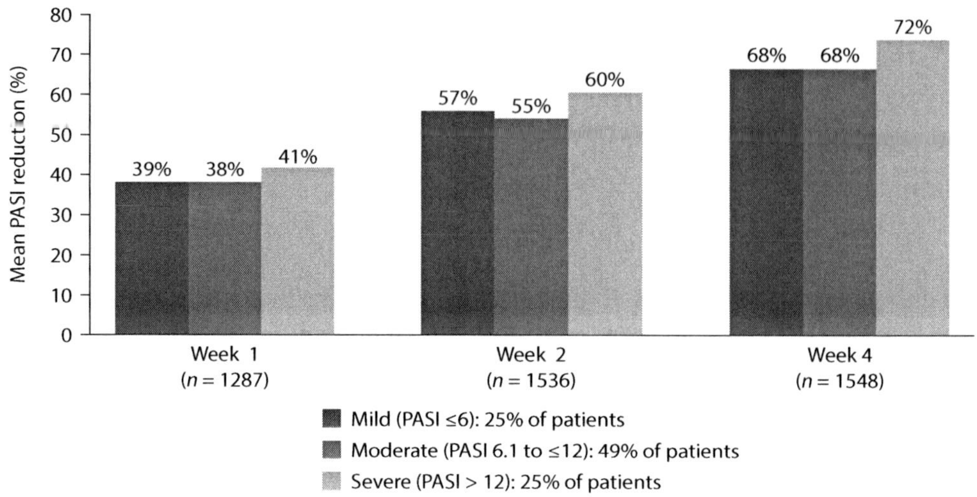

FIGURE 6.4 PASI reduction with once-daily fixed-dose combination ointment in mild, moderate, and severe psoriasis. Once-daily fixed-dose combination therapy produces consistent efficacy across all degrees of disease severity.

betamethasone dipropionate/calcipotriene combination in patients with mild (PASI ≤6), moderate (PASI 6.1–≤12), and severe (PASI >12) psoriasis. Although the analysis was somewhat limited by the use of a correlation between the Physician's Global Assessment (PGA) score and imputed PASI scores and by the failure of all investigators to report both PGA and PASI scores, it demonstrated that the fixed-dose combination used once daily produced consistent efficacy across all degrees of disease severity (Figure 6.4).

LONG-TERM, ONCE-DAILY FIXED-DOSE THERAPY IS SAFE AND EFFECTIVE

There was one large double-blind study that assessed the long-term safety of once-daily calcipotriene/betamethasone dipropionate ointment for the treatment of psoriasis up to 52 weeks [23–25]. In this study, patients used calcipotriene/betamethasone dipropionate ointment for the first month, after which time they were randomized into one of three arms for maintenance therapy through week 52: (1) fixed-dose combination therapy, (2) alternating calcipotriene ointment with fixed-dose combination therapy every four weeks, or (3) calcipotriene ointment only. The key inclusion criterion was a PGA of at least "moderate" (i.e., 4 on a 6-point scale). The key exclusion criterion was >30% body surface area (BSA) involvement. The study enrolled 634 patients, 70% of which had "moderate" psoriasis with the rest having "severe" or "very severe" disease. All treatments were used once daily on an as-needed basis to "reflect usual clinical practice" up to a maximum of 100 g/week. Patients were assessed every four weeks for adverse events and efficacy (using a 6-point PGA scale). A subset of 19 patients had adrenal function tests [adrenocorticotropic hormone (ACTH) stimulation test and 24-hour urine cortisol] performed at baseline and after 4, 12, and 52 weeks.

The clinical response observed in the initial four-week period when all patients received combination therapy reflected what was seen in the short-term studies reviewed

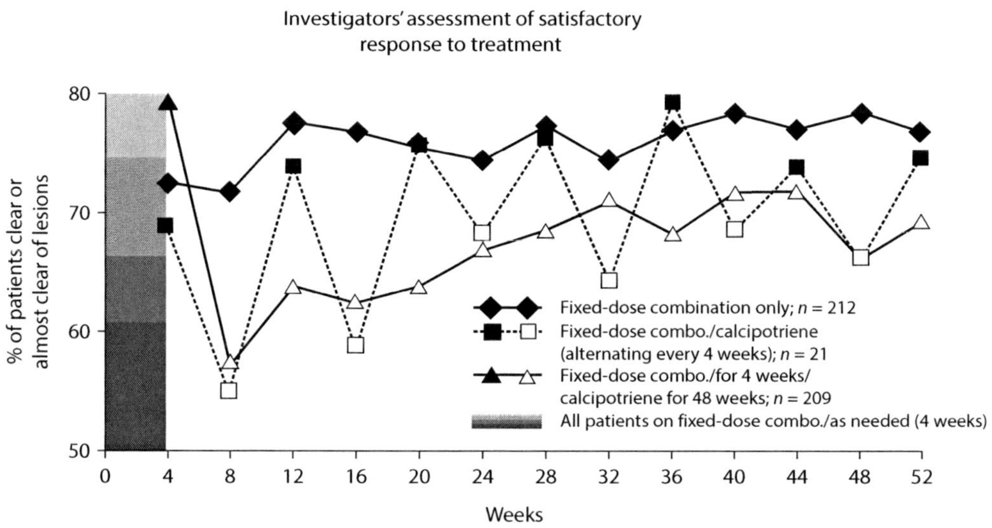

FIGURE 6.5 Efficacy of once-daily fixed-dose combination therapy up to 52 weeks. Once-daily fixed-dose combination therapy produces consistent long-term efficacy.

above—rapid onset of action and reliable lesion clearance. These clinical benefits were best maintained in the group using the combination agent only (Figure 6.5). Importantly, there was no apparent loss of efficacy or perceived tachyphylaxis in the fixed-dose combination arm. About 75% of the patients using the fixed-dose combination as needed for 52 weeks were "clear" or "almost clear" at the last assessment. On average, the patients in this group used <100 g/month of the combination ointment. The group that alternated between the combination agent and calcipotriene ointment "flip-flopped" back and forth between better control and lesser control. The patients that used calcipotriene monotherapy showed the most loss of efficacy during the maintenance period compared with the other treatment groups. However, it should be noted that calcipotriene is recommended as a twice-daily therapy in clinical practice and was used only once daily in this trial. In addition, some of the control of disease that was lost during the month after switching from combination therapy to calcipotriene monotherapy was regained by the last assessment at week 52.

The risk of an adverse drug reaction was higher in the calcipotriol monotherapy group (odds ratio [OR] 0.46, 95% CI 0.30–0.70; $p < .001$) than in the combination therapy group and was largely due to worsening of psoriasis, irritation, and pruritus. However, the risk of an adverse drug reaction in the combination therapy group was not different from the alternating therapy group (OR 0.66, 95% CI 0.42–1.03; $p = .066$).

Of greater importance was the incidence of reported adverse reactions due to corticosteroid use (e.g., adrenal insufficiency, skin atrophy, striae, folliculitis) (Table 6.1) [26]. Patients receiving combination therapy were not any more likely to have these reactions than those in the other treatment groups ($p = .445$ vs. the calcipotriene monotherapy group, $p = .317$ vs. the alternating therapy group).

TABLE 6.1 Safety of Once-Daily Fixed-Dose Combination Therapy up to 52 Weeks

	Fixed-Dose Combination Only (52 weeks; n = 207)		Fixed-Dose Combination/ Calcipotriene (alt. 4 weeks; n = 213)		Fixed-Dose Combination 4 Week/ Calcipotriene (48 weeks; n = 206)	
Event	*n*	%	*n*	%	*n*	%
Adrenal insufficiency	0	0.0	0	0.0	1	0.5
Cellulitis	0	0.0	0	0.0	1	0.5
Ecchymosis	1	0.5	0	0.0	0	0.0
Folliculitis	2	1.4	1	0.5	0	0.0
Furuncle	0	0.0	2	0.9	0	0.0
Hypertrichosis	0	0.0	0	0.0	1	0.5
Purpura	1	0.5	0	0.0	1	0.5
Rash, pustular	0	0.0	1	0.5	0	0.0
Skin atrophy	4	1.9	1	0.5	2	1.0
Skin depigmentation	2	1.0	0	0.0	0	0.0
Skin papilloma	0	0.0	1	0.5	0	0.0
Skin striae	0	0.0	1	0.5	0	0.0
Total no. of adverse events	11	7	6			
Total no. of points (%)	10	4.8	6	2.8	6	2.9

Source: Jemec GBE et al., *J Am Acad Dermatol* 59, 455–463, 2008.
Note: No statistically significant differences found between treatment groups.

Regarding the subset of 19 patients who were tested for adrenal function, none in the combination therapy group were found to have adrenal insufficiency during treatment [23]. The only patient who had evidence of adrenal insufficiency on laboratory exam (measured at week 52) was a patient in the calcipotriene monotherapy group and thus was determined not be related to study treatment. These results are consistent with prior studies that have shown safe use of high-potency topical corticosteroids as long as the quantity used and duration of therapy is not greater than the FDA-recommended limit [27]. In review of worldwide literature using calcipotriene/betamethasone dipropionate ointment, a single case report of adrenal insufficiency was found [28]. In this report, a 27-year-old woman used 60 g/day ointment (cumulative total of 1.8 kg/month, more than four times greater than the FDA-recommended limit of 400 g/month) for five months. She was admitted to the hospital for a pustular flare of psoriasis and found to have numerous clinical features of Cushing syndrome, including “buffalo” neck, large striae, and faciotruncal obesity. On stopping the combination therapy, the patient was found to have suppressed cortisol levels and was unresponsive to an ACTH stimulation test, for which she required hydrocortisone supplementation. Interestingly, despite the use of 1.8 kg/month of the combination therapy, the patient’s calcium levels were normal.

In summary, this clinical study supports the safe use of calcipotriene/betamethasone dipropionate ointment daily for one months followed by daily use as-needed for up to one year for the treatment of psoriasis. No increased risk of adrenal suppression, skin atrophy, or other adverse drug reaction was associated with the use of the fixed-dose combination therapy. It should be noted that the conclusion of this study may not apply to patients using more than the FDA maximum recommended amount of 100 g/week calcipotriene/betamethasone dipropionate ointment.

Sequential Therapy

As discussed above, combination calcipotriene betamethasone dipropionate is a safe and effective once-daily therapy for psoriasis for at least one year. Therefore, fixed-dose combination therapy may be used as sequential therapy without the need of a second topical agent for maintenance. This method is a simpler method than traditional sequential therapy that rotates a superpotent corticosteroid with a nonsteroid agent (e.g., vitamin D analogs).

Step 1 of sequential therapy with calcipotriene/betamethasone dipropionate ointment or suspension is daily use for one to two months. During this step, the goal is to decrease the intense inflammation, scaling, and thickness of psoriatic plaques that are often out of control during early stages of treatment. Once the thickness of the plaques has decreased, the patient may transition to step 2 of sequential therapy, even if the lesion is still red. For step 2, the patient may apply calcipotriene/betamethasone dipropionate ointment or suspension every other day for the next two to three months to further clear partially treated lesions. Once the plaques are macular and pink (rather than red), the patient may transition to the final step. For step 3, the patient can apply the fixed-dose combination therapy on weekends only. This maintenance strategy can be used for many months; the risk of corticosteroid-related adverse events from only two applications per week over the weekend is minimal.

In practice, the course of psoriasis is known to wax and wane depending on stressors, environmental factors, illness, and the natural history of the disease. Furthermore, improvement of psoriasis during treatment is not linear, and there may be periods of worsening after improvement. Because calcipotriene/betamethasone dipropionate is effective for clearing and safe for long-term use, the patient can fine-tune the sequential therapy to meet his or her therapeutic needs. For example, if during step 3 the patient begins to flare or if there is a special event upcoming, the patient can apply the therapy daily until better control is achieved. Thus, the patient can shift between steps 1, 2, or 3 as needed.

CORTICOSTEROID AND CALCIPOTRIENE COMBINATION FOR SCALP TREATMENT

Before being approved for body psoriasis, fixed-dose calcipotriene/betamethasone dipropionate suspension was approved for once-daily treatment of scalp psoriasis. This approval was based on two large phase III studies that demonstrated that after just one week, patients receiving the combination therapy had more improvement than those with either component alone (pooled analysis; $p < .001$ for all comparisons) [29].

In all, these double-blind studies enrolled >2900 patients with at least 10% scalp involvement with psoriasis. Subjects were randomized to one of three eight-week treatment arms:

(1) once-daily calcipotriene/betamethasone dipropionate suspension, (2) once-daily betamethasone dipropionate suspension, or (3) once-daily calcipotriene suspension [26,30]. One study also included a vehicle-only arm [26]. Both studies reported that combination therapy was more effective than the other treatment arms after just one to two weeks and was maintained throughout the study. In all, about 70% of patients achieved a PGA of 0 or 1 (on a 6-point scale) by the end of week 8. Combination therapy has also been shown to be more effective than twice-daily calcipotriene therapy [31].

The above-mentioned studies were mainly in patients who were Caucasian (about 97%) [29]. An eight-week study of scalp psoriasis in Hispanic/Latino and black/African American patients reported similar results [32]. In this study of 99 patients, 72% reached a PGA of 0 or 1 (on a 6-point scale) after eight weeks vs. 41% in vehicle only group ($p < .0001$).

Because the scalp is composed of tough, thick skin, and represents approximately 10% of body surface area, long-term use of fixed-dose combination therapy is well tolerated. This conclusion is supported by a study of 850 patients that demonstrated safe use of as needed fixed-dose combination therapy for up to 52 weeks [33]. The patients receiving combination therapy were not at increased risk of corticosteroid-associated adverse drug reactions compared with patients receiving calcipotriene monotherapy.

POTENTIAL BENEFITS OF FIXED-DOSE COMBINATION THERAPY

The new betamethasone dipropionate/calcipotriene combination appears to be more than an agent with just two-in-one convenience. The innovative preparation has two highly advantageous characteristics:

1. Well-documented synergy between the two components, allowing the combination agent to have significantly higher efficacy than the high-strength topical corticosteroid betamethasone dipropionate. The increased efficacy does not come at the expense of increased risk. Not only is the irritation risk of calcipotriene decreased by the topical corticosteroid ingredient but also the combination agent can be characterized as "high-strength topical corticosteroid that performs closer to a super high-strength topical corticosteroid." It performs better than a high-strength topical corticosteroid (i.e., betamethasone dipropionate) but is only expected to have a risk profile of high-strength rather than a super-high-strength topical corticosteroid.
2. Allowed once-daily application of a calcipotriene-containing agent to work as effectively as twice-daily application. Generally, calcipotriene is appreciated as having much better efficacy when it is applied twice daily than once daily. However, this combination agent has outstanding efficacy even though this calcipotriene-containing combination agent is only used once a day (Figures 6.6a and 6.6b). The synergistic efficacy, rapid onset of action, and once-daily administration combine to make the agent practical for use on a larger BSA than is possible with traditional topical agents.

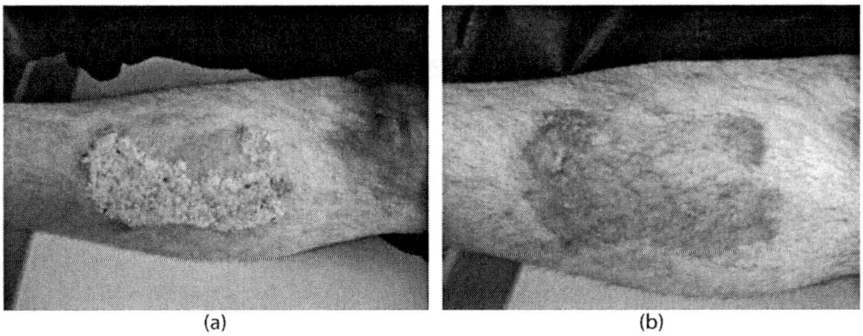

FIGURE 6.6 (See color insert.) Rapid clinical improvement in patient before (a) and after (b) treatment with fixed-dose combination therapy.

IN COMBINATION WITH BIOLOGICS

The fact that this combination agent is capable of topically treating more widespread psoriasis makes it possible to use this agent to "jumpstart" biologic agents, such as etanercept. The biologic agents that are currently approved by the FDA for psoriasis use in the United States are notable for their relative safety compared with traditional systemic agents. However, for some, the onset of action may be slow. Consequently, clinicians often have to "hold the hands" of the patient until the biologic agents reach their full efficacy. In this situation, a topical combination agent may be helpful by providing an efficacy boost to the biologic agent without increasing the risk of systemic side effects.

IN COMBINATION WITH OTHER SYSTEMIC AGENTS

There are many published studies that have established that calcipotriene can enhance the outcome of treatment modalities such as acitretin, methotrexate, cyclosporine (only low-dose cyclosporine was tested), ultraviolet B phototherapy, and psoralen plus ultraviolet A phototherapy [32,34–36]. Thus, because calcipotriene monotherapy is less efficacious than calcipotriene/betamethasone dipropionate, it is likely that the use of this combination agent in any of the above-mentioned treatments may further enhance efficacy.

POTENTIAL EFFECTS ON COMPLIANCE

Psoriasis is a chronic disease that requires compliance with treatment for successful long-term management. However, a recent meta-analysis showed that only 50%–60% of patients are compliant with topical therapy in the real-world setting (i.e., not randomized controlled clinical trials) [37]. Poor compliance may be due to several factors, including low efficacy, time constraints, and poor cosmetic characteristics of topical agents [39]. Fixed-dose betamethasone dipropionate/calcipotriene combination addresses many of these concerns and is supported by data from the clinical trials that showed compliance rates of 68% and 81% when the ointment was applied twice daily and once daily, respectively [15,40]. Another study of >2000 patients reported that around three-fourths of patients were "very satisfied" or "satisfied" with fixed-dose combination therapy over a period of six months [41]. Moreover, this level of satisfaction was consistent among patients who needed a second or third course of therapy.

CONCLUSIONS

Although corticosteroids and calcipotriene share similar antipsoriatic properties, they work by different mechanisms. Advances in drug formulation have led to the development of a fixed-dose combination of the two drugs that overcomes their inherent physiochemical incompatibilities. Both the two-compound ointment and suspension have been shown to be safe, more effective treatments than their components as monotherapy. In addition, clinical responses to the topical preparation are sustained for up to one year and are not associated with an increased risk of adrenal suppression or striae. Thus, this combination topical therapy is likely to be useful for patients with a spectrum of psoriatic skin involvement. Furthermore, it can be used as monotherapy, sequential therapy, and in combination with other treatments, such as phototherapy or systemic therapy.

REFERENCES

1. Schon MP, Boehncke WH. Psoriasis. *N Engl J Med* 2005; 352: 1899–1912.
2. Pearce DJ, Spencer L, Hu J, et al. Class I topical corticosteroid use by psoriasis patients in an academic practice. *J Dermatolog Treat* 2004; 15: 235–238.
3. Salonen S-H, for the EUROPSO Study Group. The EUROPSO psoriasis patient study: treatment history and satisfaction reported by 17,990 members of European psoriasis patient associations. Available at: http://www.psori.fi/doc/patientsurvey 1st phase (2002).pdf [Accessed May 10, 2006].
4. Miller JJ, Roling D, Margolis D, et al. Failure to demonstrate therapeutic tachyphylaxis to topically applied steroids in patients with psoriasis. *J Am Acad Dermatol* 1999; 41: 546–549.
5. Ashcroft DM, Po AL, Williams HC, et al. Systematic review of comparative efficacy and tolerability of calcipotriol in treating chronic plaque psoriasis. *BMJ* 2000; 320: 963–967.
6. Kawahara C, Okada Y, Tanikawa T, et al. Severe hypercalcemia and hypernatremia associated with calcipotriol for treatment of psoriasis. *J Bone Miner Metab* 2004; 22: 159–162.
7. Kragballe K, Barnes L, Hamberg KJ, et al. Calcipotriol cream with or without concurrent topical corticosteroid in psoriasis: tolerability and efficacy. *Br J Dermatol* 1998; 139: 649–654.
8. Lebwohl M, Siskin SB, Epinette W, et al. A multicenter trial of calcipotriene ointment and halobetasol ointment compared with either agent alone for the treatment of psoriasis. *J Am Acad Dermatol* 1996; 35: 268–269.
9. Ruzicka T, Lorenz B. Comparison of calcipotriol monotherapy and a combination of calcipotriol and betamethasone valerate after 2 weeks' treatment with calcipotriol in the topical therapy of psoriasis vulgaris: a multicentre, double-blind, randomized study. *Br J Dermatol* 1998; 138: 254–258.
10. Taclonex ointment full prescribing information [package insert]. Leo Pharma Inc. Parsippany, NJ 07054. March 2010.
11. Taclonex topical suspension full prescribing information [package insert]. Leo Pharma Inc. Parsippany, NJ 07054. October 2012.
12. Traulsen J, Hughes-Formella BJ. The atrophogenic potential and dermal tolerance of calcipotriol/betamethasone dipropionate ointment compared to betamethasone dipropionate ointment. *10th Congress of the European Academy of Dermatology and Venereology*, Munich, Oct 10–14, 2001.
13. Traulsen J. The bioavailability of betamethasone dipropionate in an ointment combination with calcipotriol (Dovobet ointment) is equal to that of betamethasone dipropionate alone in Diprosone® ointment. *10th Congress of the European Academy of Dermatology and Venereology*, Munich, Oct 10–14, 2001.
14. Hansen J. Mixing the unmixable. Verbal communication at the Leo Satellite Symposium. *10th Congress of the European Academy of Dermatology and Venereology*, Munich, Oct 10–14, 2001.
15. Douglas WS, Poulin Y, Decroix J, et al. A new calcipotriol/betamethasone formulation with rapid onset of action was superior to monotherapy with betamethasone dipropionate or calcipotriol in psoriasis vulgaris. *Acta Derm Venereol* 2002; 82: 131–135.
16. Papp KA, Guenther L, Boyden B, et al. Early onset of action and efficacy of a combination of calcipotriene and betamethasone dipropionate in the treatment of psoriasis. *J Am Acad Dermatol* 2003; 48: 48–54.

17. Guenther L, Cambazard F, van de Kerhof PCM, et al. Efficacy and safety of a new combination of calcipotriol and betamethasone dipropionate (once or twice daily) compared to calcipotriol (twice daily) in the treatment of psoriasis vulgaris; a randomized, double-blind, vehicle-controlled clinical trial. *Br J Dermatol* 2002; 147: 316–323.
18. Fleming C, Ganslandt C, Guenther L, et al. Calcipotriol plus betamethasone dipropionate gel compared with its active components in the same vehicle and the vehicle alone in the treatment of psoriasis vulgaris: a randomised, parallel group, double-blind, exploratory study. *Eur J Dermatol* 2010; 20: 465–471.
19. Langley RG, Gupta A, Papp K, et al. Calcipotriol plus betamethasone dipropionate gel compared with tacalcitol ointment and the gel vehicle alone in patients with psoriasis vulgaris: a randomized, controlled clinical trial. *Dermatology* 2011; 222: 148–156.
20. Menter A, Gold LS, Bukhalo M, et al. Calcipotriene plus betamethasone dipropionate topical suspension for the treatment of mild to moderate psoriasis vulgaris on the body: a randomized, double-blind, vehicle-controlled trial. *J Drugs Dermatol* 2013; 12: 92–98.
21. Kragballe K, Noerrelund KL. A highly effective once-daily treatment with a new calcipotriol/betamethasone ointment in psoriasis vulgaris [poster]. *J Eur Acad Dermatol Venereol* 2002; 16(Suppl 1): 276.
22. Menter A, et al. Comparative efficacy of calcipotriene/betamethasone combination product after 1, 2, 4 weeks of treatment of mild, moderate, and severe psoriasis. *63rd Annual Meeting of the American Academy of Dermatology*, 2006.
23. Fleming C, Ganslandt C, Leese GP. Short- and long-term safety assessment of a two-compound ointment containing calcipotriene/betamethasone dipropionate (Taclonex/Daivobet/Dovobet ointment): hypothalamic-pituitary-adrenal axis function in patients with psoriasis vulgaris. *J Drugs Dermatol* 2010; 9: 969–974.
24. Kragballe K, Austad J, Barnes L, et al. Efficacy results of a 52-week, randomised, double-blind, safety study of a calcipotriol/betamethasone dipropionate two-compound product (Daivobet®/Dovobet®/Taclonex®) in the treatment of psoriasis vulgaris. *Dermatology* 2006; 213: 319–326.
25. Kragballe K, Austad J, Barnes L, et al. A 52-week randomized safety study of a calcipotriol/betamethasone dipropionate two-compound product (Daivobet®/Dovobet®/Taclonex®) in the treatment of psoriasis vulgaris. *Br J Dermatol* 2006; 154: 1155–1160.
26. Jemec GBE, Ganslandt C, Ortonne J-P, et al. A new scalp formulation of calcipotriene plus betamethasone compared with its active ingredients and the vehicle in the treatment of scalp psoriasis: a randomized, double-blind, controlled trial. *J Am Acad Dermatol* 2008; 59: 455–463.
27. Castela E, Archier E, Devaux S, et al. Topical corticosteroids in plaque psoriasis: a systematic review of risk of adrenal axis suppression and skin atrophy. *J Eur Acad Dermatol* 2012; 26: 47–51.
28. Giannitelli M, Maza A, Lahfa M, et al. Iatrogenic adrenal insufficiency associated with calcipotriol-betamethasone topical combination in psoriasis. *Clin Exp Dermatol* 2010; 35: e167–168.
29. Jemec GB, van de Kerkhof PC, Enevold A, et al. Significant one week efficacy of a calcipotriol plus betamethasone dipropionate scalp formulation. *J Eur Acad Dermatol Venereol* 2011; 25: 27–32.
30. Van de Kerkhof PCM, Hoffmann V, Anstey A, et al. A new scalp formulation of calcipotriol plus betamethasone dipropionate compared with each of its active ingredients in the same vehicle for the treatment of scalp psoriasis: a randomized, double-blind, controlled trial. *Br J Dermatol* 2009; 160: 170–176.
31. Luger T, Cambazard F, Larsen FG, et al. A study of the safety and efficacy of calcipotriol and betamethasone dipropionate scalp formulation in the long-term management of scalp psoriasis. *Dermatol* 2008; 217: 321–328.
32. Tyring S, Mendoza N, Appell M, et al. A calcipotriene/betamethasone dipropionate two-compound scalp formulation in the treatment of scalp psoriasis in Hispanic/Latino and Black/African American patients: results of the randomized, 8-week, double-blind phase of a clinical trial. *Int J Dermatol* 2010; 49: 1328–1333.
33. Kragballe K, Hoffmann V, Tan J, et al. Calcipotriene plus betamethasone dipropionate gel compared to calcipotriene solution in patients with scalp psoriasis. *J Am Acad Dermatol* 2008; 58(Suppl 2): AB131.
34. Lebwohl M, Yoles A, Lombardi K, et al. Calcipotriene ointment and halobetasol ointment in the long-term treatment of psoriasis: effects on the duration of improvement. *J Am Acad Dermatol* 1998; 39: 447–450.
35. Frapazz A, Thivolet J. Calcipotriol in combination with PUVA: a randomized double-blind placebo study in severe psoriasis. *Eur J Dermatol* 1993; 3: 351–354.

36. Gossman RM, Thivolet J, Claudy A, et al. A novel therapeutic approach to psoriasis with combination calcipotriol ointment and very low-dose cyclosporine: results of a multicenter placebo-controlled study. *J Am Acad Dermatol* 1994; 31: 68–74.
37. Devaux S, Castela A, Archier E, et al. Adherence to topical treatment in psoriasis: a systematic literature review. *J Eur Acad Dermatol Venereol* 2012; 26(Suppl 3): 61–67.
38. Krueger G, Koo J, Lebwohl M, et al. The impact of psoriasis on quality of life: results of a 1998 National Psoriasis Foundation patient-membership survey. *Arch Dermatol* 2001; 137: 280–284.
39. Kauffmann R, Bibby AJ, Bissonnette R, et al. A new calcipotriol/betamethasone dipropionate formulation (Daivobet®) is an effective once daily treatment for psoriasis vulgaris. *Dermatology* 2002; 205: 389–393.
40. Clareus BW, Houwing R, Sindrup JH, et al. The DESIRE study—psoriasis patients' satisfaction with topical treatment using a fixed combination of calcipotriol and betamethasone dipropionate in daily clinical practice. *Eur J Dermatol* 2009; 19: 581–585.

Chapter 7

Tazarotene

Monica Huynh, Chai Sue Lee, and John Y. M. Koo

Tazarotene (Tazorac®) was the first topical retinoid approved for the treatment of plaque psoriasis in the United States; it was approved in 1997. It is available as a gel or cream in a concentration of either 0.1% or 0.05%. Despite its proven efficacy in the treatment of psoriasis, many patients experience significant skin irritation that limits use. In general, tazarotene is used most effectively in the treatment of psoriasis in combination with other forms of therapy, such as topical corticosteroids, calcipotriene (Dovonex®), and phototherapy to optimize efficacy and tolerability.

CHEMISTRY AND MECHANISM OF ACTION

Figure 7.1 shows the chemical structure of tazarotene. Tazarotene is a vitamin A derivative that is rapidly converted in vivo to its biologically active free-acid metabolite tazarotenic acid [1].

There are two types of retinoid receptors: retinoic acid receptors (RARs) and retinoid X receptors (RXRs). The RARs and RXRs are each composed of three distinct subtypes, labeled α, β, and γ [2]. These subtypes are found in a tissue-specific manner. RARα is primarily expressed in many embryonic and adult tissues, and RARβ is found exclusively in dermal fibroblasts. RARγ is the most ubiquitous RAR in human adult epidermis and is thought to be the key mediator of retinoid effects on keratinocytes [3]. In keratinocytes, these retinoid receptors exist as dimers, and for activation of gene regulation, RARs are always linked with RXRs. Besides RAR–RXR dimers, RXRs can exist as homodimers and as heterodimers with a wide range of other intracellular receptors, such as thyroid hormone, vitamin D_3, estradiol, and glucocorticoids [4]. These retinoid receptors belong to a large superfamily of receptors also consisting of glucocorticoid, thyroid hormone, and vitamin D_3 receptors, all of which are DNA-binding proteins that function as trans-acting transcription-modulating factors.

Tazarotenic acid, the active metabolite of tazarotene, binds to all three RAR subtypes, without having any effect on RXRs [5]. Retinoids elicit their biological effects by activating nuclear receptors and regulating gene transcription [6]. The exact molecular mechanism by which tazarotene is able to exert its effects on psoriasis is unknown, but it is thought to affect the three major pathogenic causes of psoriasis: in keratinocytes, tazarotene has antiproliferative effects, normalizes their abnormal differentiation, and decreases the expression of inflammatory markers on their cell surface [6]. Studies have shown that 0.05% tazarotene gel applied twice daily for 14 days improves keratinocyte differentiation through a reduction of hyperkeratosis and acanthosis and by reappearance

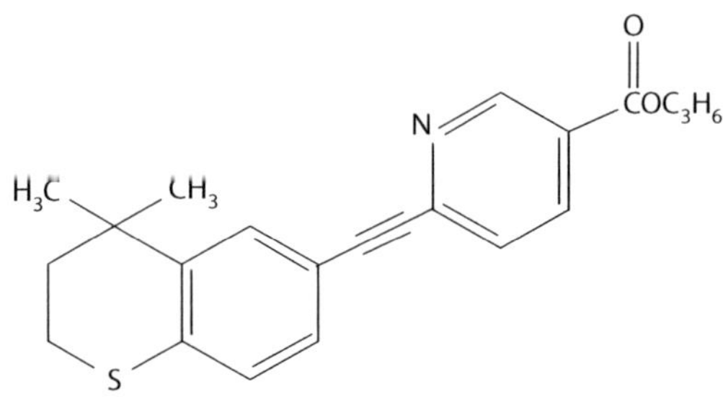

FIGURE 7.1 Chemical structure of tazarotene.

of the granular layer [7]. Histochemically, pathogenic overexpression of epidermal differentiation markers such as involucrin, keratinocyte transglutaminase, skin-derived antileukoproteinase (also known as elafin), and migration inhibitory–related factor 8 (also known as calgranulin A) are significantly reduced [6]. In addition, tazarotene elevates markers such as filaggrin in psoriatic lesions, implicating a return to a more normal and quiescent skin status [7,8].

TAZAROTENE MONOTHERAPY

Multiple clinical trials have confirmed the efficacy and safety of tazarotene gel and cream in the treatment of psoriasis [9–11]. Tazarotene 0.1% was generally more effective than the 0.05% concentration, although it was less tolerated secondary to skin irritation. In addition, the cream formulations of tazarotene (0.05% and 0.1%) might have better tolerability than gel preparations [11].

Tazarotene versus Crude Coal Tar

A single-center, bilateral comparison study investigated the efficacy and tolerability of tazarotene 0.1% gel and crude coal tar 5% ointment in patients with stable plaque psoriasis. Twenty-seven patients were instructed to apply 0.1% tazarotene gel or 5% crude coal tar ointment nightly to the limbs on different sides of the body. Assessments of erythema, scaling, and induration (ESI score) were performed at intervals of two weeks. At the end of weeks 4, 8, and 12, there was no significant difference in percentage reduction in the ESI scores between tazarotene-treated and crude coal tar–treated sides. Significant improvement (>50% reduction in ESI score) was seen on both sides in all patients at the end of week 12. At the end of eight weeks, all patients had moderate-to-marked improvement on both sides. Adverse reactions included irritation, erythema, burning sensation, and pruritus. These side effects were all considered mild and transient and were more common with tazarotene [12]. Although this study was limited in size, the results suggest that tazarotene 0.1% gel may have comparable efficacy to 5% crude coal tar in stable plaque psoriasis.

TAZAROTENE VERSUS TOPICAL STEROIDS

In a multicenter, randomized clinical trial, the safety and efficacy of 0.1% and 0.05% tazarotene gels once daily were compared with 0.05% fluocinonide cream twice daily [13];

348 psoriasis patients in total were enrolled for 12 weeks of treatment followed by a 12-week observation period. Treatment success rates, defined as improvement of 50% or more, during the treatment and posttreatment periods are shown in Figure 7.2 [12]. Although fluocinonide was more effective during the early part of the study, by the end of week 12, fluocinonide and tazarotene were similar in efficacy. During the follow-up period, relapse was most rapid with fluocinonide, especially during the first four weeks off of therapy. Signs and symptoms of skin irritation were more common with tazarotene than with fluocinonide. During the treatment period, 18%, 14%, and 11% of patients experienced pruritus, burning, and erythema, respectively, with 0.1% tazarotene; 9%, 9%, and 11%, respectively, with 0.05% tazarotene; and 1%, 7%, and 1%, respectively, with fluocinonide cream.

In a single-center, double-blind, randomized clinical trial, the clinical efficacy of tazarotene 0.1% cream was compared with clobetasol propionate 0.05% cream. Thirty-six patients with bilateral lesions applied study medication to lesions once daily for 12 weeks. At week 12, clobetasol cream had a greater reduction in erythema and scaling compared with tazarotene cream. However, tazarotene cream had a greater reduction in induration compared with clobetasol cream. Two patients using tazarotene discontinued from the study due to a severe irritation reaction. As assessed by study investigators, clobetasol had marked improvement, whereas tazarotene showed only moderate improvement; the investigators calculated the improvement as ~58% and ~75% for tazarotene at weeks 12 and 16, respectively, and ~95% and ~82% for clobetasol at weeks 12 and 16, respectively [14].

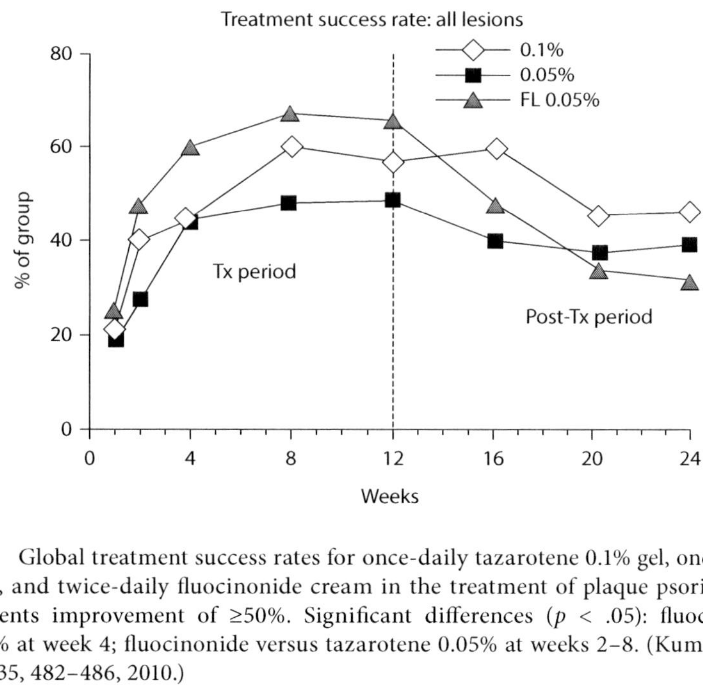

FIGURE 7.2 Global treatment success rates for once-daily tazarotene 0.1% gel, once-daily tazarotene 0.05% gel, and twice-daily fluocinonide cream in the treatment of plaque psoriasis. Treatment success represents improvement of ≥50%. Significant differences ($p < .05$): fluocinonide versus tazarotene 0.1% at week 4; fluocinonide versus tazarotene 0.05% at weeks 2–8. (Kumar U et al., *Clin Exp Dermatol* 35, 482–486, 2010.)

TAZAROTENE VERSUS CALCIPOTRIOL

In a single-center, prospective, investigator-blind, bilateral comparison study, once-daily tazarotene 0.1% gel in petrolatum versus twice-daily calcipotriol 0.005% ointment were compared. Nineteen patients were enrolled for 12 weeks of treatment followed by a four-week observation phase. Tazarotene in petrolatum was as effective as calcipotriol in both objective and subjective overall efficacy assessment. Calcipotriol had significantly greater effect in reducing erythema than tazarotene-petrolatum at weeks 2–8. Local irritation was noted with tazarotene petrolatum–treated lesions but not calcipotriol-treated lesions [15].

In another single-center, prospective, bilateral comparison study, calcipotriol 0.005% ointment was compared with tazarotene 0.05% or 0.1% gel. Seventeen adult patients with bilateral symmetrical lesions of plaque psoriasis were instructed to apply calcipotriol ointment twice daily to one side and either tazarotene 0.05% or 0.1% gel once daily to the other side for eight weeks. Assessments were made using ESI scores. Reduction in ESI scores at both weeks 4 and 8 was greater with calcipotriol than with tazarotene 0.05%. However, reduction in ESI scores was not different between calcipotriol and tazarotene 0.1%. Although not statistically significant, burning, pruritus, and irritation were observed more often in tazarotene-treated lesions [16].

COMBINATION THERAPY

To minimize unwanted side effects and improve patient's tolerability, tazarotene is optimally used in combination with mid- to high-potency topical corticosteroids, calcipotriene, ultraviolet (UV) B phototherapy, or psoralen plus ultraviolet A (PUVA).

TAZAROTENE AND TOPICAL STEROIDS

The concomitant use of tazarotene with a mid- or high-potency corticosteroid achieves a more rapid and greater efficacy and decreases irritation compared with tazarotene monotherapy, followed by a more prolonged duration of remission compared with corticosteroid monotherapy [13,17–19]. In a large-scale study to evaluate the efficacy of a combination treatment of tazarotene with a topical steroid, 300 psoriasis patients were randomly assigned to one of four treatment groups: 0.1% tazarotene gel once daily in combination with either once-daily application of placebo cream, low-potency corticosteroid (0.01% fluocinolone acetonide cream), midpotency corticosteroid (0.1% mometasone furoate cream), or high-potency corticosteroid (0.05% fluocinonide cream) [20]. Patients underwent 12 weeks of treatment, followed by four weeks of observation. It took two weeks for the tazarotene plus midpotency corticosteroid and three weeks for the tazarotene plus high-potency corticosteroid versus four weeks for the tazarotene plus low-potency corticosteroid and tazarotene plus placebo groups to obtain at least 50% improvement. At the end of 12 weeks, 91% in the tazarotene/midpotency corticosteroid group and 95% in the tazarotene/high-potency corticosteroid group versus 80% in the tazarotene 0.1% gel/placebo group obtained at least 50% improvement. The results with tazarotene/low-potency corticosteroid group were not statistically superior to the tazarotene 0.1% gel/placebo group. Local skin irritation was less frequent in the groups treated with tazarotene plus a mid- or high-potency corticosteroid.

Tazarotene plus high-potency corticosteroid had rates of burning that were almost half that of tazarotene plus placebo (12% vs. 23%, respectively). During follow-up, rebound effect, sometimes seen after discontinuation of corticosteroid monotherapy, was not observed in any of the combination tazarotene and topical steroid groups. Similarly, other studies have confirmed that the use of a mid- or high-potency corticosteroid enhances the efficacy and tolerability of tazarotene [21,22].

In addition, the efficacy and tolerability of tazarotene with a midpotency topical steroid have been further studied. The combination of 0.1% tazarotene gel once daily with 0.1% mometasone furoate cream once daily was compared with monotherapy with 0.1% mometasone furoate cream twice daily [18]. Seventy-three psoriasis patients in total were treated for 12 weeks, followed by 12 weeks of observation. At the end of 12 weeks, 74% of the patients treated with combination therapy of tazarotene with mometasone cream versus 58% of the patients treated with twice-daily mometasone furoate monotherapy achieved at least 50% global improvement in their psoriasis. During follow-up, 68% (15/22) of the mometasone furoate monotherapy group dropped out from the study during the first four weeks due to recurrence and rebound, compared with only 12% (3/26) from the combination therapy group.

Thus, the studies mentioned above show that the combination of mid- or high-potency steroid with tazarotene achieves faster and greater therapeutic effects, with less side effects and longer remission time than tazarotene monotherapy or topical corticosteroid monotherapy.

Three different mid- to high-potency topical steroids (i.e., betamethasone dipropionate 0.05% cream [Diprosone®], fluticasone propionate 0.005% ointment [Cutivate®], or diflorasone diacetate 0.05% cream [Maxiflor®]) and three different high-potency steroid ointments (i.e., fluocinonide 0.05% [Lidex®], mometasone furoate 0.1% [Elocon®], or diflorasone diacetate 0.05% [Maxiflor®]) were compared in terms of efficacy and tolerability in combination with tazarotene in a 12-week, multicenter, investigator-masked, randomized parallel-group study involving 200 patients [23]. Topical corticosteroid was applied in the morning and 0.1% tazarotene gel was applied in the evening. The best-performing steroid was betamethasone dipropionate 0.05% cream (a mid- to high-potency steroid), followed by mometasone furoate 0.1% ointment (a high-potency steroid) and diflorasone diacetate 0.05% ointment (a high-potency steroid). The best-tolerated regimen, however, was tazarotene plus mometasone furoate 0.1% ointment, and the optimal balance between efficacy and tolerability was achieved with this regimen.

The combination of betamethasone valerate foam 0.12% (Luxiq®) and 0.1% tazarotene cream was shown to be effective in a case series of 10 psoriasis patients [24]. Two patients were clear of their psoriasis by week 4 and four were clear at week 8. Most importantly, no adverse events, including irritation, were reported. The authors report the use of the corticosteroid foam may protect against tazarotene-induced skin irritation, and the cosmetic appeal of a nongreasy corticosteroid foam improved patient compliance with the resultant high efficacy that was seen.

A double-blind, randomized, vehicle-controlled study examined the efficacy of a combination of tazarotene and clobetasol both for initial efficacy and for maintenance use [19]. In total, 50 psoriasis patients were treated with a combination of 0.1% tazarotene gel and clobetasol ointment for an initial six-week "induction" phase. For the first two weeks, 0.1% tazarotene gel was applied every morning and clobetasol ointment was applied every evening. During weeks 3 and 4, 0.1% tazarotene gel was applied every morning and clobetasol ointment was applied on Tuesday, Thursday, and Saturday evenings. During the last two weeks, 0.1% tazarotene gel was applied on Monday, Wednesday, and Friday mornings and clobetasol ointment was applied on Tuesday and Thursday evenings. After the six-week induction phase, patients with at least 50% improvement were randomized into one of the following three maintenance treatment groups for five months: (1) combination therapy with 0.1% tazarotene gel applied on Monday, Wednesday, and Friday and 0.05% clobetasol propionate ointment applied on Tuesday and Thursday; (2) 0.1% tazarotene gel applied on Monday, Wednesday, and Friday and white petrolatum applied on Tuesday and Thursday; and (3) tazarotene gel vehicle applied on Monday, Wednesday, and Friday and white petrolatum applied on Tuesday and Thursday. At the end of the five-month maintenance therapy, 73% on tazarotene and clobetasol combination therapy, 47% on tazarotene thrice weekly, and 19% on vehicle retained at least 50% improvement relative to baseline. Similarly, other studies have also confirmed lengthy remissions when tazarotene is used in combination with topical steroids [25].

TAZAROTENE AND TOPICAL STEROID-INDUCED SKIN ATROPHY

Not only do tazarotene and topical steroid act synergistically but also tazarotene reduces the degree of topical steroid-induced skin atrophy [26]. In a study involving 24 healthy volunteers, subjects were randomized to apply 0.1% tazarotene gel, 0.05% diflorasone diacetate (Psorcon®), and 0.1% tazarotene gel combined with 0.05% diflorasone diacetate six days/week for four weeks [26]. The subjects who applied 0.1% tazarotene gel had a mean epidermal thickness increase of 62%. The subjects who applied 0.05% diflorasone diacetate experienced a 43% reduction in the mean epidermal thickness. However, in the subjects who used tazarotene in combination with 0.05% diflorasone diacetate, there was only a reduction of 28% in the epidermal thickness. Thus, tazarotene significantly reduced epidermal atrophy induced by topical steroid.

TAZAROTENE CHEMICAL COMPATIBILITY WITH A TOPICAL STEROID

Tazarotene and a range of topical corticosteroids (i.e., mometasone furoate 0.1% cream; fluocinonide 0.05% ointment and cream; betamethasone dipropionate 0.05% gel, ointment, cream, and lotion; clobetasol propionate 0.05% gel, ointment, cream, and scalp solution; diflorasone diacetate 0.05% ointment and cream; halobetasol propionate ointment and cream) may be applied at the same time without adversely affecting the chemical stability of either tazarotene or the corticosteroids [27]. However, chemical stability for past two weeks has not been studied; therefore, tazarotene and topical corticosteroids should not be premixed in a jar.

TAZAROTENE AND CALCIPOTRIENE

Although tazarotene and calcipotriene might not be as potent as class I topical steroids when each is used as monotherapy, they appear to have synergistic effects when combined with the same efficacy and rapidity as class I superpotent topical steroids [28]. In a prospective, open-label, left–right comparison study, combination therapy of 0.1% tazarotene gel once daily with calcipotriene ointment twice daily was comparable to clobetasol ointment twice daily [28]. The study consisted of 15 patients who underwent a two-week treatment course, followed by a four-week observation period. At the end of the two weeks, lesions treated with tazarotene and calcipotriene had the same improvement in overall lesion severity, reduction in plaque elevation, and scaling as the clobetasol-treated lesions. Not surprisingly, erythema improved more in the clobetasol-treated lesions than the combined tazarotene and calcipotriene-treated lesions. There does not seem to be any chemical incompatibility between calcipotriene ointment and tazarotene gel that is clinically significant [28].

In a multicenter, randomized, investigator-masked study involving 120 psoriasis patients, the combination of tazarotene gel once daily with mometasone furoate cream once daily was compared with calcipotriene ointment twice daily [29]. In total, 45% of patients in the combined tazarotene and mometasone group achieved ≥75% global improvement after two weeks of treatment compared with only 26% of patients in the calcipotriene group [29]. Furthermore, the combination tazarotene and mometasone group had a significantly greater reduction in scaling, erythema, plaque elevation, and body surface area involvement than calcipotriene monotherapy at the end of the four-week follow-up period.

TAZAROTENE AND UVB PHOTOTHERAPY

Tazarotene has been successfully combined with both broadband UVB phototherapy (BB-UVB) [26,27] and narrowband UVB phototherapy (NB-UVB) [30] for more effective and rapid clearing of psoriasis compared with either treatment alone.

Once-daily treatment with tazarotene 0.1% gel for two weeks followed by three times a week BB-UVB and tazarotene 0.1% gel was superior to BB-UVB monotherapy [31]. It took a median of 25 days for the tazarotene and BB-UVB group to reach at least 50% improvement versus 53 days with BB-UVB monotherapy. Combined tazarotene and BB-UVB therapy also resulted in greater improvement in plaque elevation and scaling than did BB-UVB monotherapy. In addition, tazarotene significantly reduced the amount of UV radiation required to improve psoriasis. The median cumulative BB-UVB dose was 390 mJ/cm^2 in the combined tazarotene and BB-UVB group, whereas it was approximately four times higher (i.e., 1644 mJ/cm^2) in BB-UVB monotherapy.

To evaluate the efficacy of topical tazarotene in combination with NB-UVB, 10 patients in total were treated with 0.05% tazarotene once daily to one side of the body and NB-UVB five times a week for four weeks [30]. Greater reduction in the Psoriasis Area and Severity Index (PASI) scores were noted in the tazarotene-treated side.

Tazarotene and vitamin D analogs as adjuncts to NB-UVB therapy also have been evaluated. Schiener et al. [32] studied 10 patients with widespread psoriasis and compared the combination of tazarotene gel 0.05% plus NB-UVB to calcipotriol ointment plus NB-UVB [32]. Patients received NB-UVB treatment four times weekly and applied either of the assigned topical treatments once every evening on different halves of the body. Results showed that both regimens had identical number of exposure days and identical cumulative NB-UVB dose. Calcipotriol was generally very well tolerated. One patient developed hyperpigmentation strictly limited to the area where calcipotriol ointment was applied. On the side that tazarotene 0.05% gel was applied, four patients complained of itching and dryness. Despite such complaints, a follow-up questionnaire showed that 6 of 10 patients still preferred tazarotene gel over calcipotriol ointment because it was easier to spread and less greasy.

To date, no trials have assessed efficacy or safety of tazarotene use before UVB exposure. Therefore, if used in combination with UVB, tazarotene should be applied after light treatment. Because tazarotene has been shown to reduce epidermal thickness, concerns have been expressed regarding the increased risk of burning. Some suggest reducing the UVB dosage by one-third if tazarotene is added during phototherapy [33].

No significant photosensitivity occurred when tazarotene was used with phototherapy in any of these phototherapy trials. In addition, the incidence of irritation was less than expected when tazarotene was used with phototherapy than without. Behrens et al. [30] postulated that this outcome might be the result of an enhanced barrier because UVA- and UVB-treated skin is more resistant to irritants [30].

TAZAROTENE AND PUVA PHOTOTHERAPY

To determine whether administration of topical tazarotene can increase the efficacy of systemic PUVA, Tzaneva et al. [34] compared the therapeutic response of tazarotene plus PUVA to PUVA monotherapy in 31 chronic plaque-type psoriasis patients [34]. Patients received PUVA treatment four times a week and applied 0.1% tazarotene gel every evening. To achieve complete, or near complete, clearing, the cumulative UVA dose and the number of UVA exposures were statistically lower in those receiving combined PUVA and tazarotene therapy than those with PUVA monotherapy. The median cumulative dosage was 32.3 J/cm^2 for tazarotene plus PUVA and 37.0 J/cm^2 for PUVA monotherapy. There was no difference in the observed duration of remission.

TAZAROTENE AND PALMOPLANTAR PSORIASIS

In a single-center, prospective, comparative study, 30 patients were randomized to tazarotene 0.1% cream once daily or clobetasol propionate 0.05% cream once daily for 12 weeks. Assessments were made every two weeks by using an erythema, scaling, fissures, and induration (ESFI) score and Physician's Global Assessment (PGA) scale. At week 12, there was no significant difference between the two groups. Tazarotene group showed mean ESFI reduction from 6.65 to 1.12 (83.2% improvement) and complete clearance in 53% of patients. Clobetasol propionate group showed mean ESFI reduction from 5.69 to 0.62 (89.1% improvement) and complete clearance in 62% of patients. Clobetasol was observed to have a faster onset of action in erythema, scaling, and fissuring than tazarotene. Itching and irritation were reported in the tazarotene group at weeks 2 and 4 but resolved with continued usage of study agent. More than half of the patients (53.8%) of the clobetasol propionate group reported hypopigmentation at the end of the study [35].

TAZAROTENE AND NAIL PSORIASIS

Nail psoriasis also responds to tazarotene gel. In a randomized, double-blind, vehicle-controlled study, 31 patients with fingernail psoriasis were randomized to either 0.1% tazarotene gel or vehicle gel once daily for 24 weeks [36]. The treatment was applied to two fingernails: one nail under occlusion and the other nail unoccluded. Tazarotene treatment under occlusion resulted in significant reduction of onycholysis at weeks 4 and 12 and significant reduction of pitting by week 24. Unoccluded tazarotene treatment resulted in significant reduction in onycholysis by week 24, but no improvement in pitting was noted. Tazarotene was well tolerated except for few cases of mild to moderate adverse effects of irritation and erythema. Thus, although both occluded and unoccluded tazarotene gel therapies were effective in decreasing onycholysis, the occluded tazarotene gel achieved its goal much earlier than the unoccluded tazarotene gel.

In double-blind study, 30 psoriasis patients with nail psoriasis were randomized to tazarotene 0.1% cream or clobetasol propionate 0.05% cream under occlusion nightly for 12 weeks. Fourteen patients dropped out of the study; 10 patients dropped out of the study due to urgent need for systemic therapy to address the patients' cutaneous psoriasis. The comparison of improvement between administered agents did not reach statistical significance. Three of the 16 patients in the tazarotene group reported desquamation, erythema, paronychia, and irritation. One of the 14 patients in the clobetasol group reported sensation of burning. All cases of adverse reactions were considered mild, and symptoms improved after a few days [37].

In a single-blind, bilateral comparative study, 19 patients with recalcitrant nail psoriasis treated one hand with pulsed dye laser (PDL) and tazarotene 0.1% cream (experimental group) and the other hand with tazarotene 0.1% cream only (control group). The mean decrease in nail matrix modified Nail Psoriasis Severity Index (NAPSI) score from baseline to six months was significantly greater in the experimental group than in the control group in both patients with systemic therapy and without systemic therapy. Vesicle formation after the first session of laser treatment was reported in only one patient. The energy density was adjusted, and no vesicle was noted again [38].

TAZAROTENE APPLICATION IN PSORIASIS

Proper patient instruction is essential when using tazarotene. Patients should be instructed to apply tazarotene directly on the thick and scaly psoriatic lesions, taking care to avoid surrounding unaffected skin. Once the skin has become flat and nonscaly, tazarotene should be discontinued. The gel and cream should be allowed to dry before wearing clothes, because wearing clothing immediately after application might inadvertently spread the product onto uninvolved skin and cause irritation. Only a small amount of tazarotene is required. Use of excessive amounts may result in irritation. Patients should be warned of the likelihood of

TABLE 7.1 Short-Contact Therapy

Apply tazarotene to plaques for a short time (5–20 minutes).
Wash medication off after prescribed time period with water.
Gradually increase application time by 1–5 minutes as tolerated.

TABLE 7.2 Triple Combination Therapy

Step 1. Apply a combination of superpotent topical steroid and calcipotriene in the morning.
Step 2. Apply a combination of superpotent topical steroid, calcipotriene, and tazarotene to plaques in the evening.
Step 3. Apply a combination of superpotent topical steroid and calcipotriene after short-contact therapy with tazarotene.

irritation, particularly if the agent is used on the face and neck. Intertriginous regions and genitals should be avoided. The gel preparation is preferable for scalp and nail psoriasis. If significant irritation occurs, the patient may benefit from what is termed "short-contact" therapy (Table 7.1) [39,40]. Duration of application appears to be related to the rate of improvement. For example, after a very short contact (e.g., five minutes), first signs of improvement are seen about three weeks later; after a 20-minute application, improvement is seen 7–10 days later.

Withholding treatment until irritation subsides then reintroducing therapy every other day or changing to the 0.05% cream formulation (if an alternate formulation is used) also may help to reduce irritation. For patients with sensitive skin who might be prone to irritation, treatment with tazarotene may begin with the 0.05% cream formulation and stepped up as tolerated. In addition, initiation of therapy with alternate-day application has been recommended by some studies as a method to maximize tolerability [41]. Irritation is most common during the first 1–2 weeks of therapy [42]. With time, most patients seem to be able to tolerate nightly treatment, but they may occasionally need to skip a night because of irritation.

Tazarotene may be most efficacious and best tolerated when used in combination with a mid- or high-potency topical corticosteroid, calcipotriene, UVB phototherapy, or PUVA. We favor a triple combination therapy topical regimen for treating recalcitrant thick psoriatic lesions (Table 7.2).

SIDE EFFECTS

The most common side effects of tazarotene treatment are skin irritation, including itching, burning, and erythema. These side effects occurred in 10%–23% of patients using the cream formulation and in 10%–30% of patients using the gel formulation, with 1%–5% points higher incidence correlated with the 0.1% concentration than the 0.05% concentration [43]. No other treatment-related serious adverse effects were reported.

Although the medication is not phototoxic or photoallergenic, the U.S. Food and Drug Administration (FDA)–approved package insert cautions against sunlight and sunlamp exposure. When combined with UVB, thinning of the stratum corneum has been demonstrated, predisposing patients to burn more easily [44]. If tazarotene is added to an ongoing phototherapy regimen, once there is evidence of decreased scaling and induration from the application of tazarotene, it may be prudent to lower the UVB dose by 30%–50% or UVA dose (for PUVA) by 2 J/cm^2 [41].

The FDA has classified topical tazarotene as pregnancy category X. Tazarotene should not be used in pregnancy or in women who are not practicing adequate contraception.

CONCLUSIONS

Topical tazarotene is the only topical retinoid indicated for the treatment of psoriasis in the United States. Rather than using tazarotene as a monotherapy, tazarotene should be used in combination with mid- or high-potency topical corticosteroids, calcipotriene, UVB phototherapy, or PUVA as part of a long-term maintenance regimen.

REFERENCES

1. Tang-Liu DD, Matsumoto RM, Usansky JL. Clinical pharmacokinetics and drug metabolism of tazarotene: a novel topical treatment for acne and psoriasis. *Clin Pharmacokinet* 1999; 37: 273–287.
2. Nagpal S, Chandraratna RA. Recent developments in receptor-selective retinoids. *Curr Pharm Des* 2000; 6: 919–931.
3. Fisher GJ, Talwar HS, Yiao JH, et al. Immunological identification and functional quantification of retinoic acid and retinoid X receptor proteins in human skin. *J Biol Chem* 1994; 269: 20269–20635.
4. Lefebvre P. Molecular basis for designing selective modulators of retinoic acid receptor transcriptional activities. *Curr Drug Targets Immune Endocr Metabol Disord* 2001; 1: 153–164.
5. Nagpal S, Athanikar J, Chandraratna RA. Separation of transactivation and AP1 antagonism functions of retinoic acid receptor alpha. *J Biol Chem* 1995; 270: 923–927.
6. Roeder A, Schaller M, Schäfer-Korting M, et al. Tazarotene: therapeutic strategies in the treatment of psoriasis, acne and photoaging. *Skin Pharmacol Physiol* 2004; 17: 111–118.
7. Esgleyes-Ribot T, Chandraratna RA, LewKaya DA, et al. Response of psoriasis to a new topical retinoid, AGN 190168. *J Am Acad Dermatol* 1994; 30: 581–590.
8. Nonomura K, Yamanishi K, Yasuno H, et al. Up-regulation of elafin/SKALP gene expression in psoriatic epidermis. *J Invest Dermatol* 1994; 103: 88–91.
9. Krueger GC, Drake LA, Elias PM, et al. The safety and efficacy of tazarotene gel a topical acetylenic retinoid, in the treatment of psoriasis. *Arch Dermatol* 1998; 134: 57–60.
10. Weinstein GD, Krueger GG, Lowe NJ, et al. Tazarotene gel, a new retinoid, for topical therapy of psoriasis: vehicle-controlled study of safety, efficacy and duration of therapeutic effects. *J Am Acad Dermatol* 1997; 37: 85–92.
11. Weinstein GD, Koo JY, Krueger GG, et al. Tazarotene Cream Clinical Study Group: tazarotene cream in the treatment of psoriasis: two multi-center, double-blind, randomized, vehicle-controlled studies of the safety and efficacy of tazarotene creams 0.05% and 0.1% applied once daily for 12 weeks. *J Am Acad Dermatol* 2003; 48: 760–767.
12. Kumar U, Kaur I, Dogra S, et al. Topical tazarotene vs. coal tar in stable plaque psoriasis. *Clin Exp Dermatol* 2010; 35: 482–486.
13. Lebwohl M, Aste E, Callen J, et al. Once-daily tazarotene gel versus twice-daily floucinonide cream in the treatment of plaque psoriasis. *J Am Acad Dermatol* 1998; 38: 705–711.
14. Angelo JS, Kar BR, Thomas J. Comparison of clinical efficacy of topical tazarotene 0.1% cream with topical clobetasol propionate 0.05% cream in chronic plaque psoriasis: a double-blind, randomized, right-left comparison study. *Indian J Dermatol Venereol Leprol* 2007; 73: 65.
15. Tzung TY, Wu JC, Hsu NJ, et al. Comparison of tazarotene 0.1% gel plus petrolatum once daily versus calcipotriol 0.005% ointment twice daily in the treatment of plaque psoriasis. *Acta Derm Venereol* 2005; 85: 236–239.
16. Kaur I, Dogra S, Jain R, et al. Comparative study of calcipotriol (0.005%) ointment and tazarotene (0.05% and 0.1%) gel in the treatment of stable plaque psoriasis. *Indian J Dermatol Venereol Leprol* 2008; 74: 471–474.

17. Lebwohl M. Strategies to optimize efficacy, duration of remission and safety in the treatment of plaque psoriasis by using tazarotene in combination with corticosteroid. *J Am Acad Dermatol* 2000; 43(2 Pt 3): S43–S46.
18. Koo JY, Martin D. Investigator-masked comparison of tazarotene gel q.d. plus mometasone furoate cream q.d. vs. mometasone furoate cream b.i.d. in the treatment of plaque psoriasis. *Int J Dermatol* 2001; 40: 210–212.
19. Lebwohl M, Lombardi K, Tan MH. Duration of improvement in psoriasis after treatment with tazarotene 0.1% gel plus clobetasol propionate 0.05% ointment: comparison of maintenance treatment. *Int J Dermatol* 2001; 40: 64–66.
20. Lebwohl M, Breneman D, Goffe B, et al. Tazarotene 0.1% gel plus corticosteroid cream in the treatment of plaque psoriasis. *J Am Acad Dermatol* 1998; 39: 590–596.
21. Tanghetti EA, Tazarotene Stable Plaque Psoriasis Trial Study Group. An observation study evaluating the efficacy of tazarotene plus corticosteroid in treating plaque psoriasis in patients switched from treatment with calcipotriene ± corticosteroid. *Curtis* 2000; 66(Suppl 6): 12–18.
22. Gollnick H, Menter A. Combination therapy with tazarotene plus a topical corticosteroid for the treatment of plaque psoriasis. *Br J Dermatol* 1999; 140(Suppl 54): 18–23.
23. Green L, Sadoff W. A clinical evaluation of tazarotene 0.1% gel, with and without a high- or mid-high-potency corticosteroid, in patients with stable plaque psoriasis. *J Cutan Med Surg* 2002; 6: 95–102.
24. Dhawan S, Blyumin M, Pearce D, et al. Case reports: tazarotene cream (0.1%) in combination with betamethasone valerate foam (0.12%) for plaque-type psoriasis. *J Drug Dermatol* 2005; 4: 228–230.
25. Poulin YP. Tazarotene 0.01% gel in combination with mometasone furoate in plaque psoriasis: a photographic tracking study. *Cutis* 1999; 63: 41–48.
26. Kaiddbey K, Kopper SC, Sefton J, et al. A pilot study to determine the effect of tazarotene 0.1% gel on steroid-induced epidermal atrophy. *Int J Dermatol* 2001; 40: 468–471.
27. Hecker D, Worsley J, Yueh G, et al. In vitro compatibility of tazarotene with other topical treatments of psoriasis. *J Am Acad Dermatol* 2000; 42: 1008–1011.
28. Bowman P, Maloney J, Koo J. Combination of calcipotriene (Dovonex) ointment and tazarotene (Tazorac) gel versus clobetasol ointment in the treatment of plaque psoriasis: a pilot study. *J Am Acad Dermatol* 2002; 46: 907–913.
29. Guenther LC, Poulin YP, Prasier DM. A comparison of tazarotene 0.1% gel once daily plus mometasone furoate 0.1% cream daily versus calcipotriene 0.005% ointment twice daily in the treatment of plaque psoriasis. *Clin Ther* 2000; 22: 1225–1238.
30. Koo JY, Lowe NJ, Lew-Kaya DA. Tazarotene plus UVB phototherapy in the treatment of psoriasis. *J Am Acad Dermatol* 2000; 43: 821–828.
31. Behrens S, Grundmann-Kollamn M, Schiener R, et al. Combination phototherapy of psoriasis with narrow-band UVB irradiation and topical tazarotene gel. *J Am Acad Dermatol* 2000; 42: 493–495.
32. Schiener R, Behrens-Williams SC, Pillekamp H, et al. Calcipotriol versus tazarotene as combination therapy with narrowband ultraviolet B (311 nm): efficacy in patients with severe psoriasis. *Br J Dermatol* 2000; 143: 1275–1278.
33. Hecker D, Worsley J, Yueh G, et al. Interactions between tazarotene and ultraviolet light. *J Am Acad Dermatol* 1999; 41: 927–930.
34. Tzaneva S, Seebar A, Honigsmann A. A comparison of psoralen plus ultraviolet A (PUVA) monotherapy, tacalcitol plus PUVA and tazarotene plus PUVA in patients with chronic plaque-type psoriasis. *Br J Dermatol* 2002; 147: 748–753.
35. Mehta BH, Amladi ST. Evaluation of topical 0.1% tazarotene cream in the treatment of palmoplantar psoriasis: an observer-blinded randomized controlled study. *Indian J Dermatol* 2011; 56: 40–43.
36. Scher RK, Stiller M, Zhu YI. Tazarotene 0.1% gel in the treatment of fingernail psoriasis: a double-blind, randomized, vehicle-controlled study. *Cutis* 2000; 68: 355–358.
37. Rigopoulos D, Gregoriou S, Katsambas A. Treatment of psoriatic nails with tazarotene cream 0.1% vs. clobetasol propionate 0.05% cream: a double-blind study. *Acta Derm Venereol* 2007; 87: 167–168.
38. Huang YC, Chou CL, Chiang YY. Efficacy of pulsed dye laser plus topical tazarotene versus topical tazarotene alone in psoriatic nail disease: a single-blind, intrapatient left-to-right controlled study. *Lasers Surg Med* 2013; 45: 102–107.
39. Veraldi S, Schianchi R. Short-contact therapy with tazarotene in psoriasis vulgaris. *Dermatol* 2003; 206: 347–348.

40. Persaud A, Bershad S, Lamba S, et al. *Poster presentation, short-contact tazarotene therapy for psoriasis*. Nashville, TN: American Academy of Dermatology; 2000.
41. Koo JYM, Lebwohl MG, Lowe NJ, et al. Blueprints for optimizing topical retinoid treatment of psoriasis using creative therapeutic regimens. *Skin Allergy News* 2002.
42. Guenther L. Optimizing treatment with topical tazarotene. *Am J Clin Dermatol* 2003; 4: 197–202.
43. Allergan, Inc. Tazorac® (tazarotene) package insert. Irvine, CA: Allergen, Inc. 2011.
44. Lowe NJ. Optimizing therapy: tazarotene in combination with phototherapy. *Br J Dermatol* 1999; 140(Suppl 54): 8–11.

Chapter 8

Topical Calcineurin Inhibitors

Mark G. Lebwohl and Chrystal A. Landry

Topical calcineurin inhibitors are a treatment option for individuals with certain limited manifestations of psoriasis. Although these immunomodulatory drugs were initially developed for preventing organ rejection in transplant patients, they have quickly become a mainstay of off-label treatment for psoriasis since their clinical introduction in topical formulation in 2000. The topical calcineurin inhibitors tacrolimus (Protopic®) ointment and pimecrolimus (Elidel®) cream are approved for the treatment of atopic dermatitis in the United States.

The calcineurin inhibitor cyclosporine was initially isolated from *Tolypocladium inflatum gans*, a soil fungus. Although its systemic formulation is frequently accompanied by side effects of nephrotoxicity and hypertension, it has proved to be an effective treatment for psoriasis [1]. However, it has been proven of no clinical use in topical formulation. This lack of effectiveness is mostly attributed to the inability of cyclosporine to penetrate the skin due to its large molecular weight [2]. However, novel derivatives of the cyclosporine molecule with increased penetrating capability are in development [3].

Tacrolimus and pimecrolimus, unlike cyclosporine, are macrolide xenobiotics with similar immunosuppressive properties [1]. Tacrolimus is naturally produced by and was first isolated from the bacterium *Streptomyces tsukubaensis*, whereas pimecrolimus is produced by *Streptomyces hygroscopicus* var. *ascomycetius*. Systemic tacrolimus has been shown to be effective in patients with severe recalcitrant plaque psoriasis [4,5]. Additional clinical studies show that oral pimecrolimus can also produce a dose-dependent reduction in plaque psoriasis severity [6,7].

Both macrolides have the added benefit of smaller molecular weights that eases skin penetration and thus their successful topical applications in the treatment of immune-mediated skin disease. Although tacrolimus has been shown to be less penetrative [8], macrolide-derived calcineurin inhibitors do not carry the adverse side effects associated with long-term topical corticosteroid therapy, such as cutaneous atrophy and the formation of striae. New formulations to enhance penetration of topical calcineurin inhibitors are being studied. One such vehicle, liquid crystalline nanoparticles loaded with tacrolimus, has shown some promise [9].

MECHANISM OF ACTION

Since T-helper cells have been implicated in the pathogenesis of autoimmune inflammatory skin disease, such as psoriasis, treatments that inhibit T cells and the associated inflammatory processes should theoretically be effective in the treatment of psoriasis.

When a T-helper lymphocyte interacts with an antigen-presenting cell via a major histocompatibility complex, the transmembrane CD3 complex triggers an increase in intracellular free calcium. This calcium binds and activates calmodulin, which then binds and activates the phosphatase calcineurin. Once calcineurin dephosphorylates the cytoplasmic subunit of the nuclear factor of activated T cells (NFATc), NFATc is able to move into the nucleus. Here, it combines with the nuclear subunit NFATn to form an active transcription factor that binds and promotes the transcription of a group of proinflammatory cytokine and receptor genes, including those for interleukin (IL)-2, IL-4, interferon (IFN)-γ, tumor necrosis factor (TNF)-α, and IL-2R [1,8].

Pimecrolimus and tacrolimus are both prodrugs; when they are absorbed by the skin or systemically bind to an intracellular receptor protein called FK506-binding protein, or tacrolimus-binding protein, a complex forms, which then allosterically binds and inhibits calcineurin. This complex blocks further downstream dephosphorylation of NFATc and subsequently blocks the transcription of proinflammatory cytokines and further activation of T cells [1,8]. It is believed that these drugs are successful in treating inflammatory skin disease principally by suppressing IL-2 production and IL-2R expression [1]. In a study of biopsied psoriatic lesions treated successfully with 0.3% tacrolimus gel, a significant reduction of IL-2R–positive (CD25) and CD4+ T cells in the epidermis and dermis was observed [10].

Sirolimus, another macrolide antibiotic, is in development as a topical immunosuppressive. It acts on intracellular proteins through a mechanism very similar to tacrolimus. Sirolimus, also called rapamycin, binds to the cytosolic protein FKBP12, but unlike the tacrolimus–FKBP12 complex that inhibits calcineurin, the sirolimus–FKBP12 complex inhibits the mammalian target of rapamycin (mTOR) pathway by directly binding the mTOR complex. In one preliminary double-blind study, 24 patients with chronic plaque psoriasis applied 2.2% topical sirolimus for six weeks followed by 8% sirolimus for additional six weeks to their plaques. A significant reduction in the mean clinical score, as well as CD4+ and proliferating cells in the epidermis was observed [11].

CLINICAL FINDINGS

Tacrolimus and pimecrolimus seem to be most effective in treatment of psoriasis in thin-skinned areas of the body. Since 2003, quite a few studies have supported the mounting evidence that 0.1% tacrolimus ointment is an effective and desirable treatment for recalcitrant psoriasis plaques of the face, genitals, and intertriginous areas of the body [12–17].

In one double-blind, multicenter study of 57 patients with moderate to severe inverse psoriasis, treatment with 1% pimecrolimus cream was revealed to be an effective and well-tolerated treatment. After eight weeks of twice-daily treatment, 82% of patients reported complete or good disease control compared with 41% receiving vehicle [18]. In a subsequent open-label study of 1% pimecrolimus cream with similar treatment parameters in 20 patients with facial psoriasis, 74.3% of patients improved in total symptom score. Two of the 20 patients reported transient warm sensations in their facial lesions; no additional drug-related adverse events were reported [19].

In another double-blind, parallel study, 50 patients were instructed to apply topical calcitriol (3 μg/g) or tacrolimus (0.3 mg/g) twice daily to their facial or genitofemoral psoriatic lesions for six weeks. Although both treatments were well tolerated, tacrolimus was demonstrated to provide a more advantageous clinical outcome than calcitriol by analysis of both target lesion score (67% vs. 51%) and the Physician's Global Assessment (PGA) score (60% vs. 33%). In addition, calcitriol was observed to cause perilesional erythema in significantly more patients than tacrolimus (55% vs. 16%) [20].

Corticosteroid use is associated with skin atrophy, striae, telangiectasia, and tachyphylaxis [21]. Tacrolimus and pimecrolimus may serve as an appropriate alternative to topical glucocorticoid treatment for psoriasis in areas especially prone to adverse steroid effects because calcineurin is not used in collagen synthesis [21]. In one clinical study of healthy volunteers, tacrolimus ointment was shown to have no effect on collagen synthesis in a seven-day application on buttock skin. In contrast, the same treatment with the glucocorticoid betamethasone valerate potently blocked collagen synthesis [21].

Although topical calcineurin inhibitors are quite effective in the thin skin of the face and intertriginous areas of the body, the hyperkeratotic lesions found in patients with plaque psoriasis have been less responsive to treatment. Literature suggests that more penetrative formulations of both pimecrolimus and tacrolimus could improve efficacy in treatment of plaque psoriasis.

Various formulations and methods of application of topical calcineurin inhibitors are currently in trials and development. One pilot study shows that nonocclusive application of tacrolimus ointment is not effective in treatment of plaque psoriasis [22]. However, occlusive application conditions are associated with effectiveness of topical pimecrolimus and tacrolimus treatment in psoriasis. When applied under occlusion to descaled plaques, 0.3% tacrolimus ointment was successful in decreasing both plaque erythema and induration [23]. In a study of pimecrolimus, both 0.3% and 1.0% cream concentrations were able to decrease erythema and induration scores by 82% and 63%, respectively, in a microplaque assay of psoriasis. According to Mrowietz et al. [24], 1% pimecrolimus is similar in efficacy to topical calcipotriol or clobetasol under these conditions.

In another study, 30 subjects with plaque psoriasis were treated for 12 weeks with 0.1% tacrolimus ointment in combination with 6% salicylic acid gel; the gel served as a penetration enhancer. With results based on the PGA score, 46% of patients achieved statistically significant clearing (score 0–2) of their plaque psoriasis by the end of the study [25].

Higher concentration formulations of tacrolimus have also been tested in psoriasis. Tacrolimus gel (0.3%) and tacrolimus cream (0.5%) were compared with calcipotriol ointment twice daily for 12 weeks in an open-label, observer-blinded study. All three preparations were comparably effective, but application site reactions were more common in the tacrolimus-treated sites [26].

Palmar and plantar psoriasis plaques are especially resistant to topical treatment. In a 2006 pilot study completed by Rivard et al. [27], 0.1% tacrolimus ointment was applied alone or in combination with 30 medium-dose long-wavelength ultraviolet A (UVA1) (50 J/cm^2)

treatments to the palmar or plantar plaques of five psoriasis patients. No appreciable changes were observed in palmar or plantar psoriasis plaque induration or scaling [27]. Another study did examine the benefits of tacrolimus ointment for pustular psoriasis of the palms and soles [28].

Although oral involvement of plaque psoriasis is rare, it has been successfully treated with topical tacrolimus in certain cases. In two individual cases, patients were observed to have lip and mouth psoriatic lesions in addition to widespread plaque psoriasis of the face, trunk, and extremities. After biopsies confirmed that the lip and mouth lesions were in fact psoriasis, both patients applied 0.1% tacrolimus ointment to the affected oral lesion. In both cases, marked clearing was observed within two weeks [29]. Combination therapy with topical tacrolimus, calcipotriol, and betamethasone dipropionate has been used to successfully treat psoriasis of the lips [30]. Tacrolimus ointment has also been used successfully in combination with calcipotriol ointment [31].

There have been a few observed cases of pustular psoriasis treated successfully with topical tacrolimus. In one case, a patient with generalized pustular psoriasis (GPP) applied 10 g/day of 0.1% tacrolimus to the entire body for a week after unsuccessful treatment with 5 μg/g calcipotriol. Plasma levels of tacrolimus were detected, indicating systemic absorption [32]. In another reported case, treatment with 0.1% tacrolimus ointment was initiated for a patient being treated with 3 mg/kg oral cyclosporine for GPP. Pustular lesions were cleared by day 50, and plasma levels of tacrolimus were undetectable [33]. In both cases, significant clearing of the pustular psoriasis lesions was observed. It appears that in both cases the topical tacrolimus treatment was effective due to better drug penetration; less hyperkeratosis and greater inflammation that compromise the skin barrier are characteristic of GPP.

ADVERSE EVENTS

The most common reported adverse events associated with topical tacrolimus and pimecrolimus is a mild to moderate warm or burning sensation or pruritus at the site of application. However, this usually decreases after the first few days of treatment [34]. The burning sensation and pruritus observed after topical application of calcineurin inhibitors have been attributed to their release of neuropeptides, such as substance P. The neuropeptides bind to mast cells and cause mast cell degranulation; it is thought that released histamine and tryptase bind to their receptors on sensory nerve fibers, causing pruritus and burning [35,36]. Such mild, associated treatment effects compared with other topical options, such as corticosteroids, suggest that topical calcineurin inhibitors are an optimal treatment for psoriasis of body areas where atrophy is of concern.

A more serious concern about topical calcineurin inhibitors was raised by the U.S. Food and Drug Administration (FDA) at a hearing conducted on February 15, 2005. A Pediatric Committee proposed a "black box" warning regarding the risk of lymphoma and skin cancer for the package inserts of topical tacrolimus and pimecrolimus due to the lack of long-term safety data. However, data presented at the FDA hearings largely supported the safety of topical calcineurin inhibitors. In a mouse model, 258 times the maximum human exposure of pimecrolimus had to be administered orally before lymphoma was detected [37]. In mouse models where pimecrolimus and tacrolimus were dissolved in an ethanol vehicle that increased skin penetration, it took 26 times the maximum human dose of tacrolimus and 47 times the maximum human dose of pimecrolimus before lymphomas were detected [38]. Immune-related lymphoproliferative disease was observed in a monkey model in which >35 times the maximum human exposure of oral pimecrolimus was administered [37]. However, Niwa et al. [38] demonstrated that in the presence of tacrolimus, dimethylbenzanthracene, and 12-*o*-tetradecanoylphorbol-13-acetate (TPA), there was a marked increase in skin tumor formation in mice. Tran et al. [39], however, demonstrated that topical calcineurin inhibitors filter ultraviolet B (UVB) and decrease UVB-induced thymine dimers in mice. In a large epidemiologic study, Naylor et al. [40] failed to demonstrate an increase in skin cancers in patients using tacrolimus ointment. Arellano et al. [41] found no increase in lymphomas in patients using topical calcineurin inhibitors. The safety of tacrolimus ointment has been reviewed in 8000 patients by Koo et al. [42] and for up to four years by Hanifin et al. [43]. The safety of pimecrolimus has been studied in 1133 infants for up to two years [44]. The frequency of malignancy in pivotal trials of pimecrolimus and tacrolimus was not increased in patients treated with active drug compared with those treated with placebo [37]. Importantly, topical tacrolimus is absorbed 10 times less than topical corticosteroids, and topical pimecrolimus is absorbed 70–100 times less than topical corticosteroids [45].

Despite the black box warning, the preponderance of evidence strongly suggests no increased risk of malignancy in patients treated with topical calcineurin inhibitors. Because cutaneous T-cell lymphoma (CTCL) is often misdiagnosed as eczema, many cases of CTCL attributed to topical calcineurin inhibitors most likely were misdiagnosed as eczema and incorrectly treated with calcineurin inhibitors. It is of concern that since the addition of the black box warning, physicians and patients have been reluctant to prescribe topical calcineurin inhibitors even though they are safer than treatment with chronic topical corticosteroids, systemic corticosteroids, or phototherapy. Nevertheless, for mild to moderate psoriasis, topical calcineurin inhibitors offer a valuable off-label treatment option, particularly for the face and intertriginous sites.

REFERENCES

1. Marsland AM, Griffiths, EM. The macrolide immunosuppressants in dermatology: mechanisms of action. *Eur J Dermatol* 2002; 12: 618–622.
2. Hermann RC, Taylor RS, Ellis CN, et al. Topical cyclosporin for psoriasis: in vitro skin penetration and clinical study. *Skin Pharmacol* 1988; 1: 246–249.
3. Billich A, Vyplel H, Grassberger M, et al. Novel cyclosporin derivatives featuring enhanced skin penetration despite increased molecular weight. *Bioorg Med Chem* 2005; 13: 3157–3167.
4. The European FK 506 Multicentre Psoriasis Study Group. Systemic tacrolimus (FK 506) is effective for the treatment of psoriasis in a double-blind, placebo-controlled study. *Arch Dermatol* 1996; 132: 419–423.
5. Jegasothy BV, Ackerman CD, Todo S, et al. Tacrolimus (FK 506)—a new therapeutic agent for severe recalcitrant psoriasis. *Arch Dermatol* 1992; 128: 781–785.
6. Gottlieb AB, Griffiths CEM, Ho VC, et al. Oral pimecrolimus in the treatment of moderate to severe chronic plaque-type psoriasis: a double-blind, multicentre, randomized, dose-finding trial. *Br J Dermatol* 2005; 152: 1219–1227.

7. Rappersberger K, Komar M, Ebelin M, et al. Pimecrolimus identifies a common genomic anti-inflammatory profile is clinically highly effective in psoriasis and is well tolerated. *J Invest Dermatol* 2002; 119: 876–887.
8. Nghiem P, Pearson G, Langley RG. Tacrolimus and pimecrolimus: from clever prokaryotes to inhibiting calcineurin and treating atopic dermatitis. *J Am Acad Dermatol* 2002; 46: 228–241.
9. Thapa RK, Yoo BK. Evaluation of the effect of tacrolimus-loaded liquid crystalline nanoparticles on psoriasis-like skin inflammation. *J Dermatolog Treat* 2013. [Epub ahead of print].
10. Vissers WH, van Vlijmen I, van Erp PE, et al. Topical treatment of mild to moderate plaque psoriasis with 0.3% tacrolimus gel and 0.5% tacrolimus cream: the effect on SUM score, epidermal proliferation, keratinization, T-cell subsets and HLA-DR expression. *Br J Dermatol* 2008; 158: 705–712.
11. Ormerod AD, Shah SAA, Copeland P, et al. Treatment of psoriasis with topical sirolimus: preclinical development and a randomized, double-blind trial. *Br J Dermatol* 2005; 152: 758–764.
12. Martin Ezquerra G, Sánchez Regaña M, Herrera Acosta E, et al. Topical tacrolimus for the treatment of psoriasis on the face, genitalia, intertriginous areas and corporal plaques. *J Drugs Dermatol* 2006; 5: 334–336.
13. Rallis E, Nasiopoulou A, Kouskoukis C, et al. Successful treatment of genital and facial psoriasis with tacrolimus ointment 0.1%. *Drugs Exp Clin Res* 2005; 31: 141–145.
14. Lebwohl M, Freeman AK, Chapman MS, et al. Tacrolimus ointment is effective for facial and intertriginous psoriasis. *J Am Acad Dermatol* 2004; 51: 723–730.
15. Yamamoto T, Nishioka K. Topical tacrolimus: an effective therapy for facial psoriasis. *Eur J Dermatol* 2003; 13: 471–473.
16. Clayton TH, Harrison PV, Nicholls R, et al. Topical tacrolimus for facial psoriasis. *Br J Dermatol* 2003; 149: 419–420.
17. Freeman AK, Linowski GJ, Brady C, et al. Tacrolimus ointment for the treatment of psoriasis on the face and intertriginous areas. *J Am Acad Dermatol* 2003; 48: 564–568.
18. Gribetz C, Ling M, Lebwohl M, et al. Pimecrolimus cream 1% in the treatment of intertriginous psoriasis: a double-blind, randomized study. *J Am Acad Dermatol* 2004; 51: 731–738.
19. Jacobi A, Braeutigam M, Mahler V, et al. Pimecrolimus 1% cream in the treatment of facial psoriasis: a 16-week open-label study. *Dermatology* 2008; 216: 133–136.
20. Yiao YH, Chiu HC, Tseng YS, et al. Comparison of cutaneous tolerance and efficacy of calcitriol 3 microg g(-1) ointment and tacrolimus 0.3 mg g(-1) ointment in chronic plaque psoriasis involving facial or genitofemoral areas: a double-blind, randomized controlled trial. *Br J Dermatol* 2007; 157: 1005–1012.
21. Reitamo S, Rissanen J, Remitz A, et al. Tacrolimus ointment does not affect collagen synthesis: results of a single-center randomized trial. *J Invest Dermatol* 1998; 111: 396–398.
22. Zonneveld IM, Rubins A, Jablonska S, et al. Topical tacrolimus is not effective in chronic plaque psoriasis: a pilot study. *Arch Dermatol* 1998; 134: 1101–1102.
23. Remitz A, Reitamo S, Erkko P, et al. Tacrolimus ointment improves psoriasis in a microplaque assay. *Br J Dermatol* 1999; 141: 103–107.
24. Mrowietz U, Graeber M, Brautigam M, et al. The novel ascomycin derivative SDZ ASM 981 is effective for psoriasis when used topically under occlusion. *Br J Dermatol* 1998; 139: 992–996.
25. Carroll C, Clarke J, Camacho F, et al. Topical Tacrolimus ointment combined with 6% salicylic acid gel for plaque psoriasis treatment. *Arch Dermatol* 2005; 141: 43–46.
26. Ortonne JP, van de Kerkhof PC, Prinz JC, et al. 0.3% Tacrolimus gel and 0.5% Tacrolimus cream show efficacy in mild to moderate plaque psoriasis: results of a randomized, open-label, observer-blinded study. *Acta Derm Venereol* 2006; 86(1): 29–33.
27. Rivard J, Janiga J, Lim HW. Tacrolimus ointment 0.1% alone and in combination with medium-dose UVA1 in the treatment of palmar or plantar psoriasis. *J Drugs Dermatol* 2006; 5: 505–510.
28. Laino L, DiCarlo A. Palmoplantar pustular psoriasis: clinical and video thermographic evaluation before and after topical tacrolimus treatment. *Arch Dermatol* 2011; 147(6): 760.
29. Yamamoto T, Nishioka K. Successful treatment with topical tacrolimus for oral psoriasis. *J Eur Acad Dermatol Venereol* 2006; 20: 1137–1138.
30. Sehgal VN, Sehgal S, Verma P, Singh N, Rasool F. Exclusive plaque psoriasis of the lips: efficacy of combination therapy of topical tacrolimus, calcipotriol, and betamethasone dipropionate. *Skinmed* 2012; 10(3): 183–184.

31. Tirado-Sánchez A, Ponce-Olivera RM. Preliminary study of the efficacy and tolerability of combination therapy with calcipotriene ointment 0.005% and tacrolimus ointment 0.1% in the treatment of stable plaque psoriasis. *Cutis* 2012; 90(3): 140–144.
32. Nagao K, Ishiko A, Yokoyama T, et al. A case of generalized pustular psoriasis treated with topical tacrolimus. *Arch Dermatol* 2003; 139: 1219.
33. García FR, González EF, Cabrera-Paz R, et al. Generalized pustular psoriasis successfully treated with topical tacrolimus. *Br J Dermatol* 2005; 152: 587–588.
34. Ring J, Mohrenschlager M, Henkel V. The US FDA 'black box' warning for topical calcineurin inhibitors: an ongoing controversy. *Drug Saf* 2008; 31: 185–198.
35. Ständer S, Luger TA. Antipruritic effects of pimecrolimus and tacrolimus. *Hautarzt* 2003; 54(5): 413–417.
36. Ständer S, Ständer H, Seeliger S, et al. Topical pimecrolimus and tacrolimus transiently induce neuropeptide release and mast cell degranulation in murine skin. *Br J Dermatol* 2007; 156(5): 1020–1026.
37. Anonymous. New warnings for two eczema drugs. Available at: www.fda.gov/fdac/departs/2006/206 ipd.html#eczema [Accessed April 2, 2006].
38. Niwa Y, Terashima T, Sumi H. Topical application of the immunosuppressant tacrolimus accelerates carcinogenesis in mouse skin. *Br J Dermatol* 2003; 149(5): 960–967.
39. Tran C, Lübbe J, Sorg O, et al. Topical calcineurin inhibitors decrease the production of UVB-induced thymine dimers from hairless mouse epidermis. *Dermatology* 2005; 211(4): 341–347.
40. Naylor M, Elmets C, Jaracz E, et al. Non-melanoma skin cancer in patients with atopic dermatitis treated with topical tacrolimus. *J Dermatolog Treat* 2005; 16(3): 149–153.
41. Arellano FM, Wentworth CE, Arana A, et al. Risk of lymphoma following exposure to calcineurin inhibitors and topical steroids in patients with atopic dermatitis. *J Invest Dermatol* 2007; 127(4): 808–816.
42. Koo JY, Fleischer AB Jr, Abramovits W, et al. Tacrolimus ointment is safe and effective in the treatment of atopic dermatitis: results in 8000 patients. *J Am Acad Dermatol* 2005; 53 (2 Suppl 2): S195–S205.
43. Hanifin JM, Paller AS, Eichenfield L, et al. Efficacy and safety of tacrolimus ointment treatment for up to 4 years in patients with atopic dermatitis. *J Am Acad Dermatol* 2005; 53 (2 Suppl 2): S186–S194.
44. Paul C, Cork M, Rossi AB, et al. Safety and tolerability of 1% pimecrolimus cream among infants: experience with 1133 patients treated for up to 2 years. *Pediatrics* 2006; 117(1): e118–e128.
45. Billich A, Aschauer H, Aszó di A, et al. Percutaneous absorption of drugs used in atopic eczema: pimecrolimus permeates less through skin than corticosteroids and tacrolimus. *Int J Pharm* 2004; 269(1): 29–35.

Chapter 9

Coal Tar, Anthralin, Salicylic Acid, and Lactic Acid

Sarah Fitzmaurice and John Y. M. Koo

INTRODUCTION

Topical agents for the treatment of psoriasis are indicated regardless of the body surface affected, but they are the mainstay of therapy for patients whose affected area is <10% of their body surface area. Among the traditional options of topical therapies for mild to moderate psoriasis are coal tar, anthralin, salicylic acid, and lactic acid. All four topical therapies have been used for many years and are proven safe and effective. However, newer topical agents such as calcipotriol and tazarotene, and the ever-present topical steroids, have reduced the use of these older agents. This chapter gives an overview of the use of coal tar, anthralin, salicylic acid, and lactic acid in the treatment of mild to moderate psoriasis.

COAL TAR

There are several types of tar used to treat skin conditions: wood tar, shale tar, and coal tar. Coal tar is the liquid byproduct of the distillation of bituminous coal and has a pungent smell [1]. Use of coal tar for skin conditions has been ongoing for millennia. Present-day preparations closely resemble the coal tar that Dioscorides described and called "Asphalt" almost 2000 years ago [2]. Mechanism of action is still unknown in part due to >10,000 ingredients contained in coal tar. However, its antipruritic, anti-inflammatory, and anti-psoriatic effects have been clinically evident for a very long time [3]. Coal tar's low cost, efficacy, and safety profile have made it one of the mainstays of mild to moderate psoriasis therapy during the decades preceding and following World War II. Coal tar is available in several preparations, including ointment, cream, lotion, shampoo, gel, solutions, and soaps. These products are available in multiple concentrations. Crude coal tar is often available in three concentrations—2%, 5%, and 10%—and is mainly used in Goeckerman therapy. Goeckerman therapy is named after the man who first used this treatment regimen for psoriasis in 1925 [4]. Goeckerman therapy involves the application of crude coal tar to the entire body, including unaffected areas, for several hours a day along with ultraviolet B (UVB) phototherapy. This treatment was previously an inpatient-only treatment due to the use of "black" tar, as opposed to the more elegant but less effective "gold" tar such as liquor carbonis detergens (LCD). The modern modified version involves a more convenient Monday through Friday outpatient regimen conducted in psoriasis "day treatment centers."

LCD, an alcohol extract of crude coal tar, is one of the most widely used refined preparations of coal tar that is more cosmetically acceptable and available in a solution form. The solution vehicle makes it ideal for its primary use in scalp psoriasis, but it is not as effective as black coal tar. LCD can also be compounded by specialty pharmacies in an Aquaphor base that is suitable for use on body lesions. Most preparations of topical tar are designed for once-daily application at night, but they may be used more often if the patient is willing.

Coal tar efficacy has been investigated in several trials. Goeckerman therapy efficacy was investigated in an open-label study by Lee and Koo [5]. This study examined 25 consecutive Goeckerman patients admitted to the University of California–San Francisco (UCSF) Psoriasis Treatment Center and showed that 100% of the patients reached Psoriasis Area Severity Index (PASI) score 75 by 12 weeks of treatment and 95% by eight weeks of treatment (Figures 9.1 and 9.2) [5]. This efficacy is remarkable considering that during 2003–2004 when this study was conducted, only the most recalcitrant psoriasis patients were referred to Goeckerman therapy. Most of these patients had failed many other treatment options such as etanercept, alefacept, efaluzimab, methotrexate, acitretin, outpatient phototherapy and of course, topical therapy. In fact, Goeckerman therapy is the only treatmentthat can reliably-clear patients who have failed multiple biologics, which has been reported by studies at both the University of California San Francisco and the Mayo Clinic [6,7].

Another study by Menter and Cram [8] evaluated the efficacy and remission time after Goeckerman treatment. In this study, 300 patients treated with the Goeckerman regimen were followed for one or more years. Average time to reach 90% clearing of the skin was 18 treatment days. Ninety percent of the patients remained clear for a minimum of eight months, and 73% were clear for one year or longer. It should be noted that this two-center (Dallas, Texas, and San Francisco, California) study was carried out in the early 1980s before the advent of health maintenance organizations (HMOs) and managed care, a time when

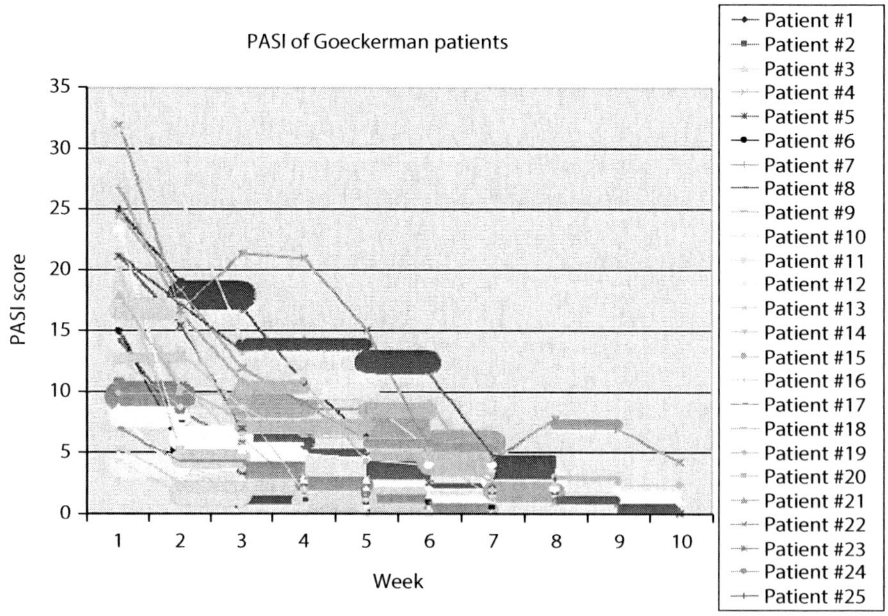

FIGURE 9.1 (See color insert.) PASI scores of 25 consecutive Goeckerman patients treated at the UCSF Psoriasis Treatment Center. (From Lee E and Koo J, *J Dermatol Treat* 16, 102–107, 2005.)

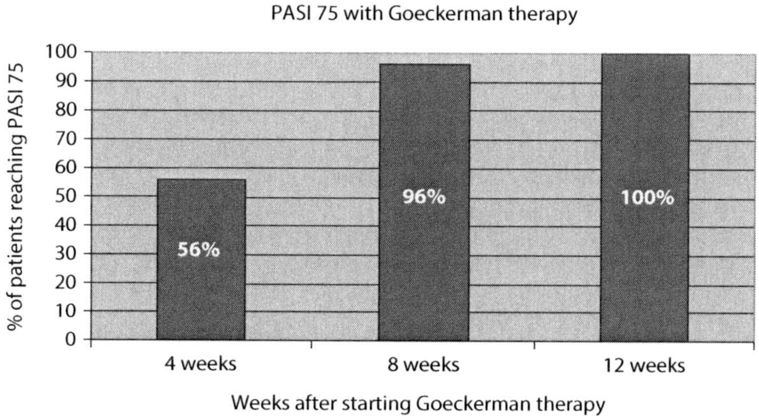

FIGURE 9.2 (See color insert.) Percentage of patients achieving PASI 75 with 4-, 8-, and 12-week Goeckerman therapy. (From Lee E and Koo J, *J Dermatol Treat* 16, 102–107, 2005.)

patients with generalized psoriasis had ready access to Goeckerman therapy. In today's practice almost two decades later, Goeckerman therapy is primarily being used by psoriasis patients who have failed multiple other treatment methods that require less commitment in time and energy. The remission time seen today can be as good as was documented by Menter and Cram [8], but primarily in those with naïve generalized psoriasis who have good insurance and gain access to Goeckerman therapy. The remission time of the more typical recalcitrant psoriasis patients referred for Goeckerman therapy today is generally shorter but still observed by us to be better than outpatient phototherapy and most biologics.

Notably, long remission times have been seen in the pediatric population treated with Goeckerman therapy. Currently, there is no systemic therapy approved by the U.S. Food and Drug Administration for pediatric psoriasis. The Mayo Clinic published results on a 21-year retrospective review of psoriasis patients from three months to 18 years who received Goeckerman treatment for a mean of 20 days in either the inpatient or outpatient day hospital setting. More than 90% of the patients were treated with 2% crude coal tar in petrolatum. The remaining patients were treated with 5% crude coal tar in petrolatum, 3% ichthyol, and 3% and 5% Zetar in Qualatum. For scalp treatment, different mixtures of LCD, salicylic acid, sulfur, topical steroids, and short-contact anthralin were used. Eighty-five percent of patients had ≥80% clearance of their psoriasis lesions and only 5% had <50% improvement. Median follow-up of 2.6 years was available for 91% of the patients treated. Of these patients, 83.3% had no relapse at one year. The only adverse side effect documented was folliculitis. They concluded that Goeckerman treatment is an effective therapy with minimal adverse effects and lasting remission in children with psoriasis [9].

Interestingly, there was some controversy about the effectiveness of coal tar in the mid-1980s. A study by Stern et al. [10] concluded that coal tar did not provide any added benefit to outpatient UVB phototherapy. This study compared 22 outpatients who applied tar oil to one side of their body and an oil vehicle to the other side of their body twice daily. They also received outpatient suberythemogenic doses of UVB phototherapy three times per week.

This study found no significant difference between the tar oil half and the oil vehicle half of the body. There was only a 9% reduction in the average UVB dose required for clearing on the body half treated with tar oil. However, it should be noted that both the tar oil and oil vehicle were applied just before phototherapy. Tar has been shown to block UVB, and this block most likely was the reason for lack of benefit of tar with suberythemogenic doses of UVB witnessed in this study. A study by Lebwohl et al. [11] confirmed tar's ability to block UVB light. For this reason, in patients treated with black tar (as opposed to brown tar or LCD) in Goeckerman therapy, UVB phototherapy is always given before the application of black tar. Since this study by Stern et al. [10] is a controversial publication, there have been many subsequent studies to validate the usefulness of coal tar with UVB. A study by Lowe et al. [12] indicated that tar is a beneficial addition to suberythemogenic doses of UVB. In this study tar was not applied before phototherapy. More rapid improvement was seen in the group treated with topical tar and suberythemogenic UVB than in the group treated with oil base and suberythemogenic UVB. This combination of topical tar and UVB effectively reduced the exposure to UVB. In general, for the ordinary psoriasis patient, erythemogenic UVB is as effective with or without tar. However, suberythemogenic UVB shows enhanced effectiveness with the addition of refined tar products such as LCD. Nevertheless, from our experience, for the rare patient with extraordinarily resistant psoriasis, Goeckerman therapy (black tar plus UVB) is much more effective than outpatient erythemogenic UVB alone. In our experience, the patient who has not cleared with maximal and optimal outpatient UVB with erythemogenic doses clears while on Goeckerman therapy.

It is widely accepted that regulatory T cells (Treg) are specialized T cells that fine-tune and abate the immune response. Psoriasis is recognized to be a T-cell-driven pathologic process with a predominance of CD8+ cells. Tregs can restrict CD8+ cells, thus theoretically diminishing the immune response in psoriasis. Kandelkova et al. demonstrated in a group of 27 psoriasis patients that the number of Treg cells in peripheral blood was higher after an average 15 days of Goeckerman treatment compared with pretreatment levels ($p = .0042$). They compared this group of psoriasis patients post-Goeckerman to healthy blood donors (no Goeckerman treatment) and found the Treg cells in psoriasis patients to be significantly higher ($p = .0019$). Mean pretreatment PASI scores of 17.5 ± 6.5 significantly decreased to 8.4 ± 4.6 post-Goeckerman treatment ($p < .0001$). This group concluded that these results support amelioration of a pathologic immune response in psoriasis via increased numbers of Treg cells subsequent to Goeckerman treatment [13].

On a similar note, a study conducted in the Czech Republic quantified the serum levels of interleukin (IL)-12 in patients pre- and post-Goeckerman therapy to assess alteration of blood levels associated with therapy. IL-12 is thought to be a proinflammatory cytokine that signals T-helper 1 (Th1) cell development. They compared the serum levels of IL-12 in 55 psoriasis patients to 47 healthy blood donors. This study by Borska et al. [14] reported statistically significant higher serum levels of IL-12 in psoriasis patients pre-Goeckerman therapy compared with controls. Post-Goeckerman therapy, there was a decrease in serum IL-12. They concluded from these results that Goeckerman had an immunosuppressive and anti-inflammatory effect. They also suggested that the study supported the belief that IL-12 is a proinflammatory mediator involved in the pathogenesis of psoriasis based on their finding of elevated IL-12 levels in psoriasis patients.

Coal tar is a safe agent to use in mild to moderate psoriasis, but it does have some obvious disadvantages and side effects that include staining of clothes and furniture, messy application, unpleasant odor, contact sensitivity, burning sensation, photosensitivity (although therapeutic in a controlled treatment setting), and tar folliculitis [2]. Generally, the higher the concentration, the more it is likely to cause skin irritation. Despite many decades of use, there seem to be no systemic side effects of topical application of coal tar. In addition, the risk of skin cancer seems to be either very small or not demonstrably different from that of the general population. A 25-year follow-up study conducted by Muller and Perry [15] in the 1980s found no difference in cancer rates between those treated with coal tar at the Mayo Clinic and that of the general population. More recent safety data on coal tar use comes from a large 2010 cohort study done in the Netherlands on 4315 psoriasis patients. Fifty-two percent of the psoriasis patients that met inclusion criteria of the study were treated with LCD, 19% with pix lithantracis (with and without LCD), and 29% had no tar treatment. The median duration of follow-up was 21 years. Multivariate proportional hazards regression analyses demonstrated no increased risk of skin cancer or nonskin cancer, including hematologic, breast, lung, gastrointestinal, bladder/urinary tract, and prostate or female genital organ malignancies [16].

A lawsuit in 2000 claiming that tar products are carcinogenic has made tar products hard to find in California. In response to this lawsuit, the FDA reviewed all available data and concluded that the therapeutic use of coal tar in concentrations and formulations used in over-the-counter drug products does not pose a risk of carcinogenicity. Despite this FDA ruling, in January 2002, California ruled that over-the-counter coal tar products that contain >0.5% coal tar are required to be labeled with cancer warnings. Due to this requirement, many companies have chosen to either change the active ingredient in their products sold in California or simply discontinue sale of their tar products in California [17,18]. Although coal tar can be inconvenient and messy, its demonstrated efficacy, low cost, and relatively safe side effect profile compared with other topicals and oral medications make it a reasonable option for long-term maintenance and treatment of mild to moderate psoriasis.

ANTHRALIN

Another option for treatment of mild to moderate psoriasis is anthralin, also known as dithranol, the most commonly used form of anthralin (Figure 9.3). This agent was initially used mistakenly as a folk remedy for fungal infections such as mycoses of the skin when it

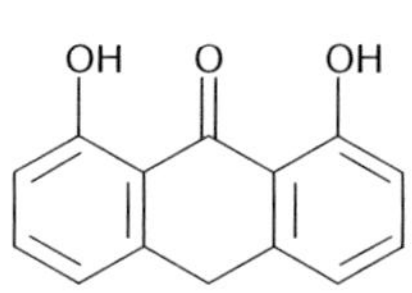

FIGURE 9.3 Structure of anthralin.

was discovered to have therapeutic effects for psoriasis in 1877. It is an antipsoriatic medication derived from a tree extract known as Goa powder. All aspects of this agent's mechanism of action are undefined; however, it has been shown to promote keratinocyte apoptosis, decrease cell respiration, and inhibit inflammation [19]. More recent evidence shows that anthralin accumulates in the mitochondria of cells, disrupting mitochondrial structure and function. It is in the mitochondria that the agent is oxidized, forming free radicals that can then interfere with cell metabolism. Subsequent DNA replication is impeded, thus slowing the excessive cell replication seen in psoriatic plaques. McGill et al. [20], in their 2005 study on the mechanism of anthralin's therapeutic effect in psoriasis, discovered that anthralin induces keratinocyte apoptosis through a novel mitochondrial pathway dependent on oxidative respiration that involves electron transfer within the ubiquinone pool. A second proposed mechanism of action is anthralin's effect on decreasing cGMP, a cyclic nucleotide that has been shown to be elevated in psoriatic lesions.

Anthralin is commercially available in the United States in cream, ointment, and paste forms, and in multiple concentrations from 0.05% to 1%. Anthralin can also be compounded by specialty pharmacies up to a concentration of 10%. Some commonly used brand names in the United States include Psoriatec, Micanol, Drithocreme, Drithocreme HP, and Dritho-scalp [21–23]. Psoriatec is a newer form of anthralin developed in an attempt to decrease the staining and inflammation associated with anthralin. Psoriatec is a 1% formulation of anthralin in a temperature-sensitive vehicle that is deliberately designed to release anthralin only at skin temperatures. The risk of staining furniture and fabrics is thought to be decreased secondary to this temperature-sensitive activation [24]. Micanol is another 1% formulation of anthralin, distinct in that it contains lipid-stabilized dithranol within a cream base. This lipid-entrapped dithranol yields an equally efficacious agent with markedly less burning and skin irritation [22].

There are several anthralin treatment regimens used for the management of plaque psoriasis both in the day-care and outpatient settings. The day-care setting involves supervised treatment of psoriasis on a daily basis at a clinical center equipped for this type of therapy. The Ingram method is designed for day-care/inpatient therapy and involves application of anthralin to the affected area, followed by covering of the area with talcum powder and then gauze or a stockinette. The anthralin is then wiped off after some time, followed by a tar bath, and finally the patient undergoes ultraviolet light therapy [25]. The day-care regimen is time-consuming and reserved for those patients with plaque psoriasis unresponsive to alternative treatment regimens.

Anthralin can also be used in a more convenient outpatient setting via two major treatment regimens—short-contact anthralin therapy (SCAT) or conventional therapy (i.e., overnight therapy). Although no optimal outpatient treatment regimen has been established, the "need for quick results in no time" mentality of Americans has led to increased popularity of SCAT. SCAT treatment involves the application of anthralin 0.1%–1% cream/ointment daily to skin or scalp that remains on the affected area for 10–30 minutes, followed by removal via bathing or shampooing [17]. A study by Runne and Kunze [26] proved the safety and efficacy of this therapy. Their study indicated that application of higher concentrations of anthralin (1%, 2%, and 3%) using SCAT for 10–20 minutes at a time is more effective than a longer exposure of three hours at a lower concentration (0.1%, 0.25%, 0.5%, 1%, and 2%). SCAT (10–20 minutes) reduced psoriasis clearing time by 6.8 days compared with longer exposure (3 hours). As opposed to SCAT, conventional therapy or overnight therapy entails anthralin application once (sometimes twice) a day to dry skin or scalp (usually at night), followed by allowing the anthralin to remain on the affected area overnight, and then removal by bathing or shampooing the next morning [21–23].

The efficacy of anthralin has been investigated in several trials. A retrospective study by Yamamoto et al. [27] examined 70 patients treated with 0.1%–2% anthralin and showed a mean improvement in PASI of 15.9 after three months of treatment. Another study compared SCAT with the Ingram regimen (inpatient regimen). The Ingram regimen showed a faster rate of improvement than the short-contact method, but it also had more irritation [28]. In general, we concluded that anthralin is most useful for thinning plaques and is associated with a remission time of 3.9–6 months [29]. Since the advent of calcipotriol ointment (a vitamin D analog), there have been some studies done comparing both this agent and anthralin in the treatment of psoriasis. A multicenter, randomized-controlled trial in the Netherlands was performed by van der Kerkhof et al. [30] to determine which agent was more efficacious. In this study, 106 patients with chronic plaque psoriasis were treated at the day-care center for 12 weeks as follows: 54 receiving calcipotriol ointment twice daily and 52 receiving dithranol cream once daily. This study concluded that dithranol was more efficacious compared with calcipotriol when used in a day-care setting. The mean percentage reduction in PASI by the end of treatment was 57.0% in the calcipotriol group versus 63.6% in the dithranol group. Approximately 15% of the patients treated with calcipotriol ointment and 25% of those treated with dithranol cream required no further treatment. Using the study subjects from the aforementioned study, de Korte et al. [31] analyzed data to assess quality-of-life parameters. Based on known dermatologic quality-of-life measurements (Skindex-29, Medical Outcomes Study, and Short Form General Health Survey-36), both the calcipotriol and the anthralin groups showed a statistically significant improvement in quality of life on all three scales. There was no statistically significant difference between the two treatment modalities. Anthralin's efficacy in adults is well studied; however, less is known about its role in pediatric patients. A single case report by Schubert et al. [32] showed efficacy of anthralin in a three-month-old infant diagnosed with exanthematous infantile psoriasis. Because many of the commonly used agents are not FDA approved in childhood psoriasis, anthralin may be a safer choice.

One of the most important disadvantages associated with anthralin is purple- to brown-yellow-colored staining of the skin and other objects (e.g., clothing, furniture) as well as skin irritation. Irritation typically improves after several days even with the same anthralin concentration [19]. There have been many interventions proposed to decrease skin irritation. Careful application to only the affected areas is important, because surrounding normal skin may become more easily irritated by anthralin contact. A study done by Schulze et al. [33] showed that patients receiving combination therapy with 5% tar and anthralin had reduced rates of irritation than patients receiving only anthralin therapy. A combination of anthralin use with the addition of corticosteroids to uninvolved perilesional skin is also commonly used. This method is most efficacious for alleviating the more severe erythema and inflammation of normal skin. In addition, application of zinc oxide paste perilesionally has been found to reduce the risk of irritation to uninvolved skin. Staining and inflammation can both be reduced with triethanolamine, a neutralizing agent. CuraStain®, a brand name for triethanolamine, is available at most pharmacies. To be most effective, it needs to be placed on unaffected skin 1–2 minutes before the anthralin is removed and should then be applied again after the area has been towel dried. Other side effects of anthralin include burning, stinging, and dryness of the skin [34]. There are no systemic or long-term side effects reported in humans. Anthralin has been used safely for many years, but staining remains a major limitation of this treatment. Newer formulations have tried to address this with some success.

SALICYLIC ACID

Salicylic acid is a keratolytic agent that is useful in the treatment of mild to moderate psoriasis (Figure 9.4). It is a good adjunct to other topical medications, but it generally is not used as monotherapy because it only removes scale. It is available in concentrations from 2% to 10% and in different vehicles, including gels, creams, and shampoos. A commonly used preparation is Keralyt gel®, a 6% salicylic acid preparation that is readily available. Salicylic acid reduces scale and therefore enhances penetration of other topical agents such as topical steroids. A study by Koo et al. [35] shows that a combination of mometasone furoate and salicylic acid ointment is more effective in treating moderate to severe psoriasis than mometasone furoate alone. In this study, 408 patients were randomized to either the treatment group with mometasone furoate alone or a combination of both mometasone furoate and salicylic acid. The topical medications were applied to target lesions twice daily for 21 days. The combination therapy of mometasone furoate and salicylic acid was significantly more effective than mometasone furoate alone, beginning at day 8. Combination therapy improvement continued through the end of the study with a more significant difference between the two study groups at day 22 than at day 8. Salicylic acid has also been used in combination with anthralin with success. However, salicylic acid should not be used in combination with calcipotriol (Dovonex®), because calcipotriol is inactivated upon contact with salicylic acid. Salicylic acid also blocks UVB and should not be applied before phototherapy.

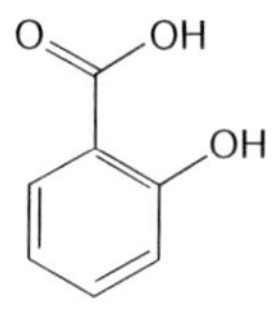

FIGURE 9.4 Structure of salicylic acid.

Although many treatment modalities exist for psoriasis, including topical, systemic, and phototherapy, a review by Lebwohl suggests that we revisit the use of salicylic acid and its role in combination therapy due to the potential toxicities of the multiple newer treatments for psoriasis. The combination of traditional therapies such as salicylic acid and topical corticosteroids may be a safe and effective alternative when other treatment modalities are too toxic or not an option. Lebwohl reported a study by Krochmal et al. [36] in which salicylic acid increased the penetration of hydrocortisone approximately threefold and that of desoximetasone, triamcinolone-acetate, and fluocinonide twofold or more. It was suggested that combination salicylic acid and topical corticosteroids could be used as first-line therapy on psoriasis plaques that are thick, scaly, or recalcitrant to topical steroids alone. The caveat to the use of salicylic acid is that it should be used with caution in patients with >20% body surface area involvement [37].

Salicylic acid may cause salicylate toxicity with application to a large body surface area (generally >20% body surface area). Early signs of salicylate toxicity such as tinnitus and fatigue should be monitored with some vigilance, because symptoms are reversible with discontinuation of salicylic acid. Other known symptoms of toxicity include nausea, vomiting, epigastric pain, blurred vision, diaphoresis, and hyperventilation. Over the past decade, there have been several case reports of acute hypoglycemia in diabetic patients treated with salicylic acid over a large body surface area. At UCSF, there was one case of a diabetic patient who became comatose after being treated with salicylic acid over a large body surface area [38]. This patient's laboratory tests showed high serum salicylate levels and low blood glucose levels. His comatose state was reversed with intravenous glucose. Due to this rare reported side effect in diabetic patients, salicylic acid should be avoided [28]. Alternate keratolytic agents such as lactic acid or urea should be considered instead.

LACTIC ACID

Lactic acid is another less common topical keratolytic agent used in the treatment of psoriasis (Figure 9.5). Lactic acid is a type of alpha-hydroxy acid mainly used as a second-line keratolytic agent when salicylate toxicity is a concern, such as in diabetic patients. Lactic acid is effective and has proven keratolytic properties as evidenced by a study on hairless mice that shows that mice treated with lactic acid demonstrate enhanced desquamation of normal skin [39]. Lactic acid can also be used on a larger surface area, because risk of salicylism is not a concern. In short, lactic acid is a beneficial second-line keratolytic agent when salicylic acid is not an option.

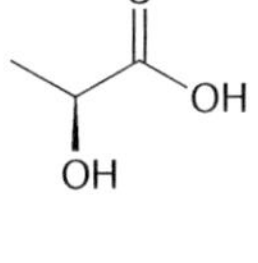

FIGURE 9.5 Structure of lactic acid.

CONCLUSIONS

The initial approach to most cases of mild to moderate psoriasis is topical therapy. Topical agents for psoriasis are usually well tolerated without serious systemic side effects. It is important not to forget the tried and true inexpensive agents such as coal tar and anthralin or the keratolytics such as salicylic acid and lactic acid.

REFERENCES

1. Thami GP, Sarkar R. Coal tar: past, present and future. *Clin Exp Dermatol* 2002; 27(2): 99–103.
2. Arnold WP. Tar. *Clin Dermatol* 1997; 15(5): 739–744.
3. Federman DG, Froelich CW, Kirsner RS. Topical psoriasis therapy. *Am Fam Phys* 1999; 59(4): 957–962, 964.
4. Gibson LE, Harold P. Goeckerman therapy. In: Henry R, Howard M, eds. *Psoriasis*. 3rd edn. Revised and expanded. New York, NY: Marcel Dekker Inc; 1998, pp. 469–477.
5. Lee E, Koo J. Modern modified "ultra" Goeckerman therapy: a PASI assessment of a very effective therapy for psoriasis resistant to both prebiologic and biologic therapies. *J Dermatol Treat* 2005; 16(2): 102–107.
6. Fitzmaurice S, Bhutani T, Koo J. Goeckerman regimen for management of psoriasis refractory to biologic therapy: the University of California San Francisco experience. *J Am Acad Dermatol*. 2013; 69(4): 648–649.
7. Serrao R, Davis MD. Goeckerman treatment for remission of psoriasis refractory to biologic therapy. *J Am Acad Dermatol* 2009; 60(2): 348–349.
8. Menter A, Cram DL. The Goeckerman regimen in two psoriasis day care centers. *J Am Acad Dermatol* 1983; 9(1): 59–65.
9. Kortuem KR, Davis MDP, Witman PM, et al. Results of Goeckerman treatment for psoriasis in children: a 21-year retrospective review. *Pediatr Dermatol* 2010; 27(5): 518–524.
10. Stern RS, Gange RW, Parrish JA, et al. Contribution of topical tar oil to ultraviolet B phototherapy for psoriasis. *J Am Acad Dermatol* 1986; 14(5 Pt 1): 742–747.
11. Lebwohl M, Martinez J, Weber P, et al. Effects of topical preparations on the erythemogenicity of UVB: implications for psoriasis phototherapy. *J Am Acad Dermatol* 1995; 32(3): 469–471.
12. Lowe NJ, Wortzman MS, Breeding J, et al. Coal tar phototherapy for psoriasis reevaluated: erythemogenic versus suberythemogenic ultraviolet with a tar extract in oil and crude coal tar. *J Am Acad Dermatol* 1983; 8(6): 781–789.
13. Kondelková K, Vokurková D, Krejsek J, et al. The number of immunoregulatory T cells is increased in patients with psoriasis after Goeckerman therapy. *Acta Medica (Hradec Kralove)* 2012; 55(2): 91–95.
14. Borska L, Andrys C, Krejsek J, et al. Serum levels of the pro-inflammatory cytokine interleukin-12 and the anti-inflammatory cytokine interleukin-10 in patients with psoriasis treated by the Goeckerman regimen. *Int J Dermatol* 2008; 47: 800–805.
15. Muller SA, Perry HO. The Goeckerman treatment in psoriasis: six decades of experience at the Mayo Clinic. *Cutis* 1984; 34(3): 265–268, 270.
16. Roelofzen JH, Aben KK, Oldenhof UT, et al. No increased risk of cancer after coal tar treatment in patients with psoriasis or eczema. *J Invest Dermatol* 2010; 130(4): 953–961.
17. National Psoriasis Foundation. Report on Internet. 2005. Available from: http://www.psoriasis.org/treatment/psoriasis/topicals/tar.php.
18. Margulies JB, Fulbright, Jaworski LLP. Calprop 65 [posting on Internet]. 1996–2004. Cited January 14, 2002. Available from: http://www.calprop65.com/coal tar.html.
19. Kraft S, Maibach HI, Shroot B. Dithranol. In: Henry R, Howard M, eds. *Psoriasis*. 3rd edn. New York, NY: Marcel Dekker Inc; 1998, pp. 435–452.
20. McGill A, Frank A, Emmett N, et al. The antipsoriatic drug anthralin accumulates in keratinocyte mitochondria, dissipates mitochondrial membrane potential, and induces apoptosis through a pathway dependent on respiratory competent mitochondria. *FASEB J* 2005; 19(8): 1012–1014.
21. Dritho-Scalp cream package insert (Dermik—US), Rev 1/97, Rec 12/98.
22. Drithocreme and Drithocreme HP package insert (Dermik—US), Rev 1/97, Rec 12/98.
23. Micanol cream package insert (Bioglan Pharma—US), Rev 3/96, Rec 10/97.

24. Thune P, Brolund L. Short- and long-contact therapy using a new dithranol formulation in individually adjusted dosages in the management of psoriasis. *Acta Derm Venereol Suppl (Stockh)* 1992; 172: 28–29.
25. Ingram JT. Approaches to psoriasis. *Br Med J* 1953; 2: 591–594.
26. Runne U, Kunze J. Short-duration ('minutes') therapy with dithranol for psoriasis: a new outpatient regimen. *Br J Dermatol* 1982; 106(2): 135–139.
27. Yamamoto T, Matsuuchi M, Irimajiri J, et al. Topical anthralin for psoriasis vulgaris: evaluation of 70 Japanese patients. *J Dermatol* 2000; 27(7): 482–485.
28. Statham BN, Ryatt KS, Rowell NR. Short-contact dithranol therapy—a comparison with the Ingram regime. *Br J Dermatol* 1984; 110(6): 703–708.
29. Lebwohl M. A clinician's paradigm in the treatment of psoriasis. *J Am Acad Dermatol* 2005; 53(1 Suppl 1): S59–S69.
30. Van de Kerkhof PC, van der Valk PG, Swinkels OQ, et al. A comparison of twice daily calcipotriol ointment with once daily short contact dithranol cream therapy: a randomized controlled trial of supervised treatment of psoriasis vulgaris in a day-care setting. *Br J Dermatol* 2006; 155(4): 800–807.
31. de Korte J, van der Valk PGM, Sprangers MA, et al. A comparison of twice daily calcipotriol ointment with once daily short contact dithranol cream therapy: quality of life outcomes of a randomized controlled trial of supervised treatment of psoriasis in a day-care setting. *Br J Dermatol* 2008; 158: 375–381.
32. Schubert B, Seitz CS, Brocker EB, et al. Exanthematous infantile psoriasis. *J Dtsch Dermatol Ges* 2007; 5(8): 680–682.
33. Schulze HJ, Schauder S, Mahrle G, et al. Combined tar–anthralin versus anthralin treatment lowers irritancy with unchanged antipsoriatic efficacy. Modifications of short-contact therapy and Ingram therapy. *J Am Acad Dermatol* 1987; 17(1): 19–24.
34. Tremblay JF, Bissonnette R. Topical agents for the treatment of psoriasis, past, present and future. *J Cutan Med Surg* 2002; 6(3 Suppl): 8–11.
35. Koo J, Cuffie CA, Tanner DJ, et al. Mometasone furoate 0.1%-salicylic acid 5% ointment versus mometasone furoate 0.1% ointment in the treatment of moderate to severe psoriasis: a multicenter study. *Clin Ther* 1998; 20(2): 283–291.
36. Krochmal L, Wang JCT, Patel B, et al. Topical corticosteroid compounding: effects on physiochemical stability and skin penetration rate. *J Am Acad Dermatol* 1989; 21: 979–984.
37. Lebwohl M. The role of salicylic acid in the treatment of psoriasis. *Int J Dermatol* 1999; 38: 16–24.
38. Maurer TA, Winter ME, Koo J, et al. Refractory hypoglycemia: a complication of topical salicylate therapy. *Arch Dermatol* 1994; 130(11): 1455–1457.
39. Kim TH, Choi EH, Kang YC, et al. The effects of topical alpha-hydroxy acids on the normal skin barrier of hairless mice. *Br J Dermatol* 2001; 144(2): 267–273.

Chapter 10

Topical Sequential Therapy

Rishu Gupta and John Y. M. Koo

INTRODUCTION

Optimal management of psoriasis, a chronically recurring disease, must include a strategy for initial rapid symptomatic relief as well as long-term maintenance therapy. Sequential therapy is a therapeutic approach that uses a deliberate sequence of specific therapies to maximize the rate of initial improvement and smoothen the transition to long-term maintenance therapy. The traditional therapeutic approach to psoriasis has been the initiation of a single treatment modality. If the chosen medication does not work effectively, it is discontinued and replaced by a new therapy. A natural consequence of this simplistic monotherapy approach is the tendency to evaluate treatments predominantly based on the rate at which they result in initial symptomatic relief. Recognizing that psoriasis is a life-long disease for most patients who are afflicted with this condition, suitability for long-term maintenance therapy, including long-term safety, duration of response, and propensity toward tachyphylaxis, should also guide treatment choice. The idea of sequential therapy is to optimize these factors by recognizing the advantages and disadvantages of each therapeutic option and then creating the most ideal pairs. Most psoriasis therapies can be categorized into "rabbits" that are fast acting and very effective but have questionable long-term safety profiles, or "turtles" that have a slower onset of action and are less effective but safer for long-term use. In sequential therapy, rabbits and turtles are paired in specific sequences to maximize both efficacy and safety.

Sequential therapy can provide rapid relief to suffering patients while also providing a strategy for safe, long-term control of disease. Sequential therapy is typically accomplished in three phases: phase 1, the clearing phase that uses a rapid-acting or quick-fix agent for fast relief; phase 2, the transition phase, the most challenging phase in which one attempts carefully, patiently, and creatively to have the turtle successfully take over from the rabbit without inciting worsening of psoriasis; and phase 3 the maintenance phase, the goal of which is long-term control with minimal side effects (Table 10.1). Because the most efficacious clearing phase agent is usually a superpotent topical steroid, there is a risk of rebound of psoriatic lesions while transitioning to the safer, less potent maintenance phase agent. The skillful combinational use of therapeutic agents and optimal timing of regimen changes during the transition phase can significantly reduce this risk.

With all of the therapeutic modalities currently available for psoriasis, the possibilities for sequential therapy schemes are endless and include systemic sequential therapy involving the newer biologic agents as well as various phototherapy options. This chapter focuses on the concept of sequential therapy using topical agents. The most common topical sequential therapy scheme in practice today is described and used to illustrate the principles that guide the clinicians in choosing among existing schemes as well as creating new schemes.

TABLE 10.1 Sequential Therapy

Clearing Phase: Ultimate goal is to achieve maximum efficacy and this phase is continued until the psoriasis lesions are flat
Transition Phase: Ultimate goal is to achieve smooth transition between phases and this phase is continued until the erythema of lesions have decreased from red to pink
Maintenance Phase: Ultimate goal is to achieve maximum safety and the treatment from this phase can be gradually tapered off

The concept of sequential therapy using systemic or phototherapy modalities are addressed in other publications.

TOPICAL SEQUENTIAL THERAPY: CALCIPOTRIENE AND HALOBETASOL PROPIONATE

The most commonly practiced topical sequential therapy scheme for psoriasis in the United States involves halobetasol propionate (Ultravate®, Bristol-Myers Squibb) ointment, a superpotent topical corticosteroid, and calcipotriene (Dovonex®, Warner Chilcott) ointment, a vitamin D analog (Table 10.2). The sequence starts with halobetasol propionate once daily in the morning and calcipotriene once daily at bedtime for approximately one month (phase 1, clearing phase); then calcipotriene twice daily on weekdays and halobetasol propionate twice daily on weekends for one month or longer (phase 2, transition phase); and finally, calcipotriene twice daily until psoriasis completely resolves, at which time therapy can be tapered off (phase 3, maintenance phase). This particular scheme has been chosen to illustrate the idea of topical sequential therapy because it is the only scheme in which the merit of each step has been validated by double-blind, randomized clinical trials directly comparing the various options.

Calcipotriene has been shown through well-controlled studies to be a safe and effective treatment for psoriasis [1–5]. For example, in a double-blind, multicenter study, calcipotriene ointment was found to be superior to fluocinonide (Lidex®, Medicis) ointment, both in rate of improvement and degree of efficacy [6]. However, many dermatologists in the United States may question the effectiveness of calcipotriene after experiencing somewhat disappointing results with the medication when it was first introduced. This less-than-expected "real-life" efficacy of calcipotriene may stem from a few issues. First, it was not realized until years after introduction that the efficacy of calcipotriene is essentially halved, and it has an even slower onset of action when it is used only once daily instead of twice daily [7]. Unfortunately, most patients were using calcipotriene once daily at bedtime, because it was initially only available in an ointment formulation, a formulation that is less conducive to morning application. Interestingly, the efficacy of once-daily calcipotriene use approaches that of twice-daily use if it is continued for eight weeks. However, most patients (and their physicians) were disappointed by the slow onset of action, especially with once-daily use, and concluded that calcipotriene was not a useful medication long before eight weeks had passed. Second, a random string of calcipotriene nonresponders may have biased some dermatologists' clinical impression of this medication. Third, calcipotriene could have caused disappointment when used abruptly in a double-blind, multicenter study replace a superpotent topical steroid only to result in rebound of psoriatic lesions. Finally, the use of calcipotriene as monotherapy is

TABLE 10.2 Example of Topical Sequential Therapy

Phase 1: halobetasol propionate q.a.m., calcipotriene q.h.s.	Phase 2: pulse therapy, calcipotriene b.i.d. on weekdays, halobetasol propionate b.i.d. on weekends	Phase 3: calcipotriene b.i.d., then taper off
Phase 1: clobetasol foam and calcipotriene b.i.d.	Phase 2: pulse therapy, calcipotriene b.i.d. on weekdays, clobetasol foam and calcipotriene b.i.d. on weekends	Phase 3: calcipotriene b.i.d., then taper off
Approximately 1 month	Approximately 1 month	Until psoriasis resolves completely

associated with a 2%–3% incidence of significant lesional and perilesional irritation, a side effect that is bothersome enough to patients that they discontinue use [8,9].

The sequential use of calcipotriene and halobetasol propionate as described previously provides a solution to many of the aforementioned concerns. Although superpotent topical steroids such as halobetasol propionate work very well, the combined use of topical steroids and calcipotriene appear to work even better. In fact, the two medications seem to be ideal partners. A double-blind, randomized, multicenter study found that, after only 14 days of therapy, the use of calcipotriene ointment in the morning and halobetasol propionate ointment in the evening was significantly more effective compared with twice-daily monotherapy with either agent and also resulted in a lower incidence of irritation from calcipotriene [10]. Additional double-blind, randomized studies have also supported the finding that calcipotriene and corticosteroids work synergistically to enhance efficacy and result in fewer side effects than treatment with either agent alone [11]. Moreover, the use of halobetasol propionate at the start of therapy can compensate for calcipotriene's slow onset of action and cover patients who might be slow responders to calcipotriene. Finally, using calcipotriene in conjunction with halobetasol propionate may decrease the incidence of skin thinning from topical steroid use [12]. Similar results were found using a combination of calcitriol, another vitamin D analog, and betamethasone valerate, another topical steroid [13].

The side effect profile of superpotent topical steroids makes them a poor choice for long-term control of psoriasis. This well-known fact is the rationale for the "weekday–weekend" or "pulse" therapy of the transition phase (phase 2). The first regimen of this kind was introduced in the late 1980s in which the patient applies a potent topical steroid daily until flattening of the plaque occurs and then uses the steroid on weekends only [14]. It has since been modified to include calcipotriene after Lebwohl et al. [15] found that the addition of calcipotriene ointment twice daily on weekdays to the use of halobetasol ointment twice daily on weekends resulted in nearly twice as many patients achieving a six-month remission and a decreased incidence of side effects associated with long-term topical steroid use. The use of this type of intermittent pulse dosing during phase 2 allows clinicians to safely extend treatment of psoriasis with superpotent topical steroids. Pulse therapy also minimizes the risk of rebound by allowing superpotent topical steroids to be gradually tapered off rather than abruptly discontinued once psoriatic plaques have become macular.

During the maintenance phase (phase 3), the twice-daily application of calcipotriene alone (phase 3) can be initiated once the lesions have not only flattened but also the degree of erythema has decreased from red to pink. This calcipotriene dose may be gradually decreased to once daily then once every other day, and ultimately, when psoriasis is no longer visible, all prescription medications can be discontinued.

Of note, the calcipotriene molecule is relatively unstable and can be inactivated when combined with some topical medications, especially if an acidic environment is created [16]. In the aforementioned study that demonstrated the superiority of using once-daily calcipotriene and halobetasol propionate to twice-daily monotherapy with either agent, the once-daily calcipotriene and halobetasol propionate ointments were applied separately, morning and night, to prevent inactivation of either agent [10]. This is also true of the phase 1 regimen presented in Table 10.2. Halobetasol propionate ointment and cream have since been found to be among the medications that are compatible with calcipotriene [17]. Therefore, because calcipotriene and halobetasol propionate are individually known to have better efficacy when applied twice a day compared with once a day, the best theoretical regimen would be to use both calcipotriene and halobetasol propionate twice daily. Patel et al. [17] recommend mixing the agents in one's palm just before each application instead of premixing agents, because inactivation can begin as soon as 50 hours after mixing. Similarly, calcipotriene can be continued on weekends during phase 2 pulse therapy, with halobetasol propionate applied in addition to calcipotriene. From common clinical experience, the simultaneous use of the two medications appears to work well, although clinical studies are yet to be performed. Recommending that patients mix calcipotriene and halobetasol propionate creams for morning application and the two ointment formulations for nighttime application may increase compliance.

OPTIMAL TIMING TO PROCEED DOWN SEQUENTIAL THERAPY SCHEME

The issue of timing of each treatment phase can be approached in two ways. The first way is to establish approximate time frames for the individual treatment phases based on clinical experience and prior studies. Generally, phase 1 takes three to four weeks, phase 2 takes another month, and phase 3 goes on indefinitely or until psoriasis has completely resolved. Needless to say, patients' lesions need to be assessed intermittently to ensure that the majority of lesions are responding appropriately to treatment. If the patients' lesions are improving faster or slower than the predicted time frames, then transitioning between phases must be adjusted accordingly. For example, some patients with chronically active lesions may require indefinite pulse therapy (phase 2). Fortunately, this weekday–weekend regimen appears to be remarkably safe. In our experience, patients do not have any significant skin atrophy with this regimen as long as superpotent topical steroids are not applied more than two days per week. Adrenal suppression should not be a concern when topical steroids are used only two days per week.

The second approach to the issue of timing is more sophisticated but also seems to be more effective. Patients are instructed to transition therapy from phase 1 to phase 2 for plaques that have flattened and from phase 2 to phase 3 for flattened lesions in which the degree of erythema has decreased from red to pink. With this approach, treatment is individualized so that faster responding lesions move quickly along the sequence and thick, recalcitrant plaques stay in phase 1 for more time, where induration obviates the concern for skin atrophy.

SEQUENTIAL THERAPY AS A FLEXIBLE THERAPEUTIC STRATEGY

The activity of psoriatic lesions is often unpredictable and therapeutic goals range from maintenance of long-term remission, control of acute flares, or even a period of treatment cessation if the severity of psoriasis decreases. Patients with this chronic disease can certainly benefit from individualized treatment plans. The advantage of sequential therapy is that the intensity of treatment can be easily adjusted to the level of activity of psoriasis. As their psoriasis improves, patients transition to the next phase, or if their psoriasis worsens (e.g., during winter), they can regress to an earlier treatment phase. Not only do patients appear to have better clinical outcomes with this flexible therapeutic strategy but they also appreciate the greater sense of control they feel over a disease that is known to unpredictably fluctuate in severity during its chronic course.

SEQUENTIAL THERAPY WITH NEW CLOBETASOL PROPIONATE STEROID FORMULATIONS

One of the new, innovative formulations of topical steroids uses a foam vehicle to deliver medication. Foam formulation is thermolabile and breaks down on contact with human skin and at body temperature. The result is drug delivery with minimal residue, quick absorption, and increased convenience of application. Furthermore, several in vitro studies have indicated that the foam formulation is a more efficient vehicle for topical drug delivery compared with traditional creams, ointments, and solutions [18–22].

Clobetasol propionate (Olux® foam) is one of the topical steroids now available in a foam formulation. Clobetasol propionate foam, like other foam formulations, is quickly absorbed and leaves minimal residue, making it ideal for use in combination with other topical agents, such as calcipotriene. The foam vehicle is absorbed so quickly that there is no theoretical concern for dilution or incompatibility when combined with other therapeutic agents. In contrast, the foam vehicle in clobetasol emollient foam (Olux-E® foam) does not rapidly evaporate, making it unsuitable for this approach.

The efficacy of clobetasol propionate foam and calcipotriene ointment when used in a topical sequential therapy scheme was recently evaluated in a clinical study [23,24]. The first part of the study evaluated the twice-daily use of clobetasol propionate foam and calcipotriene ointment as the clearing phase regimen [23]. Eighty-six subjects were randomized to three groups: twice-daily monotherapy with clobetasol propionate foam, monotherapy with calcipotriene ointment, or combination therapy. Subjects in the combination group were directed to apply calcipotriene ointment immediately after the clobetasol propionate foam was absorbed. After two weeks of treatment, reductions in psoriasis severity scores for the target lesions were significantly greater in the combination therapy group compared with either monotherapy group (clobetasol alone, $p = .0017$ [trunk lesions] and $p < .0001$ [extremity lesions]; calcipotriene alone, $p < .0001$ [both trunk and extremity lesions]). With respect to the trunk psoriatic lesions, the combination therapy group achieved a 69.3% mean reduction in psoriasis severity scores compared with 48.1% with clobetasol propionate foam alone and 36.6% with calcipotriene ointment alone. A similar pattern was seen with extremity lesions. The results also support in vitro data, as described earlier, suggesting that calcipotriene inactivation does not occur when it is applied immediately after a topical steroid foam [25].

The second phase involved 38 subjects who achieved at least a 50% reduction in their target lesion severity score during part one. Patients were randomized to one of the two groups: twice-daily calcipotriene ointment on weekdays plus twice-daily clobetasol propionate foam or placebo on weekends. Treatment groups were compared using intent-to-treat analysis. After six months of treatment, the combination therapy group showed a consistent trend toward longer maintenance of remission compared with the monotherapy group. Although the data were not found to be statistically significant, this same trend continued throughout all study assessments. The data suggested that there may be a positive effect associated with using clobetasol propionate foam and calcipotriene ointment in pulse therapy. Given the consistency of these trends, it is probable that the results would have been statistically significant if a greater number of subjects were enrolled in the study. The afore mentioned results strongly suggest that there is an advantage to using foam vehicles for drug delivery in combination sequential therapy. Once again, the foam vehicle is absorbed so quickly that calcipotriene can be applied soon thereafter without concern for dilution and incompatibility with other medications.

Clobetasol propionate 0.05% spray (Clobex spray®, Galderma) was approved by the U.S. Food and Drug Administration (FDA) in late 2005. Traditionally, class I steroid clobetasol propionate–containing agents have been approved for use up to two weeks in duration. However, the new clobetasol spray has been approved for use up to four weeks in duration without significant sacrifices in tolerability from the additional two weeks. Overall, results from the community-based research assessment (COBRA) trial investigating clobetasol propionate 0.05% spray twice daily as monotherapy or as an addition to a therapeutic regimen (ranging from topical therapy to prebiologics to biologics with inadequate symptom control) revealed that it is a well-tolerated, effective, and versatile topical therapy for plaque psoriasis [26]. Another new formulation is the clobetasol propionate 0.05% lotion (Clobex lotion®, Galderma) that provides the strength of clobetasol cream with the light consistency of a lotion.

Similar to halobetasol propionate, the use of clobetasol propionate can be combined with a vitamin D analog, such as calcipotriene, to synergistically improve the efficacy and reduce side effects of each agent. However, some topical corticosteroids may lead to degradation of the vitamin D analog when they are used together [11]. Therefore, an in vitro study was conducted to assess the stability of clobetasol propionate spray or lotion 0.05% combined with calcipotriene ointment 0.005% [27].

In this study, clobetasol propionate spray and lotion, along with halobetasol, a previously tested corticosteroid, were each mixed in a 1:1 ratio with calcipotriene ointment. Halobetasol was used as a positive control to validate the testing method because a previous study by Siskin et al. [10] had demonstrated the stability of halobetasol and calcipotriene combination. The results, measured by high-performance liquid chromatography (HPLC), demonstrated that clobetasol propionate in the spray and lotion formulations retained its potency when mixed with calcipotriene. The concentration of calcipotriene was also shown to remain stable in both mixtures over time. In the halobetasol–calcipotriene mixtures, there was a statistically significant decrease ($p = .04$) in the concentration of calcipotriene ointment when combined with halobetasol propionate cream; however, because of the small magnitude of change, Siskin et al. [10] do not believe this decrease to be clinically significant. Although there have been no clinical studies conducted, the combination of clobetasol propionate spray or lotion 0.05% with calcipotriene is likely to be stable with minimal or no loss of potency based on this study.

TOPICAL SEQUENTIAL THERAPY POSSIBILITIES BEYOND CALCIPOTRIENE

The idea of sequential therapy can also be applied to newer agents that combine a steroid and a nonsteroid such as calcipotriol and betamethasone dipropionate (Dovobet®/Daivobet®/Taclonex® [LEO Pharma A/S, Ballerup, Denmark]). In the clearing phase (step 1), combination calcipotriol/betamethasone dipropionate can be given once daily for up to eight weeks or until the lesions become flat but remain red [28]. In the transitional phase (step 2), patients can apply the agent once every other day for approximately one month or longer or until the lesions remain flat but become pink instead of red. In the maintenance phase (step 3), once the lesions are almost cleared, the patients can use once-daily application on weekends.

The use of a combined topical calcipotriol/betamethasone dipropionate formulation in sequential strategy combines three key elements of successful topical steroid therapy: (1) efficacy, (2) safety, and (3) ease of application and compliance. Studies have revealed that combination calcipotriol/betamethasone dipropionate is more effective than each of its components used alone and is much more effective then placebo [29]. In one clinical trial, investigators found that combination calcipotriol/betamethasone dipropionate once daily had the highest percent change in Psoriasis Area Severity Index (PASI) score within four weeks of use (71.3%) compared with betamethasone dipropionate once daily (57.2%) or calcipotriene once daily (46.1%) or placebo vehicle (22.7%) [29]. Regarding safety, studies have documented that combination calcipotriol/betamethasone dipropionate once daily was shown to be safe and well tolerated for up to 52 weeks ("as needed" use between weeks 8–52) [30]. Moreover, compliance is likely to be higher with the use of combination calcipotriol/betamethasone dipropionate than two separate agents. Typically, potent or superpotent topical corticosteroids require twice-daily dosing as it is more effective than once-daily dosing. However, combination calcipotriol/betamethasone dipropionate ointment has been shown to be just as effective when dosed once daily compared with twice daily [31]. Therefore, not only does combination calcipotriol/betamethasone dipropionate bring together two topical agents into one, this agent only needs to be applied once a day for maximum efficacy versus the usual twice a day application for many topical agents, such as clobetasol, fluocinonide, triamcinolone, desonide, calcipotriene, and calcitriol. For all these reasons, sequential therapy can be extremely effective when used with combination calcipotriol/betamethasone dipropionate combination agent.

THE YIN-YANG STRATEGY

The Yin-Yang strategy is a simple, yet effective strategy that alternates the use of clobetasol 0.05% spray twice daily (Yang) with calcitriol 3 μg/gointment twice daily (Yin) on a monthly basis [32]. That is, during the first month, clobetasol spray is used twice daily and during the second month calcitriol ointment is used twice daily. This sequence can be rotated as long as the patient needs treatment. The advantage of the Yin-Yang strategy is that it uses the most efficacious topical therapy (clobetasol) in a spray formulation that is easily applied to large or hard to reach areas. During the month of steroid holiday, calcitriol ointment is used to maintain the improvement achieved during the month of clobetasol use. Calcitriol has the advantage of being less irritating than other topical vitamin D preparations. Further, twice as much can be used without concern for hypercalcemia (up to 200 g/week compared with 100 g/week with calcipotriene). The merit of the Yin-Yang strategy is supported by a multi-center, open label study, in which 170 patients were treated with clobetasol spray twice daily for 4-weeks followed by calcitriol ointment twice daily for 8-weeks. At the end of 4 weeks, 94% of patients were "clear" or "almost clear". At week 8 (4-weeks after stopping clobetasol spray) 92% of patients still remained "clear" or "almost clear" [33]. Thus,the abrupt transition from clobetasol spray to calcitriol ointment during the second month of treatment resulted in essentially no deterioration in clinical benefit. And, by adhering to the Yin-Yang strategy, after 8 weeks such patients would again be ready for another month of treatment with clobetasol spray. Of note, in the above study, despite abrupt discontinuation of clobetasol spray, calcitriol ointment twice daily was able to maintain improvement for 4 weeks but not for 8 weeks. During the second 4 week period (from 4 weeks to 8 weeks after discontinuation of clobetasol spray), there was a notable deterioration in clinical status of the psoriasis research subjects.

CONCLUSION

The idea of sequential therapy can be applied to the combined use of any topical agents with rabbit (quick-fix) characteristics and turtle (safe, long-term) characteristics. For example, once-daily tazarotene (Tazorac®) 0.1% gel used in combination with mometasone furoate (Elocon®) 0.1% cream was shown in clinical trials to be more efficacious than twice-daily treatment with either agent alone [34,35]. These two medications appear to work synergistically and could possibly be used in a sequential strategy. The more traditional topical agents such as tar or anthralin might also be more effective in combination with topical steroids in a sequential therapy scheme. Thus, the possibilities with topical sequential therapy in the treatment of psoriasis are limited only by the skill and creativity of the dermatologist.

REFERENCES

1. Kragballe K, Gjertsen BT, de Hoop D, et al. Double-blind, right/left comparison of calcipotriol and betamethasone valerate in treatment of psoriasis vulgaris. *Lancet* 1991; 337: 193–196.
2. Cunliffe WJ, Berth-Jones J, Claudy A, et al. Comparative study of calcipotriol (MC 903) ointment and betamethasone 17-valerate ointment in patients with psoriasis vulgaris. *J Am Acad Dermatol* 1992; 26: 736–743.
3. Berth-Jones J, Chu AC, Dodd WAH, et al. A multi-centre, parallel-group comparison of calcipotriol ointment and short-contact dithranol therapy in chronic plaque psoriasis. *Br J Dermatol* 1992; 127: 266–271.

4. Ellis JP, Griffiths WAD, Klaber MR. Long-term treatment of chronic plaque psoriasis with calcipotriol ointment in patients unresponsive to short-contact dithranol. *Eur J Clin Res* 1995; 7: 247–257.
5. Ramsay CA, Berth-Jones J, Brundin G, et al. Long-term use of topical calcipotriol in chronic plaque psoriasis. *Dermatology* 1994; 189: 260–264.
6. Bruce S, Epinette W, Funicella T, et al. Comparative study of calcipotriene (MC903) ointment and fluocinonide ointment in the treatment of psoriasis. *J Am Acad Dermatol* 1994; 31: 755–799.
7. Ashcroft DM, Li Wan Po A, Williams HC, et al. Combination regimens of topical calcipotriene in chronic plaque psoriasis: systematic review of efficacy and tolerability. *Arch Dermatol* 2000; 136(12): 1536–1543.
8. Mason J, Mason AR, Cork MJ. Topical preparations for the treatment of psoriasis: a systematic review. *Br J Dermatol* 2002; 146: 351–364.
9. Bruner CR, Feldman SR, Ventrapragada M, et al. A systematic review of adverse effects associated with topical treatments for psoriasis. *Dermatol Online J* 2003; 9: 2.
10. Lebwohl M, Siskin SB, Epinette W, et al. A multicenter trial of calcipotriene ointment with halobetasol ointment compared with either agent alone for the treatment of psoriasis. *J Am Acad Dermatol* 1996; 35: 268–269.
11. Lamba S, Lebwohl M. Combination therapy with vitamin D analogues. *Br J Dermatol* 2001; 144: 27–32.
12. Lebwohl M. Topical application of calcipotriene and corticosteroids: combination regimens. *J Am Acad Dermatol* 1997; 37(3, pt 2): S55–S58.
13. Kowalzik L. Clinical experience with topical calcitriol (1,25 dihydroxyvitamin D_3) in psoriasis. *Br J Dermatol* 2001; 144: 21–25.
14. Katz HI, Hien NT, Prawer SE, et al. Betamethasone dipropionate in optimized vehicle: intermittent pulse dosing for extended maintenance treatment of psoriasis. *Arch Dermatol* 1987; 123: 1308–1311.
15. Lebwohl M, Siskin SB, Epinette W, et al. Calcipotriene ointment and halobetasol ointment in the long-term treatment of psoriasis: effects on the duration of improvement. *J Am Acad Dermatol* 1998; 39: 447–450.
16. Kragballe K. Vitamin D_3 analogues. *Dermatol Clin* 1995; 13: 835–839.
17. Patel B, Siskin S, Krazmien R, et al. Compatibility of calcipotriene with other topical medications. *J Am Acad Dermatol* 1998; 38: 1010–1011.
18. Lenn J, Tanojo H, Huang X. Anatomical region variations on the in vitro skin permeation of clobetasol propionate formulations. Presented at 62nd Annual Meeting of the Academy of Dermatology, Washington, DC, 2004.
19. Huang X, Tanojo H, Lenn J, et al. A novel foam vehicle for delivery of topical corticosteroids. *J Am Acad Dermatol* 2005; 53(1) (Suppl 1): S26–S38.
20. Lenn J, Madlambayan L, Huang X, et al. Comparison of clobetasol propionate skin permeation and drug distribution in vitro from various topical drug delivery vehicles (foam, lotion, and wash-off shampoo). Presented at Summer Meeting of the American Academy of Dermatology, New York, 2004–2005.
21. Deng H, Tanojo H, Lenn J, et al. Foam as a novel vehicle in topical therapy. Presented at 62nd Annual Meeting of the American Academy of Dermatology, Washington, DC, 2004.
22. Huang X, Tanojo H, Lenn J, et al. Impact of vehicle on clobetasol propionate skin permeation and drug distribution in vitro. Presented at 62nd Annual Meeting of the American Academy of Dermatology, Washington, DC, 2004.
23. Blum R, Stern D, Lebwohl M, et al. A multi-center study of calcipotriene 0.005% ointment and clobetasol propionate 0.05% foam in the sequential treatment of localized plaque-type psoriasis. Presented at Summer Meeting of the American Academy of Dermatology, New York, 2004.
24. Koo J, Blum R, Lebwohl M, et al. A 2-part, multi-center study of calcipotriene ointment, 0.005% and clobetasol propionate foam 0.05% in the sequential treatment of localized plaque-type psoriasis: long-term outcomes. Presented at 63rd Annual Meeting of the American Academy of Dermatology, New Orleans, LA, 2005.
25. Franz T, Lehman P, Spellman M. Calcipotriene stability in the presence of steroid foam. Presented at 60th Annual Meeting of the American Academy of Dermatology, New Orleans, LA, 2002.
26. Green L, Sadoff W. A clinical evaluation of tazarotene 0.1% gel, with and without a high- or mid-high-potency corticosteroid, in patients with stable plaque psoriasis. *J Cutan Med Surg* 2002; 6(2): 95–102.

27. Koo JY, Martin D. Investigator-masked comparison of tazarotene gel q.d. plus mometasone furoate cream q.d. vs. mometasone furoate cream b.i.d. in the treatment of plaque psoriasis. *Int J Dermatol* 2001; 40(3): 210–212.
28. Taclonex (Calcipotriene and Betamethasone Dipropionate) Ointment, 0.005%/0.064% [Package Insert]. Dublin, Ireland. LEO Pharma; 2012.
29. Kaufmann R, Bibby AJ, Bissonnette R, et al. A new calcipotriol/betamethasone dipropionate formulation (Daivobet) is an effective once-daily treatment for psoriasis vulgaris. *Dermatology* 2002; 205(4): 389–393.
30. Kragballe K, Austad J, Barnes L, et al. A 52-week randomized safety study of a calcipotriol/betamethasone dipropionate two-compound product (Dovobet/Daivobet/Taclonex) in the treatment of psoriasis vulgaris. *Br J Dermatol* 2006; 154: 1155–1160.
31. Guenther L, Van de Kerkhof PC, Snellman E, et al. Efficacy and safety of a new combination of calcipotriol and betamethasone dipropionate (once or twice daily) compared to calcipotriol (twice daily) in the treatment of psoriasis vulgaris: a randomized, double-blind, vehicle-controlled clinical trial. *Br J Dermatol* 2002; 147(2): 316–323.
32. Bhutani T, Zitelli KB, Koo J. Yin-yang et al. Strategy: proposing a new, effective, repeatable, sequential therapy for psoriasis. *J Drugs Dermatol.* 2011; 10: 831–834.
33. Brodell R, Bruce S, Hudson C. A Multi-center, Open-label Study to Evaluate the Safety and Efficacy of a Sequential Treatment Regimen of Clobetasol Propionate 0.05% Spray Followed by Calcitriol 3 mg/g Ointment in the Management of Plaque Psoriasis. *J Drugs Dermatol.* 2011; 10: 158–164.
34. Koo JY. Relevance of the COBRA trial in current psoriasis practice. *Cutis* 2007; 80: 4–11.
35. Colon L, Lehman P, Johnson L, et al. Chemical stability of commonly combined topical psoriasis medications. Presented at 65th Annual Meeting of the American Academy of Dermatology, Washington, DC, 2007.

Chapter 11

Phototherapy and Laser

Mio Nakamura, Holly A. Kerr, and Iltefat Hamzavi

INTRODUCTION

Phototherapy has long been a mainstay therapy for psoriasis. In the past 5–10 years, there have been exciting developments in new light sources for the treatment of psoriasis. These newer technologies have increased the efficacy of phototherapy and hopefully will decrease the long-term adverse events.

The ultraviolet (UV) spectrum is divided into three spectral regions: UVC, UVB, and UVA. UVC (200–290 nm) is rarely present on earth because it is absorbed by the ozone layer. UVB (290–320 nm) is a mainstay in the treatment of psoriasis; it is known as the sunburn spectrum. UVA (320–400 nm) is divided into UVA1 (340–400 nm) and UVA2 (320–340 nm). UVA2, being of shorter wavelength range, has biologic properties that are closer to UVB. UVA1 has only recently been evaluated for the treatment of psoriasis. The combination of psoralen and UVA (PUVA) is a well-established psoriasis therapy. Pulsed dye laser (PDL) and photodynamic therapy (PDT) have been investigated for the treatment of psoriasis, with varying results.

Ideal phototherapy for localized psoriasis would be localized treatment, sparing the healthy skin from the side effects of UV radiation. There are now a few targeted phototherapy devices that deliver UVB, UVA, or both. In addition, an excimer laser light source, delivering 308-nm radiation to targeted psoriatic lesions, has been shown to be another effective therapeutic modality for psoriasis.

Although phototherapy is generally not used as first-line therapy for the treatment of localized psoriasis, it is a safe and effective second-line therapy, either as a monotherapy or as a combination therapy for many patients.

MECHANISM OF ACTION

T cells play a central role in the pathogenesis of psoriasis. The induction of T-cell apoptosis is felt to be the main mechanism by which phototherapy is effective in the treatment of psoriasis. T-cell apoptosis has been shown with the treatment of broadband UVB (BB-UVB) [1], narrowband UVB (NB-UVB) [2], PUVA [3], the 308-nm excimer laser [4], and UVA1 [5]. The excimer laser has been shown to be more effective than NB-UVB in inducing apoptosis of T cells [6]. Other effects of UV include suppression of DNA synthesis and generation of prostaglandins and cytokines. The cutaneous immunomodulation induced by phototherapy is an effective mode of treatment without systemic immunosuppression and its associated side effects. With PUVA, an additional mechanism of action is the formation of cross-links between psoralen and the pyrimidine bases in the DNA, inhibiting DNA replication.

ULTRAVIOLET B

UVB phototherapy as monotherapy, or in combination with other therapies, is an effective treatment for psoriasis. Clearance rates with UVB can be ≥80% in combination with topical therapy. The potential to induce remission is also an attractive feature.

BB-UVB has been one of the mainstay therapies in the past for psoriasis. In 1981, Parrish and Jaenicke [7] identified that 313 nm is the most effective wavelength for the treatment of psoriasis; this identification lead to the development of NB-UVB (a novel fluorescent lamp, TL-01, that emits 311–312 nm), the new standard of care. Booth, hand and foot, and comb phototherapy machines are available.

Efficacy

Studies have compared BB-UVB to NB-UVB for the treatment of psoriasis, all of which demonstrate superiority of NB-UVB [8]. In a randomized, double-blind study comparing the efficacy of NB-UVB to PUVA, 88 patients were either treated with twice weekly NB-UVB or PUVA therapy, starting at 70% of the minimum phototoxic or erythema dose, with 20% dose increases as tolerated until clearance, or up to a maximum of 30 sessions [9]. Skin types V and VI had a lower rate of clearance than those with skin types I through IV (24% vs. 75%). In skin types I through IV, PUVA was significantly more effective than NB-UVB at achieving clearance (84% vs. 65%). The median number of treatments to clearance was significantly lower in the PUVA group (17.0 vs. 28.5). Six months after therapy, 68% of PUVA-treated patients were still in remission versus 35% of NB-UVB-treated patients.

Several other studies have compared the efficacy of NB-UVB with PUVA and have demonstrated similar results [10–13]. In the only randomized, double-blind, placebo-controlled study of systemic PUVA, 86% of subjects achieved Psoriasis Area and Severity Index (PASI) 75 after 12 weeks of three times per week PUVA exposure (vs. 0% in placebo) [14]. One study favored NB-UVB over bath PUVA. This randomized controlled trial compared the efficacy of NB-UVB and 4,5,8-trimethoxypsoralen (TMP) bath PUVA for chronic plaque psoriasis in 28 patients (skin types I–III). Each body half was treated with either NB-UVB or bath PUVA. The NB-UVB-treated half achieved clearance a median of 11 days more quickly than PUVA [15]. Remission durations did not differ.

In practice, NB-UVB should be considered as the first-line UV-based therapy, especially in Caucasians, due to its lower risk for skin cancer. However, in patients with skin type V or VI, or in patients with very thick or large psoriatic lesions, PUVA may offer an advantage over NB-UVB due to the deeper penetration of UVA radiation.

"Selective" broadband sources are fluorescent lamps (UV6 lamps) with relatively little emission below 290 mm. The photocarcinogenesis action spectrum predicts that NB-UVB is 1.5 times more carcinogenic than selective BB-UVB [16]. One hundred patients with psoriasis were treated with either selective BB-UVB or NB-UVB in a randomized, observer-blinded study. The mean number of treatments for clearance was 28.4 for NB-UVB and 30.4 for selective BB-UVB, with a statistically significant difference. There were no significant differences in the proportion of patients achieving clearance. The side effect profiles were similar. These two lamps appear to have similar efficacy; however, the NB-UVB may be more carcinogenic and selective BB-UVB may be a safer option for the treatment of psoriasis. Further studies are needed in this area.

Combination Therapy

NB-UVB in combination with anthralin [17] or topical tazarotene [18] has been shown to be more effective than monotherapy. Topical tazarotene applied three times per week significantly enhances the efficacy of BB-UVB compared with BB-UVB monotherapy. Furthermore, patients receiving combination therapy had much lower cumulative exposure to BB-UVB [19]. There are conflicting reports of the efficacy of the combination of NB-UVB and calcipotriol; however, it appears to have some added benefit [20–23]. The addition of topical corticosteroids to BB-UVB has not shown any added benefit compared with BB-UVB monotherapy and may even induce a higher relapse rate [24]. Systemic retinoids in combination with NB-UVB is more effective than NB-UVB alone [25]; with the added anticarcinogenic effects of retinoids, this combination is a very useful treatment option. Acitretin in combination with NB-UVB results in faster improvement even in difficult-to-treat patients. The combination of the two treatments appears to have synergistic effects [26]. Isotretinoin appears to have similar results and accelerates therapeutic response to NB-UVB, reducing the cumulative dose of NB-UVB [27]. Practitioners should be careful to reduce light doses when using phototherapy in conjunction with retinoids [28].

Recent randomized, placebo-controlled trials comparing methotrexate plus NB-UVB versus NB-UVB alone [29,30] confirmed prior studies [31] that methotrexate in combination with NB-UVB is an effective combination therapy. Methotrexate was initiated three weeks before NB-UVB phototherapy. The combination clears more patients with psoriasis in significantly fewer treatments than NB-UVB alone. However, in view of the potentiating effect of methotrexate in PUVA-induced photocarcinogenesis [32], the combination of methotrexate and NB-UVB should be used with caution.

In cultured keratinocytes, calcineurin inhibitors (cyclosporine, tacrolimus, and pimecrolimus) have been shown to decrease apoptosis and DNA repair after exposure to UVB radiation [33]. As such, until additional long-term studies are complete, it is prudent not to combine UVB phototherapy with topical calcineurin inhibitors.

Recent studies have suggested greater efficacy of biologic therapies in combination with NB-UVB compared with biologic monotherapy. In a prospective study, 13 patients were treated with etanercept 25 mg twice daily. Two marker lesions were selected on each patient for determination of the modified PASI (M-PASI). NB-UVB was applied to one of the two marker lesions three times weekly, and the other maker lesion was covered and used as nonirradiated control. After six weeks of therapy, the relative M-PASI reduction was significantly higher in etanercept- plus NB-UVB-treated lesions compared with control lesions [34]. NB-UVB may also have the potential to accelerate the therapeutic response to monoclonal antibody therapies such as adalimumab [35] and ustekinumab [36]. However, due to risk of malignancy and immunosuppression with some biologic therapies, it may be beneficial to avoid long-term treatment. Further research is needed to assess malignancy potential, as well as remission rates of such combination therapies.

Indications

The indications for UVB therapy include stable plaque psoriasis, history of rapid clearance with exposure to sunlight, resistant plaques to topical therapy, the ability of the patient to comply with treatment regimen, and patient preference. UVB is safe in patients who are pregnant, breast feeding, or planning to become pregnant when topical agents, such as retinoids, are not a treatment option. In patients with skin type I or II, or a past history of X-ray therapy, arsenic exposure, and the use of immunosuppressive agents, UVB would be a better phototherapy option than PUVA. Should it be necessary, it is generally considered safer to treat patients with known history of nonmelanoma skin cancer, or melanoma, with UVB compared with treatment with PUVA. Patient preference for avoiding oral medications is also an important factor in the decision-making process. Compared with PUVA, NB-UVB does not use photosensitizing agents; therefore, it is better tolerated and is more cost-effective.

Contraindications

There are very few *absolute* contraindications to UVB phototherapy; these contraindications include patients with xeroderma pigmentosum, systemic lupus erythematosus, and basal cell nevus syndrome. *Relative* contraindications include photosensitive disorders, use of photosensitizing medications with an action spectrum in the UVB range, and history of skin cancer. Photodermatoses whose action spectrum may include the UVB range include polymorphous light eruption, chronic actinic dermatitis, and solar urticaria. It should be noted that the action spectrum of the majority of drug-induced photosensitivity is UVA; because NB-UVB emits at 311 to 312 nm, it is a safe light source to use. Due to the thin skin in the genital region and the historically reported increased risk of cutaneous malignancies, it is preferable not to treat this area with phototherapy.

In a study involving a small number of subjects, UVB irradiation was shown to result in activation of human immunodeficiency virus (HIV) in the skin [37]. However, multiple other studies showed effectiveness of UVB for many HIV-related dermatoses without any adverse side effects [38].

Advantages and Disadvantages

NB-UVB is well tolerated. The advantages of NB-UVB are ease of administration and potential to induce remission. For localized disease, hand and foot, comb, and targeted units are available. NB-UVB can be used safely in pregnancy and in childhood psoriasis. The major disadvantage of NB-UVB phototherapy, which can be generalized to all forms of office-based phototherapy, is the time commitment of one to three office visits per week. In addition, both BB-UVB and NB-UVB generally require more frequent maintenance treatments compared with PUVA; this obviously needs to be balanced with the apparently higher photocarcinogenicity of PUVA, especially in fair-skinned individuals. If the patient is responsive to UVB, home phototherapy units can be considered as an option.

Dose and Administration

The initial dose of UVB can be determined by minimal erythema dose (MED) testing, the preferred test, or by Fitzpatrick skin type, a test that is less accurate. MED is the dose of UVB that produces minimally perceptible erythema covering the entire irradiated area. The guideline that we use for MED testing at Henry Ford Hospital is shown in Table 11.1. The initial fluence is usually 70% of the patient's MED. In both methods, the dose is increased by 10%–15% at each visit, guided by the patient's side effects of the previous dose. Ideally, phototherapy should be dosed based on the individual's ability to photoadapt. Photoadaptation is defined as the diminished future response to equivalent doses of irradiation [39], which in part is due to a persons' facultative pigmentation and an increase in epidermal thickness. Palmer et al. [40] retrospectively reviewed 352 psoriasis patients with skin types I–IV who received NB-UVB phototherapy twice weekly—starting dose of 70% MED and increased by 20% as tolerated. They found that patients with higher skin types photoadapt almost equally per unit of UVR compared with patients with lower skin types but that they have a greater overall absolute photoadaptation. They felt that differences in MED are not associated with tendency to erythema and that the accepted protocol of phototherapy starting at 70% MED and increasing by 20% as tolerated is suitable for skin types I–IV.

Despite accepted protocols of starting dose of 70% of MED, various studies have shown similar clinical outcomes regardless of starting dose. A recent randomized, double-blind clinical trial showed no difference in outcome when comparing starting dose by 70% of individual MED, 50% of individual MED, and fixed dose in subjects with skin phototypes I–III [41]. The subjects were treated three times per week with a 20% followed by 10% incremental reduction in dose. Another study had similar results with starting dose of 35% of MED in subjects with skin phototypes I–III [42]. Regardless, MED assessment is important for patient safety, and starting dose of 70% of MED remains the accepted protocol. NB-UVB three times per week has been shown to clear psoriasis significantly faster than twice weekly treatment and therefore is preferable for most patients [43]. It also may produce a longer period of remission. Once satisfactory clearing of the psoriatic lesions has occurred, at our institution, the frequency of therapy is usually decreased to twice a week for four weeks, and finally maintained once a week for a few weeks and then stopped if the patient remains clear. Some patients

TABLE 11.1 Guidelines for Determination of NB-UVB MED

1. Using MED testing template, expose five sites to 100, 200, 400, 600, and 800 mJ/cm^2.
2. Read at 24 hours.
3. MED is defined as the minimal dose of NB-UVB that produces perceptible erythema covering the entire irradiated area.

may require long-term treatment with UVB therapy because their psoriasis will relapse if phototherapy treatments are discontinued.

Goggles for eye protection are routinely used during the treatment session. In addition, as discussed previously, male genitalia should be shielded during treatment [44]. Thick application of creams and ointments can actually block the transmission of UVB. Several topical treatments for psoriasis have been shown to block UVB. Anthralin can be found in a base containing salicylic acid, the latter absorbs UVB, hence limiting UVB transmission. Tar should also be removed before phototherapy because it physically blocks UV transmission. Clear liquid emollients such as mineral oil can be applied before phototherapy. Topical and systemic retinoids can decrease the MED due to their property of thinning the epidermis; therefore, if a retinoid is added to a treatment regime, at our center, we decrease the UVB dose by 30%.

If the patient's psoriasis is limited to a few areas of the body, one should consider shielding the unaffected skin from UV radiation. The articles that are used to shield healthy tissue should be kept consistent to prevent UV-induced erythema in previously shielded sites. Physical barriers such as drapes are preferred to sunscreens due to inconsistent application of sunscreen.

Adverse Effects

The acute side effect of UVB is erythema that appears 4–6 hours after radiation and peaks at 12–24 hours. If the fluence is too high, acute phototoxicity can occur that would result in blistering over large body surfaces. Patients will become tanned. UVB can induce a keratitis if proper eyewear is not used.

The long-term side effects of UVB include photoaging. Animal studies show that the carcinogenicity of NB-UVB is approximately two to three times that of BB-UVB at equivalent doses. Extrapolation of this data suggests that NB-UVB is two to three times more carcinogenic than BB-UVB per MED [45]. However, the MED equivalent of NB-UVB required to clear psoriasis is about one-third of that for BB-UVB; theoretically, there should be no greater risk of skin cancer for patients treated with NB-UVB compared with BB-UVB [46]. The concerns are at the molecular level that NB-UVB maybe more carcinogenic than BB-UV [47], but those findings have not translated to a clinical increase in cutaneous malignancies. The role of BB-UVB or NB-UVB therapy in skin carcinogenesis of humans with psoriasis is not clear. The incidence of skin tumors in 195 psoriasis patients receiving BB- or NB-UVB phototherapy with up to nine years of follow-up did not provide evidence for an increased skin cancer risk [48]. In a review of the literature, treatment with UVB phototherapy did not show an increased skin cancer risk in all studies reviewed but one; this study showed an increased risk of genital tumors with UVB [44].

An ongoing study of 3867 patients treated with NB-UVB in Dundee, Scotland, with the median cumulative number of NB-UVB treatments of 29 and 24,753 person-years of follow-up showed no significant association between NB-UVB treatment and basal cell carcinoma (BCC), squamous cell carcinoma (SCC), or melanoma [49]. Therefore, based on currently available data, both BB- and NB-UVB are safe treatment modalities.

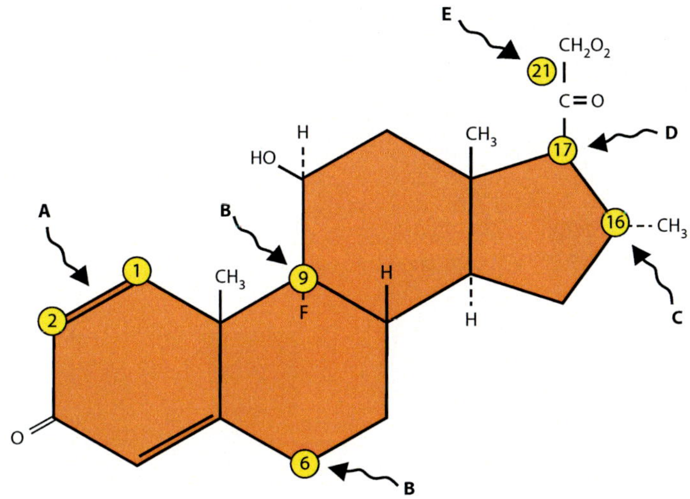

FIGURE 4.1 Functional effects of changing corticosteroid structural elements. The steroid base contains four rings. Corticosteroids have a dihydroxyacetone side chain attached to the carbon atom at position 17. The addition of a double bond between the C-1 and C-2 atoms of the cholesterol backbone (A) increases potency by increasing the lipophilicity of the molecule. Halogenation (with fluoride or chlorine) at the C-6 or C-9 structural positions (B) increases corticosteroid potency through interactions with the corticosteroid receptor. Reduced polarity of the molecule, and therefore greater lipophilicity, can also be achieved by removal of the C-16 α-hydroxyl group (C) or the C-17 dihydroxyacetone side chain (D), or by masking hydrophilic side groups via esterification of the C-17 or C-21 positions (E).

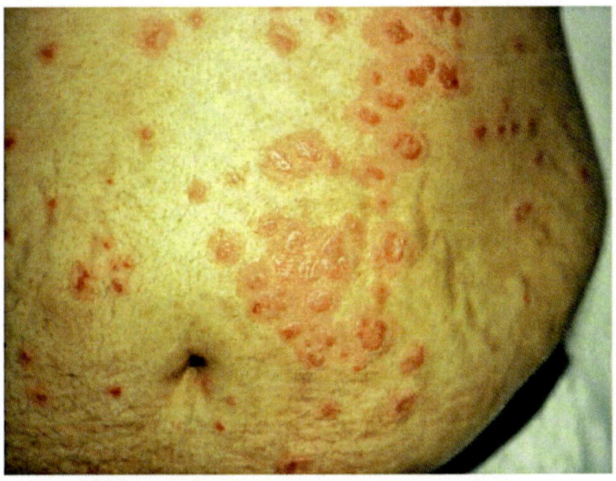

FIGURE 5.2 Abdominal skin irritation from calcipotriene.

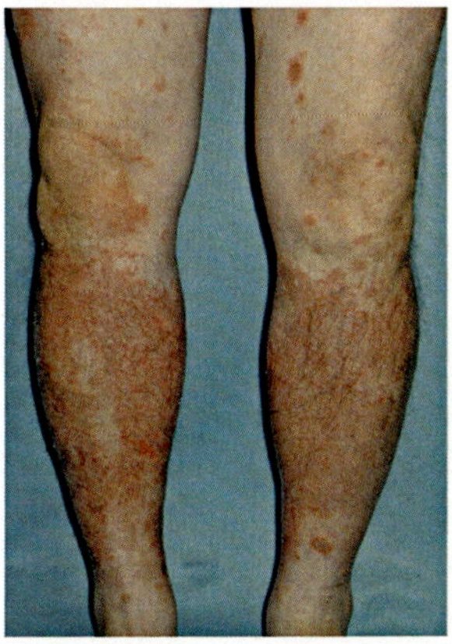

FIGURE 5.3 Lower extremities skin irritation from calcipotriene.

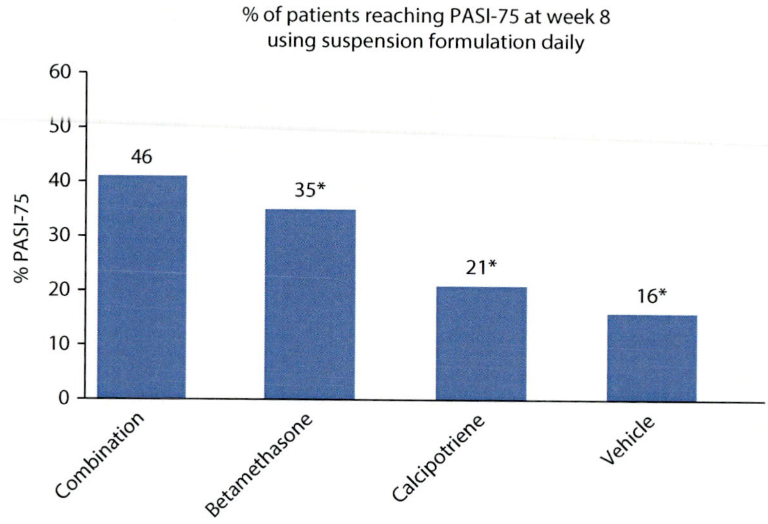

FIGURE 6.1 All patients treated with once-daily topical suspension. Combination = calcipotriene/betamethasone dipropionate ointment. *$p < .001$ for comparison with combination therapy. (Data from Kragballe K and Noerrelund KL, *J Eur Acad Dermatol Venereol* 16, 276, 2002.)

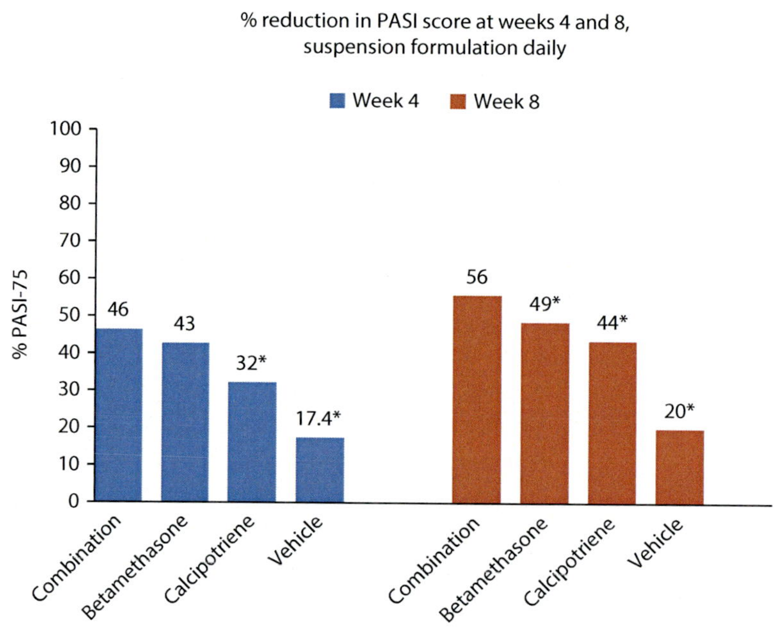

FIGURE 6.2 All patients treated with once-daily topical suspension. Combination = calcipotriene/betamethasone dipropionate suspension. *$p \leq .004$ for comparison with combination therapy. (Data from Kragballe K and Noerrelund KL, *J Eur Acad Dermatol Venereol* 16, 276, 2002.)

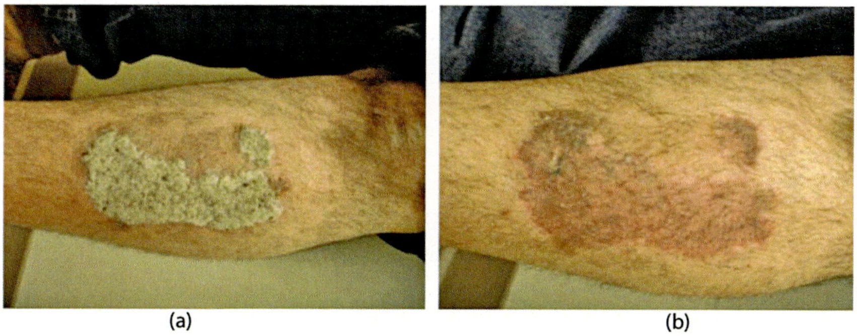

FIGURE 6.6 Rapid clinical improvement in patient before (a) and after (b) treatment with fixed-dose combination therapy.

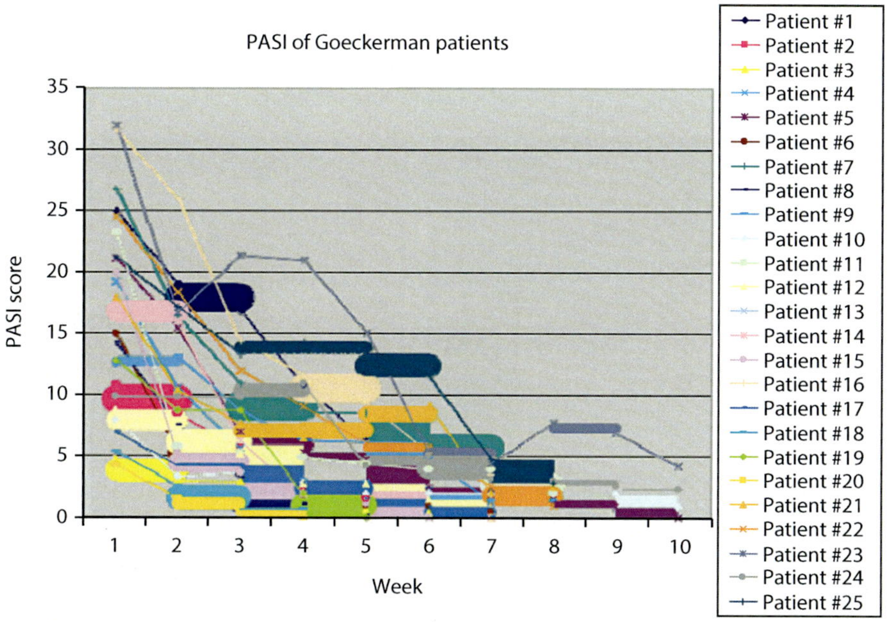

FIGURE 9.1 PASI scores of 25 consecutive Goeckerman patients treated at the UCSF Psoriasis Treatment Center. (From Lee E and Koo J, *J Dermatol Treat* 16, 102–107, 2005.)

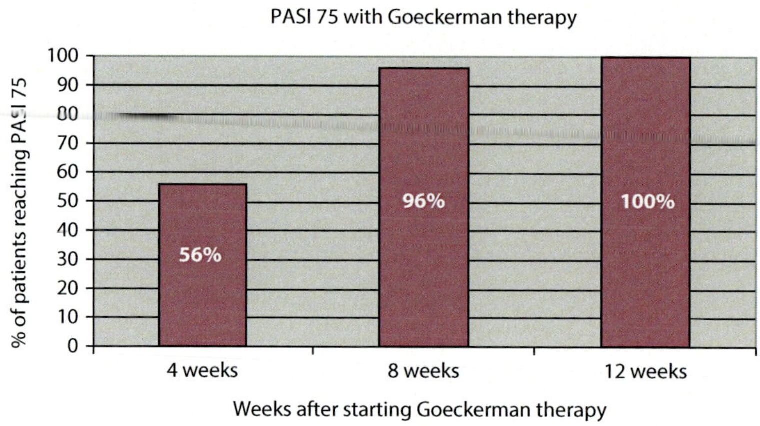

FIGURE 9.2 Percentage of patients achieving PASI 75 with 4-, 8-, and 12-week Goeckerman therapy. (From Lee E and Koo J, *J Dermatol Treat* 16, 102–107, 2005.)

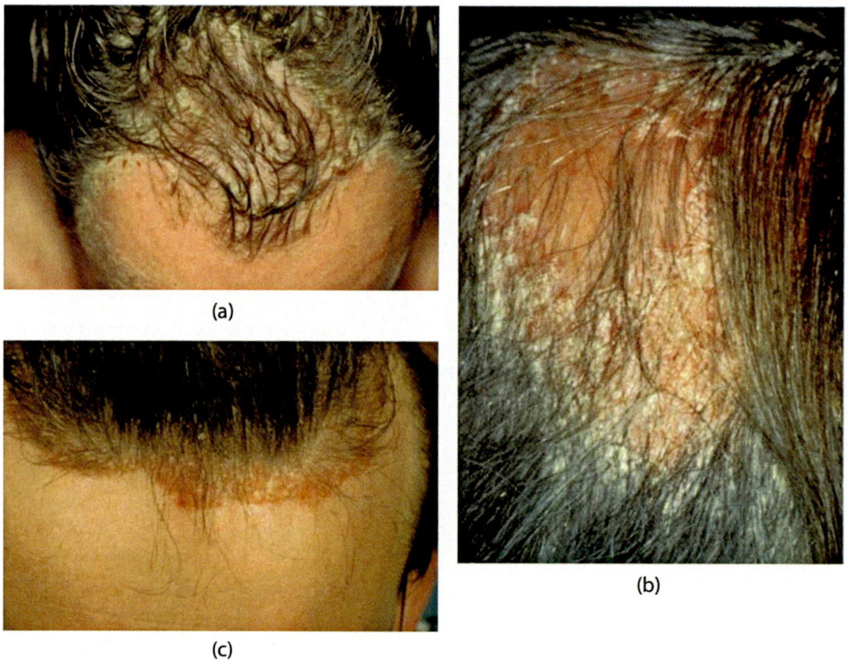

FIGURE 14.1 Classical manifestations of scalp psoriasis. (a) Psoriasis of the scalp. (b) Scarring psoriatic alopecia. (c) Hairline psoriasis.

PSORALEN AND UVA

PUVA photochemotherapy can be considered the gold standard of UV-based therapy for the treatment of psoriasis. The absorption spectrum of 8-methoxypsoralen (8-MOP) is 315–350 nm, with the maximum absorption occurring at 330–335 nm. The spectral output of the UVA light bulb used in PUVA ranges from 320 to 400 nm, with a peak emission at 352 nm.

The efficacy of PUVA is probably due to a few mechanisms. Psoralens intercalate into double-stranded DNA; with the absorption of a photon in the UVA range, 3,4- or 4′,5′-cyclobutane monoadducts with pyrimidine bases are formed. When a second photon of light is absorbed by either of these two monoadducts, a bifunctional adduct is formed that cross-links the DNA double helix. This adduct inhibits DNA replication, ultimately causing arrest of the cell cycle and decreasing epidermal proliferation. This is likely the main mechanism of action in the treatment of psoriasis. Psoralens in an excited state can also react with molecular oxygen, resulting in reactive oxygen species and mitochondrial dysfunction leading to apoptosis of both keratinocytes and lymphocytes [50]. Direct effects on the cell surface membrane and inhibition of epidermal growth factor binding by PUVA also decrease epidermal proliferation.

Psoralen can be administered orally or topically. 8-MOP is the only form of psoralen available in the United States; it is used for systemic and topical therapy. Systemic 8-MOP currently comes in a hard gelatin capsule and a soft gelatin capsule (encapsulated liquid preparation, Oxsoralen-Ultra). The soft capsule reaches peak levels in the blood faster compared with the hard capsule (mean, 1.8 vs. 3 hours). It also demonstrates a shorter time to peak photosensitivity (mean, 2.1 vs. 3.9 hours). MED is also substantially less in the soft capsule than that required for the hard capsule (mean, 7.1 vs. 12.9 J/cm^2) [51]. Unfortunately, the soft capsules cost four to five times more than the hard capsules. 5-Methoxypsoralen (5-MOP) is used primarily in Europe. TMP, 8-MOP, and 5-MOP can be used for bath PUVA. UVA can be administered by booth phototherapy, hand and foot units, or targeted phototherapy.

Efficacy

PUVA is a very effective therapy, and responses range from 74% to 100% [52]. Patients treated with PUVA are able to achieve long remissions without requiring maintenance therapies [53]. After 20–30 treatments two to three times per week, up to 90% of patients achieve marked improvement or clearing [54,55].

Combination Therapy

PUVA can be combined with other therapies to improve its efficacy, to decrease the cumulative dose of UVA, and ultimately to minimize its adverse effects. Topical therapies such as anthralin, calcipotriol [56], and tazarotene [57] can be effectively used in combination with PUVA. Tar, with an action spectrum in the UVA range, is not widely used in combination with PUVA due to its photosensitizing potential. Studies on efficacy of topical corticosteroids in combination with PUVA have yielded conflicting results. Five studies comparing PUVA alone to PUVA and topical corticosteroids showed more rapid rates of clearing with the combination regimen; however, one of the five studies showed a more rapid relapse rate in the combination group [58]. In a recent study of 40 patients, there was no significant difference in clinical improvement of psoriasis treated either by PUVA plus topical steroids or PUVA plus bland emollients [59].

PUVA combined with systemic retinoids (RePUVA) is one of the most effective combination therapies. In a randomized, double-blind study, patients with severe, widespread psoriasis were treated either with PUVA as monotherapy or in combination with acitretin. Eighty percent of patients achieved marked or complete clearance with PUVA monotherapy compared with 96% of the patients with adjunctive acitretin administration. The cumulative UVA dose in the acitretin–PUVA group was 42% less than the PUVA only group [60]. Similar results have been seen in other studies. In a study performed by Lauharanta et al. [61], 34 patients with plaque psoriasis were treated with either acitretin or etretinate and bath PUVA, and all patients achieved remission. There were no differences in the clinical response of the two groups, suggesting that acitretin is as effective as etretinate in combination with bath PUVA for the treatment of psoriasis. The combination of methotrexate and PUVA can be an effective treatment, however, due to the immunosuppressive properties of both treatment modalities; this combination should only be considered after the use of retinoids. Retinoids or methotrexate should be started one to three weeks before the initiation of PUVA, and continued until the psoriasis is almost clear. The retinoids or methotrexate can be tapered and then stopped, and PUVA should be continued as maintenance therapy; the latter is then tapered as appropriate.

The combination of NB-UVB whole-body irradiation followed by topical PUVA therapy using cream preparation of psoralen for selected psoriatic plaques has been shown to have significantly higher efficacy compared with either monotherapy [62]. The cumulative UV doses were significantly lower in the combination therapy group. It should be noted that this study, performed in Germany, used 0.001% 8-MOP in a cream base; whether the 0.1% 8-MOP lotion commonly used in the United States would have the same synergistic effect with NB-UVB remains to be evaluated.

Indications

PUVA has been shown to be more effective in clearing psoriasis in darker skin types, probably due to the longer wavelength that results in deeper UV penetration. Thick plaques as well as the hands and soles of the feet are generally more effectively treated with PUVA. Additional indications include failure to respond to UVB phototherapy and aggressive disease, such as pustular psoriasis.

Contraindications

Absolute contraindications to PUVA include xeroderma pigmentosum, basal cell nevus syndrome, personal history of melanoma, and photosensitive disorders, such as lupus erythematosus and dermatomyositis. Other absolute contraindications include young age (<10 years, because of the known chronic side effects of PUVA), aphakia, and nursing mothers (because of the presence of 8-MOP in breast milk). Although psoralens are not considered to be teratogenic, it is not advisable to use PUVA in pregnant patients. Relative contraindications include family history of melanoma, history of nonmelanoma skin cancer or dysplastic nevi, ingestion of photosensitizing medications, significant solar damage, and current or previous treatment with ionizing radiation, arsenic, methotrexate, cyclosporine, and systemic tacrolimus. PUVA should be used with caution in patients between the age of 10 and 18 years due to its long-term side effects. Caution should be used in patients with hepatic insufficiency as the metabolism of systemic psoralen may be delayed, resulting in prolonged photosensitivity. Renal insufficiency can slow down psoralen excretion.

Advantages and Disadvantages

In light-skinned individuals with thinner psoriatic plaques, PUVA has a role as a second-line light-based therapy after NB-UVB. PUVA is preferable to NB-UVB in dark-skinned patients and for thick lesions. The disadvantages of oral PUVA are its acute and chronic side effects (see "Side Effects"). Bath PUVA provides uniform psoralen distribution to the skin with low plasma levels, and it results in a shortened duration of photosensitivity. Moreover, available data so far have shown no evidence for increased risk of skin cancer of any type with bath PUVA. However, to administer this treatment, one needs to have a bathtub, and because of the rapid decline of phototoxicity, the patient has to be exposed to UVA within 10–15 minutes after soaking in psoralen-containing bath water, the latter needs to be freshly prepared for each patient. It is a resource-intensive therapy to administer. Topical psoralens in the form of creams or lotions avoid most of the systemic side effects of psoralens, and they are convenient to administer; however their nonuniform distribution can result in unpredictable phototoxicity. Furthermore, topical PUVA has a narrow therapeutic window, that is, with a slight increase in UVA, there could be a significant increase in phototoxicity. The areas that receive localized topical PUVA may become quite tanned and the uneven pigmentation may be a cosmetic concern.

Dose and Administration

With the newer Oxsoralen-Ultra formulation, 8-MOP is taken 1–1.5 hours before phototherapy, at a dose of 0.4–0.6 mg/kg, with a maximum of 70 mg/kg. After oral administration, there are significant inter- and intraindividual variations in the absorption of 8-MOP. Therefore, it is very important that the psoralen dose, type, and amount of food intake and timing of phototherapy after ingestion of psoralen are kept constant. It is preferable that psoralen be taken on an empty stomach, because food intake slows absorption and reduces the peak blood levels. However, due to gastrointestinal side effects, especially with 8-MOP, nonfat small meals may be taken to alleviate some of these symptoms. In some patients, the capsules may have to be ingested 10 minutes apart to minimize the gastrointestinal side effects. Antiemetics may have to be given to some patients.

In patients who are unable to tolerate systemic PUVA, psoralen can be administered in a bath or cream/lotion, avoiding the gastrointestinal tract. In our institution, topical PUVA is administered using 0.1% 8-MOP solution in Lubriderm® lotion, applied 20 minutes before exposure to UVA. The topical PUVA protocol is shown in Table 11.2. Bath PUVA is only performed in very few centers in the United States because of the need for a bathtub. A bath

TABLE 11.2 Topical PUVA Protocol

1. 0.1% Methoxypsoralen in Lubriderm lotion is applied to the affected areas 20–30 minutes before treatment. This topical is only applied in the medical office.
2. The initial dose of UVA is 0.25–0.5 J/cm².
3. The dose increase is based on side effects. If tolerated, increase by 0.25–0.5 J/cm².
4. Photochemotherapy is given three times per week.
5. The maximum dose is 8 J/cm².
6. Once the condition has improved, treatment frequency can be decreased to twice per week for 4–8 weeks, then once per week for 4–8 weeks, and then discontinued.

containing 0.5–5.0 mg/L 8-MOP, or 0.33 mg/L TMP, needs to be freshly prepared; the patient will then soak in it for 15–30 minutes. At some phototherapy facilities (e.g., University of California–San Francisco [UCSF]), effective bath PUVA is being conducted simply by dissolving 50 mg of Oxsoralen-Ultra in a hot cup of water first and then added to 100 liters of bath water. Exposure to the UVA needs to be performed within 30 minutes after the patient steps out of the bathtub.

In Europe, oral 5-MOP is commonly used. It is less phototoxic than 8-MOP; therefore, it requires a higher cumulative UVA dose. The dose range used is 1.2–1.8 mg/kg. It has less gastrointestinal side effects, thus it is better tolerated. It is not available in the United States.

Avoidance of prolonged sun exposure and wearing UVA-absorbing sunscreens and photoprotective clothing on the days of PUVA therapy are necessary to prevent significant phototoxicity. Unlike UVB-induced erythema, PUVA-induced phototoxicity begins approximately 24 hours after exposure and peaks at 48–72 hours after exposure. This is the reason why PUVA should not be administered two days in a row. If PUVA is administered on consecutive days, a treatment protocol more often used in Europe, the dose is kept constant on the first two days of the week, followed by a nontreatment third day; an increased but identical dose may be given on the fourth and fifth day of the week [57].

The initial dose of UVA can either be determined by minimal phototoxicity dose (MPD) or by Fitzpatrick skin type. The MPD is the minimal dose of PUVA that produces well-defined erythema. These readings are performed at 48–72 hours. The dose of UVA should be adjusted, usually decreased by 25%, if patients are taking photosensitizing medications. UVA doses should also be decreased if topical or systemic retinoids are added during a course of PUVA because they thin the stratum corneum, reducing the amount of light required for phototoxicity.

Before, during, and after UVA exposure, protective eyewear should be used. Male genitalia are particularly sensitive to the development of SCC [63]; therefore, male genitals should be shielded during all of the UVA exposure. If PUVA is required for limited disease, careful shielding of unaffected skin is recommended.

Therapy is usually administered twice to three times per week until the psoriasis is well controlled; it then can be decreased to twice and eventually once a week. Maintenance therapy has been shown to increase the duration of remission; however, it will increase the patient's cumulative dose of UVA. The British Phototherapy Group recommends that long-term PUVA maintenance therapy should only be considered in patients with a history of rapid relapses [64]. Whether this applies to non-Caucasians is not clear.

To better define the frequency of PUVA therapy, a prospective, randomized, half-side study was performed in Austria, using 18 patients with chronic plaque psoriasis who received paired PUVA regimens [65]. It was shown that reducing the number of treatments while maintaining the same UVA dose per week did not reduce efficacy. Reducing the number of treatments from four times per week to twice a week and reducing the UVA dose from 1 MPD to 0.75 or 0.5 MPD per treatment only slightly affected therapeutic efficacy and had no effect on final clearance rates or time to complete clearance. The mean cumulative UVA dose was significantly lower for the least intensive dose regimen (0.5 MPD twice/week) than for the more intensive regimens.

Because of the increased development of cutaneous malignancies with PUVA therapy, one should strongly consider the combination with other drugs such as retinoids or in rotation with other treatments to minimize total cumulative dose of PUVA.

Adverse Effects

The acute side effects can be due to either the psoralen or the UVA radiation. Systemic psoralen causes nausea and occasionally vomiting in up to 30% of patients taking 8-MOP. 5-MOP has less gastrointestinal symptoms and is better tolerated. Most drug-induced photosensitivities are due to UVA; therefore, a careful medication history will help prevent this adverse event. PUVA-induced phototoxic reactions, such as erythema and vesiculation, appear at 24–36 hours and peak at 48–72 hours; they can persist for a week or longer. Subacute side effects can be an intractable pruritus known as "PUVA itch." In some patients, therapy may have to be stopped until the pruritus resolves, and one can then consider restarting the treatment at a lower UVA dose. Tanning is a constant feature, especially in patients with darker skin. Other known side effects include photo-onycholysis, melanonychia, and friction blisters.

Long-term side effects include photoaging, the development of small brown to black macules in PUVA-exposed sites known as PUVA lentigines, and photocarcinogenesis. Many of these long-term side effects have been reported by the U.S. PUVA Follow-Up Group, a 16-center prospective cohort study of 1380 patients first treated with PUVA in 1975–1976 in the United States [66]. In a study on photoaging, actinic damage was observed on the hands of 61% of patients and on the buttocks of 21% of patients. Pigmentary changes were seen on the hands of 59% of patients and on the buttocks of 25% of the patients [67].

Increased risk of SCCs is a well-documented, dose-dependent adverse effect in Caucasians. In a study from the PUVA Follow-Up Group, there was no increase in nonmelanoma skin cancer in the first 15 years of the study. However, after 25 years, 50% of patients who had received >400 treatments had SCC, and 33% of patients who had received greater than 200 treatments had BCC [66]. In another study by the PUVA Follow-Up Group in which >1000 patients were treated with PUVA, UVB exposure (≥300 treatments vs. <300 treatments) was associated with a modest but significant increase in SCC and BCC risk [68]. These carcinomas occurred on body sites typically exposed to UVB therapy but not on chronically sun-exposed sites typically covered during therapy. A Swedish study followed where 4799 patients who had received PUVA between 1974 and 1985 with an average follow-up period of 15.9 years for men and 16.2 for women showed an increase in the risk for SCC; the relative risk for SCC was 5.6 for men and 3.6 for women [69]. In contrast, a meta-analysis of all available long-term data on non-Caucasians with respect to nonmelanoma skin cancer so far revealed no increase in risk in nonmelanoma skin cancer in non-Caucasians [70].

Using the U.S. PUVA Follow-Up database, 135 patients who had used oral retinoids for >26 weeks in one year were studied. The development of SCC and BCC for each patient during retinoid use years was compared with the nonretinoid use years. It was found that oral retinoids reduced the risk of SCC but did not significantly alter BCC incidence [71]. However, a recent study looking at cytotoxic and genotoxic effects of acitretin alone or in combination with psoralen-UVA or NB-UVB on blood from psoriatic patients found that although acitretin alone or acitretin in combination with NB-UVB did not show genotoxic effects, combination therapy with acitretin and PUVA induced slight genotoxic effects [72]. Further studies are needed to clarify its genotoxic potential and clinical application.

There is a significant dose-dependent increase in genital SCC of PUVA-treated male patients. The incidence of invasive penile and scrotal SCCs was increased by 52.6-fold. This dose-dependent increase in the risk of genital tumors is persistent long after PUVA therapy has been stopped, especially among those with high-dose exposures to both PUVA and tar or UVB [63].

There are conflicting results of long-term studies on the incidence of melanoma after PUVA therapy. The PUVA Follow-Up Study reported an increased risk of melanoma, greatest in patients exposed to high doses of PUVA (≥250 treatments), beginning 15 years after first exposure to PUVA. The incidence rate ratio was 8.4 [73]. In contrast, the Swedish follow-up study of 4799 patients who had received PUVA between 1974 and 1985, with an average follow-up period of 15.9 years for men and 16.2 for women, did not find an increased risk for melanoma, nor in a subcohort comprising 1867 patients followed for 15–21 years [69].

Since 1977, the PUVA follow-up study has monitored the ocular status of 1237 cohort members with psoriasis using structured eye examinations [74]. Based on their data, the age-adjusted incidence of cataract did not increase significantly. They concluded that exposure to PUVA does not increase the cataract risk among persons using appropriate eye protection.

TARGETED (LOCALIZED) PHOTOTHERAPY

The appeal of targeted, or localized, phototherapy is its ability to spare healthy skin from the side effects of UV radiation. In addition, the affected areas can usually tolerate a higher dose than unaffected skin, as the rate determining factor for generalized phototherapy is usually erythema of uninvolved skin. It is known that normal skin can be exposed to up to three MEDs without blistering, whereas psoriatic skin may be exposed up to three times this dose (9 MEDs) without blistering [75,76]. The recent commercial introduction of fiber-coupled

TABLE 11.3 Targeted UVA and UVB Phototherapy Units

Phototherapy Unit	Company	UV Type	Wavelength (nm)	Spot Size (cm)	Other Features
XTRAC®, XL +, Ultra®	PhotoMedex, Inc.	Xenon chloride laser	308	1.8 × 1.8 circular	
PHAROS EX-308™	Ra™ Medical Systems, Inc.	Xenon chloride laser	308	Adjustable beam, range from 1.8 × 1.8 to 2 mm round	
VTRAC®	PhotoMedex, Inc.	Xenon chloride lamp	308	6.1 × 3.1 rectangular	Water-cooled handpiece
BClear™/ ReLume™	Lumenis®	UVB	290–320	1.6 × 1.6 square	Portable
DuaLight™	Theralight™, Inc.	UVB and UVA	290–330; 330–400	1.9 × 1.9 square	Can switch from UVB to UVA, compact
MultiClear®	CureLight, Ltd.	UVB, UVA-1, and visible	295–315; 360–370; 405–450	2.3 × 2.3	
Lumera	Daavlin	UVB Lamp	290–320; 330–400	1.5 × 1.5 square	Compact, portable, Brush
308 Excimer System	Alma Lasers, Ltd.	UVB Lamp	308 nm	16 × 16	Small, portable

UVB phototherapy systems facilitates the use of this treatment modality for localized psoriasis plaques.

The mechanism of action of targeted phototherapy is similar to that of the other UV-based therapy, that is, by inducing T-cell apoptosis, suppression of DNA synthesis, and generation of prostaglandins and cytokines. It has been reported that 308-nm excimer laser is more effective in the induction of T-cell apoptosis compared with NB-UVB [6].

At the time of this writing, there are several targeted phototherapy systems available (Table 11.3). XTrac™ and the PHAROS™ EX-308 lasers are the only laser-targeted phototherapy systems; the rest are nonlaser light sources.

Efficacy

Most of the published studies on targeted phototherapy have been performed with the 308-nm excimer laser system; this system is the focus of the discussion in this section.

Initial case reports and subsequent larger studies [77] have shown significant improvement and even remission of psoriatic lesions after exposure to 308-nm excimer laser. In a multicenter study of 80 patients, stable mild to moderate plaque-type psoriasis was treated twice per week for a total of 10 treatments or clear disease [78]. The initial dose was based on MED testing and the following treatments were based on plaque response. Seventy-two percent achieved at least 75% clearing in an average of 6.2 treatments. Eighty-four percent of patients reached improvement of at least 75% after 10 or fewer treatments. Fifty percent reached improvement of at least 90% after 10 or fewer treatments. In a follow-up study, 55% of patients reported an overall satisfaction with their treatments, and 25% reported that their treatment was better than other therapies they had tried for localized disease [79]. A recent retrospective study of 98 patients treated with 308-nm excimer laser showed similar results [80].

Higher doses can be used on psoriatic plaques with faster clearing and decreased cumulative dose compared with conventional booth phototherapy [81]. A single administration with 10 times MED has been shown to induce apoptosis and consequently decrease PASI [82]. A dose–response study showed clearance of psoriasis with high fluences (8–16 times MED) in as little as one treatment [76]. Koebner reactions were not observed despite the side effects of transient painful blistering. Treatment with higher fluences was more effective than low and medium fluences. In addition, the lesions treated with high fluences remained in remission longer. The four-month relapse-free outcome is comparable or better than the standard topical or systemic therapy for psoriasis [76]. In a study with four children with psoriasis, mean age 11 years, excimer laser was found to be a safe and effective treatment for localized psoriasis in these children [83]. Two studies have compared the excimer laser to incoherent UVB phototherapy with similar outcomes. Tanghetti et al. [84] compared the clinical outcome of treatment with excimer laser to a continuous-wave, incoherent UVB light source. Both systems cleared the treated psoriasis plaques equivalently, requiring no more than two to five weeks of treatment. When used at equally erythemogenic high doses, both systems produced rapid plaque clearance with minimal side effects. Köllner et al. [85] treated 15 patients with plaque psoriasis. Three different psoriatic lesions were treated with the xenon chloride 308-nm excimer laser, the 308-nm excimer lamp, or 311-nm narrowband UVB three times per week. UVB doses were increased slowly and stepwise. There was no statistically significant difference among the three groups after 10 weeks. The mean number of treatments needed to achieve clearance was 24. Both 308-nm light sources treated psoriasis with a similar efficacy to standard NB-UVB phototherapy.

There are a few published studies demonstrating the effectiveness of targeted nonlaser UV phototherapy units in the treatment of psoriasis. The targeted UVB lamp (BClear™) was evaluated in the treatment of plaque-type psoriasis in 28 patients. Treatment was given twice weekly for 6–18 sessions (median, 10) [86]. The mean psoriasis severity index (PSI) improvement during treatment peaked at 73% after six weeks and declined to 63% at 16 weeks. Kaur et al. [87] used nonlaser localized NB-UVB phototherapy in subjects with localized psoriasis. Treatments were given two to three times weekly. Of the 6 of 10 patients that completed the study, all reached >90% clearing of their disease.

Combination Therapy

Ten patients with stable psoriasis were randomized to receive either targeted NB-UVB alone or 8-MOP and NB-UVB. Two areas within the same lesion of stable psoriasis were treated.

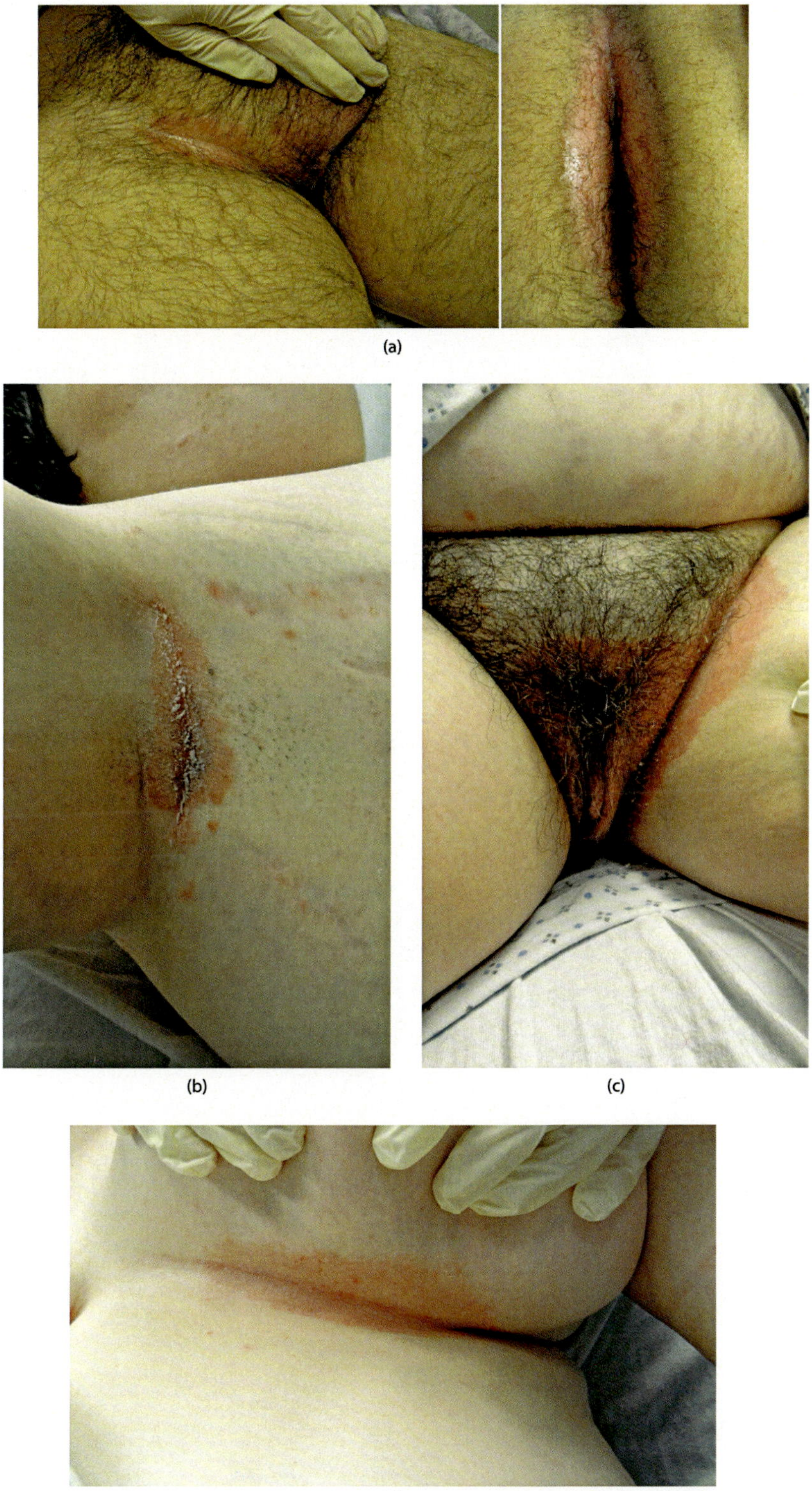

FIGURE 15.1 Well-demarcated, red plaques in the inguinal crease and intergluteal cleft (a), axilla (b), inguinal crease (c) and inframammory fold (d) of patients with inverse psoriasis.

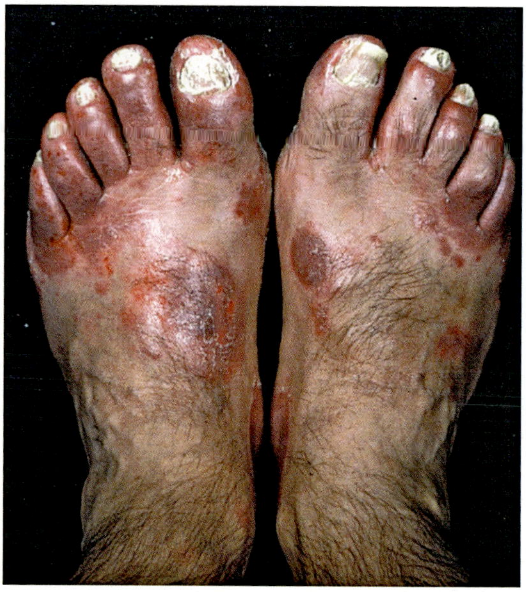

(a)

FIGURE 16.1 (a) Plaque psoriasis with nail involvement.

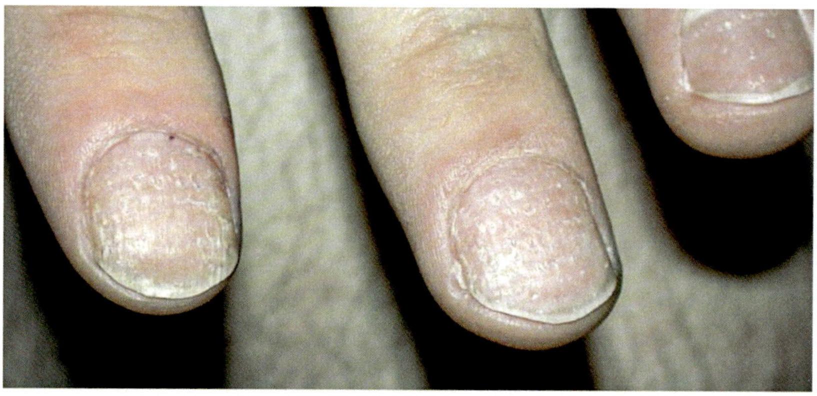

FIGURE 16.2 Pitting in nail psoriasis.

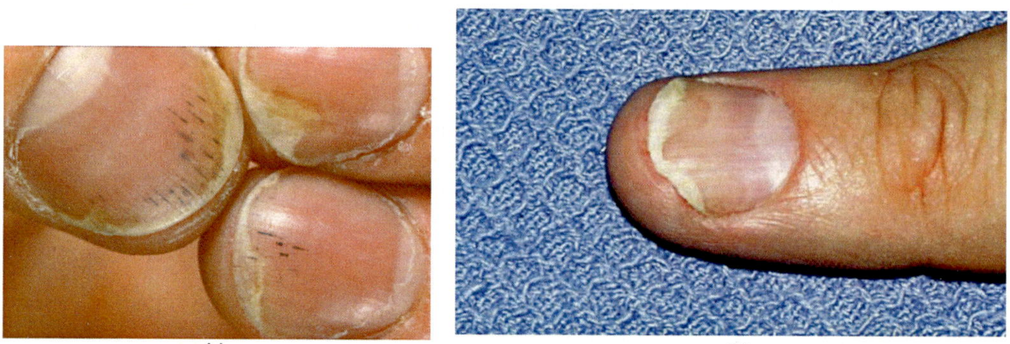

(a) (b)

FIGURE 16.3 (a) Splinter hemorrhages and oil spots in nail psoriasis. (b) Oil spot in nail psoriasis.

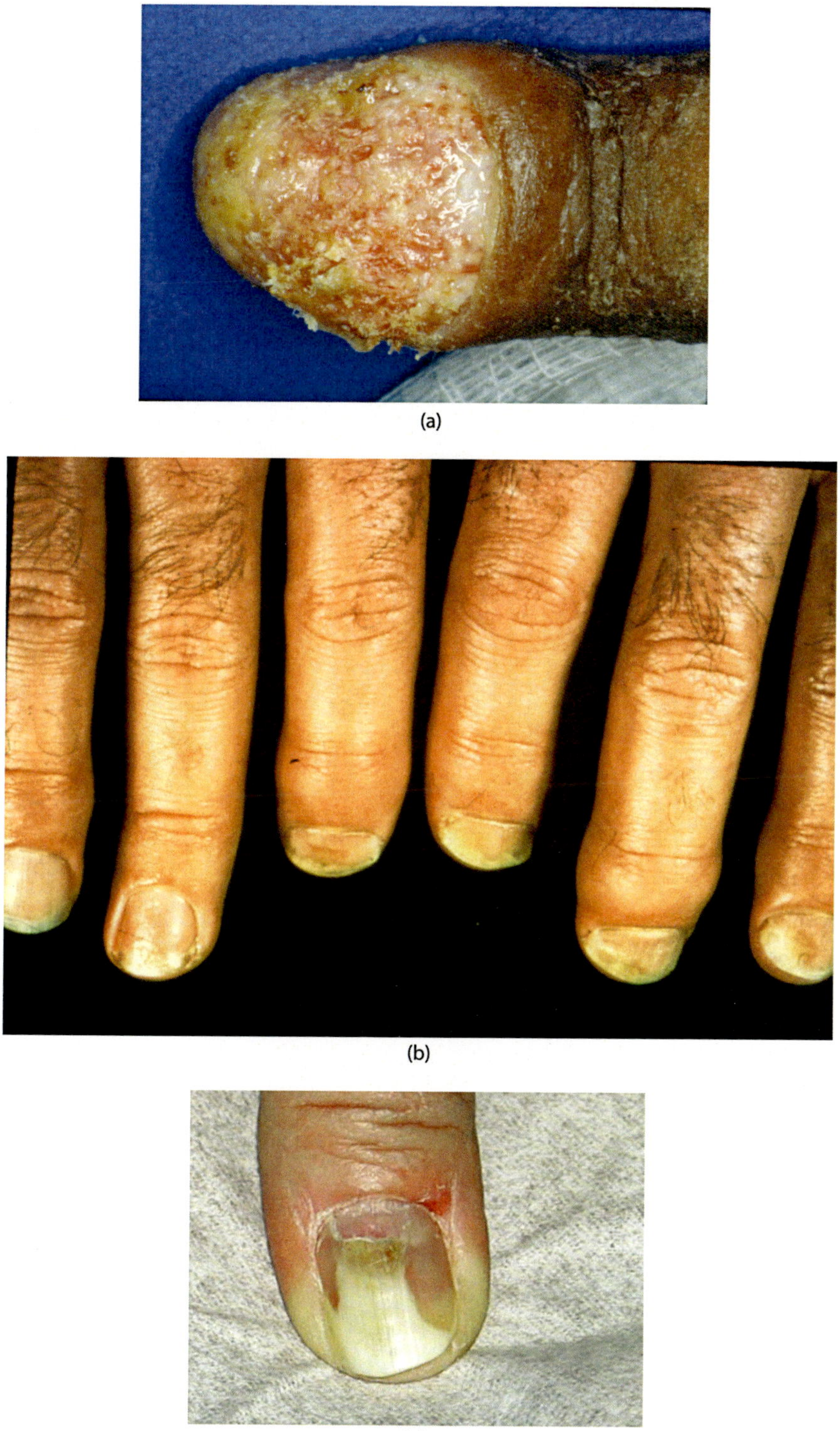

FIGURE 16.4 (a) Severe pustular psoriasis (acrodermatitis continua of Hallopeau) in a patient with HIV. (b) Enthesitis in a patient with psoriatic arthritis. (c) Onycholysis in nail psoriasis.

Four lesions were cleared by 8-MOP and NB-UVB, whereas three were cleared by NB-UVB alone. The decrease in PASI score was statistically significantly better in the combination group. There was also an increase in the mean remission time in the combination group that was eight weeks, whereas that for lesions that were cleared by NB-UVB alone was 4.67 weeks [88].

A prospective randomized study of 272 patients with moderate to severe plaque-type psoriasis treated patients with either PUVA plus up to four UVB308-nm radiations or PUVA monotherapy. There was no statistically significant difference when comparing the efficacy of PUVA and PUVA plus excimer, but patients treated with the combination method went into remission in half the treatment time and with half the cumulative UVA dose [89].

Recent studies have also shown effectiveness of 308-nm excimer laser in combination with corticosteroid ointment [90].

Indications

Targeted phototherapy is ideal for localized mild to moderate psoriasis, including lesions on the palms and soles, and on the scalp.

Contraindications

There are no absolute contraindications. Contraindications are related to the corresponding wavelength.

Advantages and Disadvantages

The advantages of targeted phototherapy include sparing healthy tissue from UV radiation and the ability to deliver high fluences to affected areas. This results in faster rate of response and a lower cumulative dose. However, the time to administer therapy is greatly increased as compared to booth phototherapy. One can spend up to 20 minutes per session two to three times per week. Under appropriate supervision, the therapy can be delivered by an experienced nurse, or phototherapy technician.

Dosage and Administration

Treatments are usually delivered two to three times per week. The initial dosing is usually based on a predetermined MED as well as plaque thickness and location. Fluences should be adjusted according to symptoms and response to treatment. The initial dose is usually maintained until the plaques flatten at which point the dose is decreased. Likewise, if there is no improvement with the initial dose, the fluence should be increased.

Housman et al. [91] showed that twice weekly excimer laser treatments promote clearance of psoriatic plaques and that tapering the treatments may be beneficial in maintaining the level of plaque clearance. After improvement of disease, they tapered the dose as follows: one treatment per week for four weeks, one treatment every other week for four weeks, and one final treatment four weeks later, for a total of seven treatments. No flares after the first month of tapering. No flares were noted in four out of five patients after the second month of treatment.

Köllner et al. [85] treated 16 patients with the 308-nm excimer laser or with the 308-nm lamp with an accelerated scheme three times per week. They compared this treatment with UVB therapy in which the dose was increased after every second treatment. With the accelerated scheme, clearance was achieved with fewer treatments and with half the cumulative dose of a slow and stepwise regime. The side effects such as blistering and crusting were also increased.

Adverse Effects

The adverse effects of targeted phototherapy are related to the wavelength administered. The lesional and perilesional skin can develop erythema, tanning, vesiculation, erosion, or crusting and result in an uneven skin tone that may be a cosmetic concern for some patients. This dyspigmentation fades gradually with time once phototherapy is stopped. Interestingly, koebnerization has not been reported with vesiculation. In fact, just the opposite has been reported, faster clearance in the vesiculated areas—a "reverse" Koebner phenomenon. There are no long-term studies on carcinogenesis.

UVA1

UVA1 is a relatively new type of phototherapy in the United States; however, it has been used since the early 1990s in Europe. Its main indications are for the treatment of atopic dermatitis and sclerosing disorders.

Efficacy

There are two small studies published on the use of UVA1 for the treatment of psoriasis. Kowalzick et al. [92] performed a paired controlled trial in three patients using medium-dose UVA1 and BB-UVB for three weeks. Both the UVA1- and BB-UVB-treated lesions improved. A review cited three HIV-positive psoriatic patients who benefited from UVA1 phototherapy [93]. However, in a review of Mang and Krutmann's personal experience, there is little to no efficacy of UVA1 for the treatment of psoriasis [94].

It has been suggested that UVA1 is the phototherapy of choice for HIV-positive patients with psoriasis [94]. Three HIV patients with psoriasis were treated with high-dose (130 J/cm^2) UVA1 with benefit. A quantitative polymerase chain reaction (PCR)–based assay was performed in both lesional and nonlesional skin after one UVB or UVA1 exposure. The UVB-treated skin showed a 6- to 15-fold increase in the HIV copy number, whereas the UVA1-treated skin did not show any increase [93]. Further studies are clearly needed.

Combination Therapy

Forty-five patients with psoriasis were divided into three treatment groups, namely calcipotriol monotherapy, calcipotriol plus UVA1, or calcipotriol plus NB-UVB [95]. The responses to UVA1 and NB-UVB with calcipotriol were superior to calcipotriol monotherapy.

In a pilot study of five patients with palmer or plantar psoriasis, the combination of medium-dose UVA1 (50 J/cm^2) and tacrolimus ointment versus tacrolimus ointment monotherapy for the treatment of psoriasis was evaluated [96]. No dramatic changes were noted in either group.

Indications

The indications for UVA1 for psoriasis are not clear; further investigations are necessary to determine its efficacy.

Contraindications

Contraindications include photodermatoses with action spectrum in the UVA1 range. In patients taking photosensitizing medications, UVA1 needs to be used with caution.

Advantages and Disadvantages

Further studies are necessary.

Dosage and Administration

Until further studies with psoriasis show good efficacy, there is no established dose for this treatment. For atopic dermatitis and localized scleroderma, studies have been done using low dose (20 J/cm^2), medium dose (50–60 J/cm^2), and high dose (120 J/cm^2). The low and medium doses are the more commonly used regimens currently.

Adverse Effects

UVA1 is generally well tolerated. Exposed skin will become tanned. There is a significant amount of heat generated by the equipment throughout the treatment. Other possible side effects include xerosis, pruritus, and rarely skin burning. The long-term side effects are not known. In the animal model, UVA1 has induced squamous cell cancers [97].

LASER

PDL is considered the gold standard treatment for vascular lesions. Because the development of psoriasis is partially dependent on the vasculature that serves as the delivery system for lymphocytes, PDL have been studied for the treatment of psoriasis.

Efficacy

PDL treatment is associated with decreased microvessel count that is shown to have a strong positive correlation to PASI [98]. Destruction of the superficial capillary vasculature bed in a psoriatic lesion is probably how the PDL improves psoriasis, and secretion of angiogenic cytokines in treated lesions are responsible for endothelial reproliferation and return of psoriasis [99]. However, PDL is not a commonly used therapy.

There are several small studies [100–102] that report clinical improvement of psoriasis after one to five treatments with PDL. Although it is shown to be less efficacious than excimer laser, PDL is effective in a small subset of patients [103]. A prospective study using PDL as treatment for therapy-resistant psoriasis of the hands and feet showed average duration of remission of 11 months [104]. In a randomizer, double-blind study, pulse duration had no effect on efficacy for nail psoriasis [105].

Combination Therapy

As noted above, salicylic acid was used in combination as a keratolytic agent. Calcipotriol ointment was also used in combination with PDL. Further studies are necessary.

Indications

The benefits of PDL are not established, and its role in the treatment of psoriasis needs to be better defined. It may have a role in managing persistent patches of erythema that remain after clearance of induration and scale.

Contraindications

None identified.

Advantages and Disadvantages

The advantages of targeted phototherapy include sparing healthy tissue from therapy. However, the time to administer therapy is greatly increased compared with booth phototherapy.

Adverse Effects

Side effects of the PDL include transient purpura, moderate discomfort during treatment, transient dyspigmentation, transient crusting, and atrophy.

PHOTODYNAMIC THERAPY

PDT has many well-established indications in dermatology. Its use in the treatment of psoriasis is currently being investigated. PDT causes a photochemical reaction that requires the presence of a photosensitizing molecule, such as 5-aminolaevulinic acid, photoactivating wavelengths of light, and tissue oxygen.

Efficacy

Accumulated protoporphyrin IX (PpIX) has been shown in psoriatic lesions, but it has a highly variable distribution within plaques. Kleinpenning et al. [106] incubated psoriatic plaques with 20% 5-aminolaevulinic acid (ALA) ointment for three hours after keratolytic treatment in 14 patients with stable plaque psoriasis. By using fluorescence to determine the uptake of PpIX, they were able to show that a thicker stratum corneum has a lower fluorescence. Fluorescence intensity and thickness of the stratum corneum proved to be negatively correlated. The variable clinical response seen after PDT in psoriasis could be explained by this and that optimal desquamation prior to PDT is required for more favorable results.

In a prospective randomized, double-blind phase study, 12 patients with chronic plaque psoriasis were treated with topical ALA-PDT [107]. In each patient, three psoriatic plaques were treated with a light dose of 20 J/cm2 and 0.1%, 1%, and 5% ALA, respectively. Treatment was conducted twice a week until complete clearance or to a maximum of 12 treatments.

The mean percentage improvement was 37.5%, 45.6%, and 51.2% in the 0.1%, 1%, and 5% ALA-treated groups, respectively.

There are a few studies that show similar modest therapeutic outcomes [108–110]. There are only five case reports of PDT's benefits in the treatment of palmopustular psoriasis [111,112], and further studies are needed.

Combination Therapy

The use of a keratolytic agent should be considered to decrease epidermal thickness.

Indications

Although not a first- or second-line therapy, PDT may be considered in limited circumstances for the treatment of localized psoriasis.

Advantages and Disadvantages

Further studies are necessary to confirm the effectiveness of topical PDT and optimizing the treatment protocol may increase clinical efficacy. It is a time-consuming treatment and has an unfavorable, adverse event profile.

The unsatisfactory clinical response and frequent occurrence of pain during and after irradiation renders topical ALA-based PDT an inadequate treatment option for psoriasis.

Adverse Effects

PDT can cause stinging, burning, or pain during irradiation. In most studies, there is a subset of patients that interrupt treatment or drop out of the study due to discomfort.

CONCLUSIONS

Phototherapy and photochemotherapy have a role in the treatment of localized and generalized psoriasis. Patient compliance and the ability for the patient to come to the office regularly for the treatment are factors that need to be considered. Targeted phototherapy sparing uninvolved skin is a new development that is beneficial for selected patients. The side effects of PUVA are well established. UVB, when judiciously administered, has minimal side effects. NB-UVB has become the preferred treatment modality for most patients with psoriasis.

REFERENCES

1. Krueger JG, Wolfe JT, Nabeya RT, et al. Successful ultraviolet B treatment of psoriasis is accompanied by a reversal of keratinocytes pathology and by selective depletion of intraepidermal T cells. *J Exp Med* 1995; 182(6): 2057–2068.
2. Ozawa M, Ferenczi K, Kikuchi T, et al. 312-nanometer ultraviolet B light (narrowband UVB) induces apoptosis of T cells within psoriatic lesions. *J Exp Med* 1999; 189(4): 711–718.
3. Johnson R, Staiano-Coico L, Austin L, et al. PUVA treatment selectively induces a cell cycle block and subsequent apoptosis in human lymphocytes. *Photochem Photobiol* 1996; 63(5): 566–571.
4. Bianchi B, Campolmi P, Mavilia L, et al. Monochromatic excimer light (308 nm): an immunohistochemical study of cutaneous T cells and apoptosis-related molecules in psoriasis. *J Eur Acad Dermatol Venereol* 2003; 17(4): 408–413.
5. Morita A, Werfel T, Stege H, et al. Evidence that singlet oxygen-induced human T helper cell apoptosis is the basic mechanism of ultraviolet-A radiation phototherapy. *J Exp Med* 1997; 186(10): 1763–1768.

6. Novak Z, Bonis B, Baltas E, et al. Xenon chloride ultraviolet B laser is more effective in treating psoriasis and in inducing T cell apoptosis than narrow-band ultraviolet B. *J Photochem Photobiol B* 2002; 67(1): 32–38.
7. Parrish JA, Jaenicke KF. Action spectrum for phototherapy of psoriasis. *J Invest Dermatol* 1981; 76(5): 359–362.
8. Coven TR, Burack LH, Gilleaudeau R, et al. Narrowband UV B produced superior clinical and histopathological resolution of moderate to severe psoriasis in patients compared with broadband UV-B. *Arch Dermatol* 1997; 133(12): 1514–1522.
9. Yones SS, Palmer RA, Garibaldinos TT, et al. Randomized double-blind trial of the treatment of chronic plaque psoriasis: efficacy of psoralen-UV-A therapy vs narrowband UV-B therapy. *Arch Dermatol* 2006; 142(7): 836–842.
10. Gordon PM, Diffey BL, Matthews JNS, et al. A randomized comparison of narrow-band TL-01 phototherapy and PUVA chemotherapy for psoriasis. *J Am Acad Dermatol* 1999; 41: 728–732.
11. Tanew A, Radakovic-Fijan S, Schemper M, et al. Narrowband UV-B phototherapy vs. photochemotherapy in the treatment of chronic plaque-type psoriasis: a paired comparison study. *Arch Dermatol* 1999; 135(5): 519–524.
12. Markham T, Rogers S, Collins P. Narrowband UV-B (TL-01) phototherapy vs 8-methoxypsoralen psoralen-UV-A for the treatment of chronic plaque psoriasis. *Arch Dermatol* 2003; 139(3): 325–328.
13. Salem SA, Barakat MA, Morcos CM. Bath psoralen + ultraviolet A photochemotherapy vs. narrow band-ultraviolet B in psoriasis: a comparison of clinical outcome and effect on circulating T-helper and T-suppressor/cytotoxic cells. *Photodermatol Photoimmunol Photomed* 2010; 25(5): 235–242.
14. Sivanesan SP, Gattu S, Hong J, et al. Randomized, double-blind, placebo-controlled evaluation of the efficacy of oral psoralen plus ultraviolet A for the treatment of plaque-type psoriasis using the Psoriasis Area Severity Index score (improvement of 75% or greater) at 12 weeks. *J Am Acad Dermatol* 2009; 61(5): 793–798.
15. Dawe RS, Cameron H, Yule S, et al. A randomized controlled trial of narrowband ultraviolet B vs. bath-psoralen plus ultraviolet A photochemotherapy for psoriasis. *Br J Dermatol* 2003; 148(6): 1194–1204.
16. Kirke SM, Lowder S, Lloyd JJ, et al. A randomized comparison of selective broadband UVB and narrowband UVB in the treatment of psoriasis. *J Invest Dermatol* 2007; 127: 1641–1646.
17. Storbeck K, Holzle E, Schurer N, et al. Narrow-band UVB (311 nm) versus conventional broad band UVB with and without dithranol in phototherapy for psoriasis. *J Am Acad Dermatol* 1993; 28(2, pt 1): 227–231.
18. Behrens S, Grundmann-Kollmann M, Schiener R, et al. Combination phototherapy of psoriasis with narrow-band UVB irradiation and topical tazarotene gel. *J Am Acad Dermatol* 2000; 42(3): 493–495.
19. Koo JY, Lowe NJ, Lew-Kaya DA, et al. Tazarotene plus UVB phototherapy in the treatment of psoriasis. *J Am Acad Dermatol* 2000; 43(5 Pt 1): 821–828.
20. Bourke JF, Iqbal SJ, Hutchinson PE. The effects of UVB plus calcipotriol on systemic calcium homeostasis in patients with chronic plaque psoriasis. *Clin Exp Dermatol* 1997; 22(6): 259–261.
21. Rim JH, Choe YB, Youn JI. Positive effect of using calcipotriol ointment with narrow-band ultraviolet B phototherapy in psoriatic patients. *Photodermatol Photoimmunol Photomed* 2002; 18(3): 131–134.
22. Woo WK, McKenna KE. Combination TL01 ultraviolet B phototherapy and topical calcipotriol for psoriasis: a prospective randomized placebo-controlled clinical trial. *Br J Dermatol* 2003; 149(1): 146–150.
23. Brands S, Brakman M, Bos JD, et al. No additional effect of calcipotriol ointment on low-dose narrow-band UVB phototherapy in psoriasis. *J Am Acad Dermatol* 1999; 41(6): 991–995.
24. Meola T, Jr, Soter NA, Lim HW. Are topical corticosteroids useful adjunctive therapy for the treatment of psoriasis with ultraviolet radiation? *Arch Dermatol* 1991; 127(11): 1708–1713.
25. Green C, Lakshmipathi T, Johnson BE, et al. A comparison of the efficacy and relapse rates of narrowband UVB (TL-01) monotherapy vs. etretinate (re-TL-01) vs. etretinate-PUVA (re-PUVA) in the treatment of psoriasis patients. *Br J Dermatol* 1992; 127(1): 5–9.
26. Spuls PI, Rozenblit M, Lebwohl M. Retrospective study of the efficacy of narrowband UVB and acitretin. *J Dermatolog Treat* 2003; 14(Suppl 2): 17–20.

27. Mortazavi H, Khezri S, Hosseini H, Khezri F, Vasign M. A single-blind randomized clinical study: the efficacy of narrow band ultraviolet B in the treatment of psoriasis vulgaris. *Photodermatol Photoimmunol Photomed* 2011; 27(3): 157–161.
28. Busse K, Koo J. Introducing the delayed retinoid burn: a case report and discussion of this potential risk of retinoid-phototherapy combination management. *J Am Acad Dermatol* 2011; 64(5): 1011–1012.
29. Asawanonda P, Nateetongrungsak Y. Methotrexate plus narrowband UVB phototherapy versus narrowband UVB phototherapy alone in the treatment of plaque-type psoriasis: a randomized, placebo-controlled study. *J Am Acad Dermatol* 2006; 54: 1013–1018.
30. Mahajan R, Kaur I, Kanwar AJ. Methotrexate/narrowband UVB phototherapy combination vs. narrowband UVB phototherapy in the treatment of chronic plaque-type psoriasis – a randomized single-blinded placebo-controlled study. *J Eur Acad Dermatol Venereol* 2010; 24(5): 595–600.
31. Paul BS, Momtaz K, Stern RS, et al. Combined methotrexate-ultraviolet B therapy in the treatment of psoriasis. *J Am Acad Dermatol* 1982; 7(6): 758–762.
32. Stern RS, Laird N. The carcinogenic risk of treatments for severe psoriasis. Photochemotherapy Follow-up Study. *Cancer* 1994; 73(11): 2759–2764.
33. Canning MT, Nay SL, Pena AV, et al. Immunosuppressive drugs that inhibit calcineurin decrease DNA repair and reduce apoptosis after UVB exposure in human keratinocytes. *J Invest Dermatol* 2005; 124: A19.
34. Gambichler T, Tigges C, Scola N, et al. Etanercept plus narrowband ultraviolet B phototherapy of psoriasis is more effective than etanercept monotherapy at 6 weeks. *Br J Dermatol* 2011; 164(6): 1383–1386.
35. Wolf P, Hofer A, Wolfgang W, et al. 311 nm ultraviolet B-accelerated response of psoriatic lesions in adalimumab-treated patients. *Photoderm Photoimmunol Photomed* 2011; 27(4): 186–189.
36. Wolf P, Weger W, Legat FJ, et al. Treatment with 311-m, ultraviolet B enhances response of psoriatic lesions in ustekinumab-treated patients: a randomized intraindividual trial. *Br K Dermatol* 2012; 166(1): 147–153.
37. Breuer-McHam J, Simpson E, Dougherty I, et al. Activation of HIV in human skin by ultraviolet B radiation and its inhibition by NFkappaB blocking agents. *Photochem Photobiol* 2001; 74(6): 805–810.
38. Akaraphanth R, Lim HW. HIV, UV and immunosuppression. *Photodermatol Photoimmunol Photomed* 1999; 15(1): 28–31.
39. Oh C, Hennessy A, Ha T, et al. The time course of photoadaptation and pigmentation studied using a novel method to distinguish pigmentation from erythema. *J Invest Dermatol* 2004; 123: 965–972.
40. Palmer RA, Aquilina S, Milligan PJ, et al. Photoadaptation during narrowband ultraviolet-B therapy is independent of skin type: a study of 352 patients. *J Invest Dermatol* 2006; 126: 1256–1263.
41. Dawe RS, Cameron H, Yule S, et al. A randomized comparison of methods of selecting narrowband UV-B starting dose to treat chronic psoriasis. *Arch Dermatol* 2011; 147(2): 168–174.
42. Akaraphanth R, Kittipavara Y, Voravutinon N, Wachiratarapadorn U, Gritiyarangsan P. Efficacy of a far erythemogenic dose of narrow-band ultraviolet B phototherapy in chronic plaque-type psoriasis. *J Dermatol* 2010; 39(2): 140–145.
43. Cameron H, Dawe RS, Yule S, et al. A randomized, observer-blinded trial of twice vs. three times weekly narrowband ultraviolet B phototherapy for chronic plaque psoriasis. *Br J Dermatol* 2002; 147(5): 973–978.
44. Lee E, Koo J, Berger T. UVB phototherapy and skin cancer risk: a review of the literature. *Int J Dermatol* 2005; 44(5): 355–360.
45. Man I, Crombie IK, Dawe RS, et al. The photocarcinogenic risk of narrowband UVB (TL-01) phototherapy: early follow-up data. *Br J Dermatol* 2005; 152(5): 755–757.
46. Young AR. Carcinogenicity of UVB phototherapy assessed. *Lancet* 1995; 345(8962): 1431–1432.
47. Kunisada M, Kumimoto H, Ishizaki K, et al. Narrow-band UVB induces more carcinogenic skin tumors than broad-band UVB through the formation of cyclobutane pyrimidine dimer. *J Invest Dermatol* 2007; 127(12): 2865–2871.
48. Weischer M, Blum A, Eberhard F, et al. No evidence for increased skin cancer risk in psoriasis patients treated with broadband or narrowband UVB phototherapy: a first retrospective study. *Acta Derm Venereol* 2004; 84(5): 370–374.
49. Hearn RMR, Kerr AC, Rahim KF, Ferguson J, Dawe RS. Incidence of skin cancers in 3867 patients treated with narrow-band ultraviolet B phototherapy. *Br J Dermatol* 2008; 159: 931–935.

50. Stern RS. Psoralen and ultraviolet A light therapy for psoriasis. *N Engl J Med* 2007; 357: 682–690.
51. Levins PC, Gange W, Momtaz TK, Parrish J, Fitzpatrick T. A new liquid formulation of 8-methoxypsoralen: bioactivity and effect of diet. *J Invest Derm* 1984; 82: 185–187.
52. Griffiths CE, Clark CM, Chalmers RJ, et al. A systematic review of treatments for severe psoriasis. *Health Technol Assess* 2000; 4: 1–125.
53. Koo J, Lebwohl M. Duration of remission of psoriasis therapies. *J Am Acad Dermatol* 1999, 41(1). 51–59.
54. Melski JW, Tanenbaum L, Parrish JA, et al. Oral methoxsalen photochemotherapy for the treatment of psoriasis: a cooperative clinical trial. *J Invest Dermatol* 1977; 68(6): 328–335.
55. Henseler T, Hoenigsmann H, Wolff K, et al. Oral 8-methoxypsoralen photochemotherapy of psoriasis: The European PUVA study: a cooperative study among 18 European centers. *Lancet* 1981; 317(8225): 853–857.
56. Torras H, Aliaga A, Lopez-Estebaranz JL, et al. A combination therapy of calcipotriol cream and PUVA reduces the UVA dose and improves the response of psoriasis vulgaris. *J Dermatolog Treat* 2004; 15(2): 98–103.
57. Behrens S, Grundmann-Kollmann M, Peter RU, et al. Combination treatment of psoriasis with photochemotherapy and tazarotene gel, a receptor-selective topical retinoid. *Br J Dermatol* 1999; 141(1): 177.
58. Meola T, Soter NA, Lim HW. Are topical corticosteroids useful adjunctive therapy for the treatment of psoriasis with ultraviolet radiation? A review of the literature. *Arch Dermatol* 1991; 127(11): 1708–1713.
59. Tahir R, Mujtaba G. Comparison of psoralen ultraviolet A (PUVA) photochemotherapy plus topical corticosteroids with PUVA plus bland emollients in the treatment of psoriasis. *J Ayub Med Coll Abbottabad* 2005; 17(1): 34–36.
60. Tanew A, Guggenbichler A, Honigsmann H, et al. Photochemotherapy for severe psoriasis without or in combination with acitretin: a randomized, double-blind comparison study. *J Am Acad Dermatol* 1991; 25(4): 682–684.
61. Lauharanta J, Geiger JM. A double-blind comparison of acitretin and etretinate in combination with bath PUVA in the treatment of extensive psoriasis. *Br J Dermatol* 1989; 121(1): 107–112.
62. Grundmann-Kollmann M, Ludwig R, Zollner TM, et al. Narrowband UVB and cream psoralen-UVA combination therapy for plaque-type psoriasis. *J Am Acad Dermatol* 2004; 50(5): 734–739.
63. Stern RS, Bagheri S, Nichols K. PUVA Follow-up Study. The persistent risk of genital tumors among men treated with psoralen plus ultraviolet A (PUVA) for psoriasis. *J Am Acad Dermatol* 2002; 47(1): 33–39.
64. Anonymous. British Photodermatology Group guidelines for PUVA. *Br J Dermatol* 1994; 130(2): 246–255.
65. Legat FJ, Hofer A, Quehenberger F, et al. Reduction of treatment frequency and UVA dose does not substantially compromise the antipsoriatic effect of oral psoralen-UVA. *J Am Acad Dermatol* 2004; 51(5): 746–754.
66. Nijsten TE, Stern RS. The increased risk of skin cancer is persistent after discontinuation of psoralen + ultraviolet A: a cohort study. *J Invest Dermatol* 2003; 121(2): 252–258.
67. Stern RS. Actinic degeneration and pigmentary change in association with psoralen and UVA treatment: a 20-year prospective study. *J Am Acad Dermatol* 2003; 48(1): 61–67.
68. Lim JL, Stern RS. High levels of ultraviolet B exposure increase the risk of non-melanoma skin cancer in psoralen and ultraviolet A-treated patients. *J Invest Dermatol* 2005; 124(3): 505–513.
69. Lindelof B, Sigurgeirsson B, Tegner E, et al. PUVA and cancer risk: the Swedish follow-up study. *Br J Dermatol* 1999; 141(1): 108–112.
70. Murase JE, Lee EE, Koo J. Effect of ethnicity on the risk of developing non-melanoma skin cancer following long-term PUVA therapy. *Online Int J Dermatol* 2004; 44(12): 1016–1021.
71. Nijsten TE, Stern RS. Oral retinoid use reduces cutaneous squamous cell carcinoma risk in patients with psoriasis treated with psoralen-UVA: a nested cohort study. *J Am Acad Dermatol* 2003; 49(4): 644–650.
72. Silva FS, Oliveira H, Moreiras A, et al. Cytotoxic and genotoxic effects of acitretin, alone or in combination with psoralen-ultraviolet A or narrow-band ultraviolet B-therapy in psoriatic patients. *Mutat Res* 2013; 753(1): 42–47.
73. Stern RS, PUVA Follow-up Study. The risk of melanoma in association with long-term exposure to PUVA. *J Am Acad Dermatol* 2001; 44(5): 755–761.

74. Malanos D, Stern RS. Psoralen plus ultraviolet A does not increase the risk of cataracts: a 25-year prospective study. *J Am Acad Dermatol* 2007; 57(2): 231–237.
75. Bonis B, Kemeny L, Dobozy A, et al. 308 nm UVB excimer laser for psoriasis. *Lancet* 1997; 350(9090): 1522.
76. Asawanonda P, Anderson RR, Chang Y, et al. 308-nm excimer laser for the treatment of psoriasis: a dose-response study. *Arch Dermatol* 2000; 136(5): 619–624.
77. Gerber W, Arheilger B, Ha TA, et al. Ultraviolet B 308-nm excimer laser treatment of psoriasis: a new phototherapeutic approach. *Br J Dermatol* 2003; 149(6): 1250–1258.
78. Feldman SR, Mellen BG, Housman TS, et al. Efficacy of the 308-nm excimer laser for the treatment of psoriasis: results of a multicenter study. *J Am Acad Dermatol* 2002; 46: 900–906.
79. Rodewald EJ, Housman TS, Mellen BG, et al. Follow-up survey of 308-nm laser treatment of psoriasis. *Lasers Surg Med* 2002; 31(3): 202–206.
80. Hadi SM, Al-Wuran H, deSa Earp AP, Hadi AS, Lebwohl M. The use of 308-nm excimer laser for the treatment of psoriasis. *Photomed Laser Surg* 2010; 28(5): 693–695.
81. Trehan M, Taylor CR. High-dose 308-nm excimer laser for the treatment of psoriasis. *J Am Acad Dermatol* 2002; 46(5): 732–737.
82. Kagen M, Cao LY, Oyetakin-White P, Tacastacas JD. Single administration of lesion-limited dose (TURBO) ultraviolet B using eximer laser: clinical clearing in association with apoptosis of epidermal and dermal T cell subsets in psoriasis. *Photodermatol Photoimmunol Photomed* 2012; 28(6): 293–298.
83. Pahlajani N, Katz BJ, Lozano AM, et al. Comparison of the efficacy and safety of the 308 nm excimer laser for the treatment of localized psoriasis in adults and in children: a pilot study. *Pediatr Dermatol* 2005; 22(2): 161–165.
84. Tanghetti E, Gillis PR. Photometric and clinical assessment of localized UVB phototherapy systems for the high-dosage treatment of stable plaque psoriasis. *J Cosmet Laser Ther* 2003; 5(2): 101–106.
85. Kollner K, Wimmershoff MB, Hintz C, et al. Comparison of the 308-nm excimer laser and a 308-nm excimer lamp with 311-nm narrowband ultraviolet B in the treatment of psoriasis. *Br J Dermatol* 2005; 152(4): 750–754.
86. Lapidoth M, Adatto M, David M. Targeted UVB phototherapy for psoriasis: a preliminary study. *Clin Exp Dermatol* 2007; 32(6): 642–645.
87. Kaur M, Oliver B, Hu J, Feldman SR. Nonlaser UVB-targeted phototherapy treatment of psoriasis. *Cutis* 2006; 78(3): 200–203.
88. Amornpinyokeit N, Asawanonda P. 8-Methoxypsoralen cream plus targeted narrowband ultraviolet B for psoriasis. *Photodermatol Photoimmunol Photomed* 2006; 22(6): 285–289.
89. Trott J, Gerber W, Hammes S, et al. The effectiveness of PUVA treatment in severe psoriasis is significantly increased by additional UV 308-nm excimer laser sessions. *Eur J Dermatol* 2008; 18(1): 55–60.
90. Dong J, He Y, Zhang W, Wang Y, Tian Y, Wang J. Clinical efficacy of flumetasone/salicylic acid ointment combined with 308-nm excimer laser for treatment of psoriasis vulgaris. *Photodermatol Photoimmunol Photomed* 2012; 28(3): 133–136.
91. Housman TS, Pearce DJ, Feldman SR. A maintenance protocol for psoriasis plaques cleared by the 308 nm excimer laser. *J Dermatolog Treat* 2004; 15(2): 94–97.
92. Kowalzick L, Suckow M, Waldmann T, et al. Mitteldosis-UV-A1 versus UV-B-Therapie bei Psoriasis. *Z Dermatol* 1999; 185: 92–94.
93. Krutmann J, Stege H, Morita A. Ultraviolet-A1 phototherapy: indications and mode of action. In: Krutmann J, Hönigsmann H, Elmets CA, Bergstresser PR, eds. *Dermatological Phototherapy and Photodiagnostic Methods*. Berlin, Germany: Springer-Verlag; 2001, pp. 261–276.
94. Mang R, Krutmann J. UVA-1 Phototherapy. *Photodermatol Photoimmunol Photomed* 2005; 21(2): 103–108.
95. Roussaki-Schulze AV, Kouskoukis C, Klimi E, et al. Calcipotriol monotherapy versus calcipotriol plus UVA1 versus calcipotriol plus narrow-band UVB in the treatment of psoriasis. *Drugs Exp Clin Res* 2005; 31(5–6): 169–174.
96. Rivard J, Janiga J, Lim HW. Tacrolimus ointment 0.1% alone and in combination with medium-dose UVA1 in the treatment of palmar or plantar psoriasis. *J Drugs Dermatol* 2006; 5(6): 505–510.
97. Sterenborg HJ, van der Leun JC. Tumorigenesis by a long wavelength UV-A source. *Photochem Photobiol* 1990; 51(3): 325–330.

98. Noborio R, Kurokawa M, Kobayashi K, Morita A. Evaluation of the clinical and immunohistological efficacy of the 585-nm pulsed dye laser in the treatment of psoriasis. *J Eur Acad Dermatol Venereol* 2009; 23(4): 420–424.
99. Hern S, Allen MH, Sousa AR, et al. Immunohistochemical evaluation of psoriatic plaques following selective photothermolysis of the superficial capillaries. *Br J Dermatol* 2001; 145(1): 45–53.
100. Hacker SM, Rasmussen JE. The effect of flash lamp-pulsed dye laser on psoriasis. *Arch Dermatol* 1992; 128: 853–855.
101. Zelickson BD, Mehregan DA, Wendelschfer-Crebb G. Clinical and histological evaluation of psoriatic plaques treated with a flashlamp pulsed dye laser. *J Am Acad Dermatol* 1996; 35: 64–68.
102. Ros AM, Garden JM, Bakus AD, et al. Psoriasis response to the pulsed dye laser. *Lasers Surg Med* 1996; 19: 331–335.
103. Taibjee SM, Cheung ST, Laube S, et al. Controlled study of excimer and pulsed dye lasers in the treatment of psoriasis. *Br J Dermatol* 2005; 153: 960–966.
104. de Leeuw J, Tank B, Bjerring PJ, et al. Concomitant treatment of psoriasis of the hands and feet with pulsed dye laser and topical calcipotriol, salicylic acid, or both: a prospective open study in 41 patients. *J Am Acad Dermatol* 2006; 54(2): 266–271.
105. Treewittayapoom C, Singvahanont P, Chanprapaph K, Haneke E. The effect of different pulse durations in the treatment of nail psoriasis with 595-nm pulsed dye laser: a randomized, double-blind, intrapatient left-to-right study. *J Am Acad Dermatol* 2012; 22(5): 807–812.
106. Kleinpenning MM, Smits T, Ewalds E, et al. Heterogeneity of fluorescence in psoriasis after application of 5-aminolaevulinic acid: an immunohistochemical study. *Br J Dermatol* 2006; 155(3): 539–545.
107. Schleyer V, Radakovic-Fijan S, Karrer S, et al. Disappointing results and low tolerability of photodynamic therapy with topical 5-aminolaevulinic acid in psoriasis. A randomized, double-blind phase I/II study. *J Eur Acad Dermatol Venereol* 2006; 20(7): 823–828.
108. Smits T, Kleinpenning MM, van Erp PE, et al. A placebo-controlled randomized study on the clinical effectiveness, immunohistochemical changes and protoporphyrin IX accumulation in fractionated 5-aminolaevulinic acid-photodynamic therapy in patients with psoriasis. *Br J Dermatol* 2006; 155(2): 429–436.
109. Fransson J, Ros AM. Clinical and immunohistochemical evaluation of psoriatic plaques treated with topical 5-aminolaevulinic acid photodynamic therapy. *Photodermatol Photoimmunol Photomed* 2005; 21(6): 326–332.
110. Radakovic-Fijan S, Blecha-Thalhammer U, Schleyer V, et al. Topical aminolaevulinic acid-based photodynamic therapy as a treatment option for psoriasis? Results of a randomized, observer-blinded study. *Br J Dermatol* 2005; 152(2): 279–283.
111. Yim YC, Lee ES, Chung PS, et al. Recalcitrant palmoplantar pustular psoriasis successfully treated with topical 5-aminolaevulinic acid photodynamic therapy. *Clin Exp Dermatol* 2005; 30(6): 723–724.
112. Kim JY, Kang HY, Lee ES, et al. Topical 5-aminolaevulinic acid photodynamic therapy for intractable palmoplantar psoriasis. *J Dermatol* 2007; 34(1): 37–40.

Chapter 12

Combination Therapy

Maya G. Debbaneh and Alice B. Gottlieb

THE RATIONALE FOR COMBINATION THERAPY

Even in mild cases of psoriasis, therapy with a single topical agent often fails to provide patients with adequate disease control for a large portion of patients. According to a study using data from the National Ambulatory Medical Survey from 1990 to 2010, almost half of psoriasis patients surveyed were taking two or more medications for treatment of psoriasis [1]. Topical agents can be used in combination with other topical medications, systemic therapies, and phototherapy. Different strategies for combining therapies include simultaneous use, sequential therapy, and rotational therapy. The treatment of mild to moderate psoriasis may warrant this approach for refractory disease, acute flares, poor quality of life, or an upcoming major life event for which total clearance is desired. Combination therapy may be most useful in treating patients who have failed monotherapy, who are taking a medication that has dose-related toxicity, or who require tapering from a single therapeutic agent [2]. This approach frequently involves using smaller doses of each agent for a limited period, with the more potent agent discontinued as clinical improvement allows. Just as there is no single topical agent that can be used to treat all patients with psoriasis, flexibility with combinational therapeutics is also necessary to achieve disease control. Guidelines on when to consider combination therapy can be found in Table 12.1.

PHOTOTHERAPY COMBINATIONS

Many phototherapy combinations exist, including therapy with ultraviolet B light (UVB) and Oxsoralen plus ultraviolet A light (PUVA), as well as numerous combinations of ultraviolet phototherapy and topical and systemic medications.

UVB and PUVA

A study by Momtaz and Parrish [3] found that the simultaneous administration of UVB and PUVA in patients with psoriasis led to more rapid clearing than either therapy used alone. The investigators administered UVB and PUVA to patients who had previously failed phototherapy. All 42 of the study subjects tolerated the treatments well and cleared in an average of 11.3 treatments, half the number of treatments usually required with either therapy alone. In addition, the cumulative UVB dose was decreased by 18% compared with UVB monotherapy. The mean cumulative PUVA dose was less than half of that used in monotherapy.

TABLE 12.1 Combination Therapy Guidelines

Factors in considering the switch to combination therapy	
	Monotherapy is not or no longer effective
	Cumulative and/or acute toxicity is projected to be less
	Side effects are projected to be fewer
	Improved therapeutic outcomes (e.g., time, likelihood of clearing)
	Increased possibility of tailoring therapy to individual needs
Factors in choosing a particular combination of agents	
	Severity of disease
	Patient's expectations and ease of use
	History, relative to use of agents in the combination
	Response
	Side effects
	Reported efficacy and cost

Source: Menter MA et al., *Journal of the American Academy of Dermatology*, 1996, 34(2 Pt 1), 315–321.

Narrowband UVB and Bath PUVA

In a more recent study of 12 patients, the combined use of bath PUVA and narrowband UVB (NB-UVB) cleared the psoriatic lesions with fewer total exposures as well as lower cumulative ultraviolet A (UVA) doses [4]. However, the small number of patients and lack of long-term follow-up were limitations. There is limited information of the carcinogenic potential of simultaneous PUVA and NB-UVB.

NB-UVB and Cream PUVA

It is well known that the systemic absorption of oral psoralens is associated with certain risks, including the risk of developing cutaneous malignancies after long-term or high-dose therapy [5]. To reduce these side effects, bath PUVA was developed, which has similar efficacy and fewer side effects. In a study of 30 patients with moderate to severe plaque psoriasis, Grundmann-Kollman et al. [6] examined the use of cream PUVA, a newer and less burdensome and costly modality compared with bath PUVA, in combination with NB-UVB. In the study, 8-methoxypsoralen in Dorithin® cream (25% oil-in-water emulsion, Astra Medica, Vienna, Austria) at a concentration of 0.001% was applied four times a week in an even layer for 30 minutes on psoriatic lesions. After this period, the remaining cream was removed and followed by UVA administration after 30 minutes. Although both therapies induced clearance in all patients within five to seven weeks, combination therapy induced complete clearance of lesions in all patients within three to four weeks. In addition, the cumulative UV doses were greatly reduced in the combination regimens versus either therapy alone. The study strongly suggests that cream PUVA in conjunction with NB-UVB would be useful in psoriasis, especially for stubborn lesions.

Not all studies demonstrated benefits of dual UVB and PUVA therapy. A study involving 19 patients in which combination PUVA and UVB was compared with PUVA monotherapy did not show a difference in the mean number of treatments, the mean UVA dose at clearing, or the mean cumulative UVA dose [7].

UV PHOTOTHERAPY AND TOPICAL MEDICATIONS

UVB and Topical Vitamin D

Studies testing combination therapy with UVB and topical vitamin D analogs, such as calcipotriol and calcipotriene (Dovonex), generally show more effective clearance with decreased cumulative UVB exposure [8–14].

A study of 20 patients using calcipotriol in combination with UVB phototherapy suggests that combination therapy may be superior to calcipotriol monotherapy. Although there were too few patients to show statistical significance. 39% of patients in the combination group showed clearance after 8 weeks as compared to 17% in the monotherapy group [9].

In a bilateral comparison study of 12 patients, calcipotriol twice daily combined with NB-UVB five times per week significantly reduced Psoriasis Area Severity Index (PASI) scores by almost twice as much as calcipotriol monotherapy after two weeks of treatment (68% vs. 36%) [10].

Molin [11] conducted a large multicenter trial that examined 101 patients treated with both UVB and calcipotriol or calcipotriol alone over the course of eight weeks. By the end of the study, the combined therapy group had an 82% mean reduction in the PASI score versus 70% in the calcipotriol monotherapy group which was statistically significant. During study follow-up, those patients who had received combination calcipotriol and UVB had a longer duration of therapeutic effect.

Another study performed by Hecker and Lebwohl [8] examined a total of 20 patients with symmetric plaque-type psoriasis. Patients were treated with a combination of calcipotriene ointment and UVB on one side of the body and with UVB and mineral oil on the other side of the body. Of the 20 patients, 11 (55%) showed a greater decrease in severity of their psoriasis with combined therapy versus UVB with mineral oil. These differences were found to be statistically significant as early as the first week. Another study by Ramsay and colleagues [12] examining twice weekly UVB plus calcipotriene cream versus three times a week UVB plus placebo cream found that efficacy was generally comparable. However, patients with combination therapy required fewer exposures and cumulative UVB therapy to achieve total clearance than those patients receiving UVB alone.

Calcitriol (vertical), another vitamin D derivative, may also have increased efficacy when used in combination with broadband (BB)-UVB phototherapy. In one study, there was a 65% improvement in PASI score in patients using calcitriol twice daily with phototherapy versus 43% improvement in patients on UVB phototherapy plus placebo ($p = .0014$). As with other studies, there was a decrease in total UVB exposure in the combination group [13].

Woo and McKenna [14] aimed to determine whether the combination of NB-UVB and topical calcipotriol produced the same UVB-sparing effects that were seen in previous studies with BB-UVB. Fifty patients with psoriasis were randomized into two groups: one group received NB-UVB with calcipotriol and the other group received NB-UVB and placebo topical emollient. The mean cumulative UVB dose for the NB-UVB-calcipotriol group was significantly lower than that of the NB-UVB group, confirming that NB-UVB with topical calcipotriol cream has a UVB-sparing effect.

In summary, topical vitamin D analogs combined with UVB phototherapy may decrease the cumulative amount of UV light needed for treatment and are usually well tolerated [8–14].

UVA and Topical Vitamin D

Topical vitamin D derivatives are also useful when applied in combination with PUVA. The first study exploring calcipotriol with PUVA phototherapy involved 103 patients. The patients were randomized to receive twice-daily calcipotriol or placebo in combination with PUVA for 10 weeks. At the end of the study, there was a mean reduction in PASI scores of 91.4% for patients treated with calcipotriol and PUVA and 75.7% for patients treated with PUVA and placebo. In addition, the cumulative UVA dose for the combination group was lower compared with the PUVA and placebo group [15]. A second study using the left–right body comparison method examined 11 patients with plaque psoriasis receiving calcipotriene with PUVA versus PUVA alone. The study showed that patients with plaques treated with calcipotriene needed fewer treatments as well as lower cumulative doses of UVA to clear their lesions [16].

In a randomized, double-blind comparative study (n = 120) comparing the use of calcipotriol plus PUVA versus PUVA plus placebo over a period of 12 weeks, 69% of the patients in the combination group had a >90% improvement in PASI scores compared with 36.4% in the PUVA plus placebo group. Mean PASI scores were significantly lower ($p < .01$) in the combination group compared with the PUVA plus placebo group (2.65 and 7.03, respectively) [17].

As demonstrated, faster clearing is observed with the simultaneous use of PUVA light therapy along with topical vitamin D derivatives, because fewer overall PUVA treatments are required.

Recommendations regarding UVB and Topical Vitamin D

In 1997, Lebwohl and colleagues [18] studied the interactions between calcipotriene and ultraviolet light. The minimal erythema dose (MED) was determined for UVB, and immediate pigment darkening was measured for UVA. Calcipotriene was applied to a small patch of skin before UVB, PUVA, UVA, or no phototherapy. The study found that the observed MED for UVB and immediate pigment darkening for UVA were not affected by calcipotriene. In contrast, the thick application of calcipotriene resulted in an increased MED with UVA phototherapy. UVA phototherapy also resulted in a significant decrease in the concentration of calcipotriene present in the ointment after therapy, as tested by high-performance liquid chromatography. Therefore, when using calcipotriene/calcipotriol with phototherapy, it should be applied after UVA light administration. In addition, calcipotriene should be applied more than two hours before UVB exposure to prevent a burning sensation in sensitive patients [19].

UVB and Tazarotene

Tazarotene (Tazorac) is a topical retinoid that mediates cell differentiation and proliferation [20]. Studies examining the use of tazarotene and light therapy suggest improved efficacy and safety when combining these therapies. Behrens et al. [20] performed a whole-body right–left comparison of NB-UVB plus tazarotene compared with NB-UVB alone in 10 patients with plaque psoriasis. After two weeks, both treatments markedly reduced PASI scores, and after four weeks, the median PASI reduction with combination therapy was 64% versus 48% with NB-UVB alone ($p < 0.05$).

A study by Koo and colleagues [21] examined whether the addition of topical tazarotene to BB-UVB phototherapy improved efficacy without causing adverse events such as photosensitivity. A randomized, investigator-blinded study of 40 patients evaluated the outcomes of subjects treated with UVB alone or UVB in addition to 0.1% tazarotene gel applied three times per week. Plaques treated with tazarotene and UVB achieved 75% improvement or better in a median of 28 days earlier than did lesions treated with UVB monotherapy ($p < 0.01$). Cumulative UVB dose was significantly lower in patients using combination therapy with tazarotene.

Tazarotene and PUVA

Behrens and colleagues [22] evaluated the efficacy of tazarotene in combination with PUVA bath therapy in a total of 12 patients with plaque psoriasis. This study was a left–right comparison, with plaques on one-half of the body treated either with tazarotene or placebo once daily, as well as both sides of the body treated with PUVA bath therapy four times a week. After three weeks, mean PASI reduction was significantly greater in the combination therapy group (76% vs. 58% in PUVA monotherapy).

Concerns regarding the Use of Tazarotene and Phototherapy

The most common side effects of tazarotene include local pruritus, erythema, and burning. These effects are generally well tolerated [23]. As the studies exemplify, combination therapy with tazarotene and phototherapy is beneficial, allowing for improved efficacy and fewer cumulative phototherapy doses, but it should be used with caution. Applying tazarotene three times a week for two weeks does cause thinning of the stratum corneum, permitting patients to burn more readily. Doses of UVB should be reduced approximately one-third when tazarotene is added in the middle of a course of phototherapy [24]. It has also been recommended to initiate PUVA therapy at slightly lower doses than usual [25]. In addition, tazarotene is classified as pregnancy category X and should be avoided in women of child-bearing age [23].

UVB and Tar/Anthralin

The Goeckerman regimen involves the use of topical crude coal tar under occlusion combined with daily UVB phototherapy. A variant known as Ingram therapy uses anthralin instead of crude coal tar. Although effective, these therapies are time-consuming and messy. Furthermore, they are usually administered in a supervised medical setting, which can be expensive.

There are some studies that use modified variants of these methods to determine whether similar effectiveness is possible with a less demanding schedule. A bilateral comparison study by Lebwohl and colleagues compared combination therapy with anthralin and UVB phototherapy to UVB monotherapy. Two of 11 patients had a more rapid response on the side treated with combination therapy [26]. In another study, 4 of 15 patients had improved clearance on the side treated with combination anthralin plus UVB (vs. UVB monotherapy) [27].

Other variations of the Goeckerman and Ingram methods have shown promise in reducing treatment time and increasing efficacy. Swinehart and colleagues [28] used high-pressure, high-output metal halide UVA–UVB lamps, along with short-contact tar and more potent short-contact anthralin to examine whether time of therapy could be reduced while maintaining effectiveness. At the end of the study, there was a mean clearance of 89%, with about 75% of these patients maintaining clearance for six months without the need for further therapy. Compared with the more traditional methods, this technique required fewer hours in contact with the medications, as well as less cost, time, and UV exposure. When anthralin was compared to calcitriol, a vitamin D derivative, along with UVB phototherapy, no difference in effectiveness was found, although patients did feel that calcitriol was easier to use and caused less irritation [29].

Lee and Koo [30] published the results of 25 patients with severe psoriasis who received a modern modified "ultra" Goeckerman regimen in which various low-risk adjunctive therapies such as anthralin, acitretin, bath PUVA, or calcipotriene/tazarotene were added to improve response in recalcitrant cases. After eight weeks of treatment, 95% achieved PASI-75, and at 12 weeks, 100% achieved PASI-75.

In a three-month study of 12 patients, coal tar combined with NB-UVB was more effective than NB-UVB monotherapy ($p < .05$) as measured by physicians' global assessment (PGA) [31]. As in other studies, greater efficacy of combination therapy is associated with decreased total doses of ultraviolet light when UVB is combined with coal tar [32].

In summary, coal tar combined with UVB phototherapy is well tolerated and can help patients achieve clearance at lower cumulative doses of phototherapy. However, many patients are not able to use coal tar or anthralin preparations due to the inconvenience or messiness associated with these agents.

PUVA and Tar/Anthralin

Several years ago, a study by Morison and colleagues [33] examined combination therapy of PUVA with anthralin. Although they found that the combination did clear the subjects' lesions more readily than PUVA alone, the study participants largely disliked the therapy mainly due to staining.

UVB and Topical Steroids

Dover and colleagues [34] examined the effect of potent topical steroid cream used together with UVB phototherapy on clearing of psoriatic lesions and duration of remission. A randomized, double-blind, placebo-controlled study was performed with patients being treated with UVB three times a week, with approximately half of the patients applying topical corticosteroids twice daily and the other half applying placebo. The study found that there was no statistical significance between clearance rates. In addition, there were no statistically significant differences in the number of treatments or dosages of UVB required to achieve clearance. This study is in agreement with other earlier studies that found no advantageous effects of combining UVB and topical steroids.

PUVA and Topical Steroids

Findings of studies on the use of topical steroids in combination with PUVA, in contrast to studies with UVB, have indicated some benefit. In a comparison of studies by Meola et al. [35], five studies examining PUVA alone versus PUVA with topical steroids showed more rapid rates of clearing and fewer doses of UVA when using combination therapy. One of the studies in the review did show a higher relapse rate with corticosteroid use [33].

COMBINING SYSTEMIC AGENTS WITH TOPICAL THERAPIES IN THE TREATMENT OF MILD TO MODERATE PSORIASIS

Although systemic therapies are often reserved for patients with moderate to severe psoriasis, there are several capacities in which these potent medications may play a role in the management of mild to moderate disease. According to the American Academy of Dermatology Consensus Statement on psoriasis therapies, systemic therapy may be used in the treatment of mild to moderate psoriasis when the disease is unresponsive to topical agents or if there is lifestyle and/or employment disturbance [36]. Patients meeting these qualifications may still demonstrate a limited affected body surface area, because treatment decisions ultimately involve the combined consideration of lesion severity and the patient's quality of life and comorbidities, as well as the cost, risks, and benefits of treatment relative to the patient's desires [37]. Cases initially perceived as mild may have a substantial impact on a patient's quality of life and may therefore merit the consideration of a more vigorous treatment plan than originally envisioned by the physician [38].

Patients with mild to moderate disease who have not responded to topical monotherapy are typically introduced to a combination of topical agents or phototherapy. Systemic therapy is considered if a patient's lesions continue to resist these therapeutic measures or if an adverse reaction to phototherapy occurs. In some cases, systemic therapy may be indicated earlier due to widespread disease, involvement of areas severely impacting quality of life, frequent relapse, or joint involvement [36,39]. Furthermore, patients with moderate disease may request systemic therapy in an effort to avoid the excessive usage of topical agents or to ease the administration of therapy. For these reasons, as well as to increase compliance, there is currently a demand to develop systemic medications for the treatment of moderate disease [39].

The systemic medications traditionally used in the treatment of psoriasis are methotrexate, cyclosporine, and acitretin. Novel developments in the immunopathogenesis of psoriasis have led to the introduction of biologic therapies such as etanercept, infliximab, adalimumab, and ustekinumab. Less conventional systemic treatments that are not approved by the Food and Drug Administration (FDA) for the treatment of psoriasis include pimecrolimus, mycophenolate mofetil, hydroxyurea, and 6-thioguanine. Use of these agents may either follow or accompany topical therapy. An approach to treatment is generally governed by the physical characteristics of lesions, the locations affected, relapse frequency, and convenience of treatment modality [40]. Although many systemic medications are oral, the newer biologics are dispensed by subcutaneous injection or intravenous infusion. Using topical therapy in combination with systemic agents often allows for a reduction in the amount of systemic therapy administered as well as a decrease in associated toxicities.

Combining topical and systemic therapies is commonplace in the treatment of psoriasis. In a retrospective analysis of 650 patients treated for psoriasis in an academic setting, more than one-third of the patients receiving systemic therapy were simultaneously treated with a class I steroid [41]. Although not used as first-line agents in the treatment of mild to moderate disease, systemic therapy plays an integral role in general psoriatic therapy and therefore is important to all physicians treating patients with this disease. This chapter does not focus on the treatment of moderate to severe psoriasis, discussion of systemic therapy is limited to the following questions:

- What systemic therapies are available for use with topical medications?
- What are the advantages of the use of systemic therapies and what are the most effective combinations?
- How should systemic medications be used with topical treatment and what are the associated toxicities?

Not all combinations are effective and some are even associated with increased toxicity. It is important to recall that although several combination therapies may be presented here, therapy for psoriasis is designed on an individual basis.

Methotrexate

Methotrexate is among the oldest systemic medications used in the treatment of psoriasis; however, its role in treating mild to moderate disease involves only those cases that are unresponsive to topical therapy [42]. A decision to administer methotrexate to patients with mild to moderate disease should be carefully considered because of the associated immunosuppression, and possible liver or bone marrow toxicity. Phototherapy and systemic retinoids should be considered prior to starting methotrexate [43]. Combination therapy with topicals such as coal tar, anthralin, and vitamin D analogs may be helpful [43,44]. A study conducted in India demonstrated that disease could be adequately controlled with short-term methotrexate interspersed by topical coal tar, anthralin, or calcipotriene. In many patients, remission was facilitated by the application of aggressive topical therapy to residual lesions during the tapering of methotrexate [45].

In a multicenter, double-blind study ($n = 97$), the addition of calcipotriol to methotrexate decreased the dose of methotrexate needed to obtain clearance and increased the duration of remission by three months [46]. In studies where methotrexate was added to BB-UVB or PUVA, the number of phototherapy sessions and the cumulative dosage of ultraviolet light were reduced by more than half [47–52]. However, the use of methotrexate with PUVA was associated with a subacute phototoxicity reaction in some patients [48].

In summary, methotrexate serves as a cost-effective alternative to retinoids, cyclosporine, and biologics and can be used effectively in conjunction with topicals and phototherapy.

Cyclosporine

In the treatment of psoriasis, cyclosporine is usually used in patients with moderate to severe disease. In mild to moderate psoriasis, cyclosporine is only used for unique cases of refractory or particularly life-altering disease (e.g., palmoplantar disease) because of the potential of serious side effects such as nephrotoxicity and hypertension [49]. Unlike methotrexate, cyclosporine is not associated with acute bone marrow toxicity and may be a safer alternative for short-term use.

Short courses of cyclosporine monotherapy rapidly clear chronic plaque psoriasis [50]. When combined with topical agents such as anthralin, corticosteroids, and vitamin D analogs, a lower required dosage of cyclosporine may be sufficient [36,51,52]. There are two approaches to using cyclosporine in combination regimens. First, cyclosporine can be used as monotherapy to rapidly clear psoriasis at a dosage of up to 5 mg/kg/day. Topical preparations, including tar, anthralin, retinoids, or calcipotriene, can be added for use on resistant areas. The immunosuppressive nature of the drug tends to diminish cutaneous irritation caused by these agents. Alternatively, the same topical agents can be used at the onset of treatment with a low starting dose of cyclosporine, such as 2 mg/kg/day. This dose can then be titrated up to the desired therapeutic efficacy, not surpassing 5 mg/kg/day [36]. Studies using both calcipotriol and anthralin have demonstrated the increased efficacy of cyclosporine when combined with topical therapy [52].

Although cyclosporine is very effective at rapidly clearing psoriatic plaques, relapses often occur after the discontinuation of therapy. This observation led to trials investigating the use of the drug in combination with topical clobetasol propionate. The addition of clobetasol to a daily cyclosporine dose of 3 mg/kg daily cleared psoriasis in 3.5 weeks rather than in six weeks in patients treated with cyclosporine alone. However, there was no significant difference in relapse rates. These data suggest that when used in combination with clobetasol, a lower cumulative dose of cyclosporine may be used to achieve clearance [53].

Acitretin

Acitretin (Soriatane) is an oral retinoid effective in treating pustular as well as plaque-type psoriasis. Often, acitretin is used in combination agents for enhanced efficacy, such as UVB or PUVA phototherapy, topical calcipotriene, cyclosporine, or methotrexate [54]. Acitretin is the metabolite of etretinate, a molecule that is approximately 50 times more lipophilic and thus accumulates in adipose tissue and exhibits an extended half-life. Both are highly teratogenic; however, the lengthy half-life of etretinate led to its replacement by acitretin in June 1997 [55]. The ingestion of alcohol with acitretin leads to its enzymatic conversion to etretinate and subsequently to the clinically significant accumulation of the teratogenic compound. It is therefore imperative that all women treated with acitretin are educated of the risks associated with concurrent alcohol ingestion and acitretin therapy [55,56].

As with all systemic medications, the use of acitretin is most often reserved for moderate to severe disease but may still have a role in combination with other agents in mild to moderate disease. As a class, oral retinoids are not as efficacious as phototherapy or methotrexate [57]. In plaque-type psoriasis, acitretin is used in combination with topical steroids, anthralin, or phototherapy [58]. These regimens tend to decrease the dose of acitretin required for clinical improvement while maximizing efficacy and decreasing adverse effects.

Combinations of oral retinoids with PUVA, anthralin, topical steroids, and topical vitamin D derivatives have been extensively studied, although largely with etretinate [59–61]. A retinoid in combination with betamethasone valerate cream 0.1% applied twice daily was found to be more effective than either agent alone [62]. The effectiveness of acitretin for plaque-type psoriasis is markedly improved with UVA or UVB treatment [63–65].

In a double-blind comparison study, 34 patients were randomized to receive UVB phototherapy plus 50 mg/day acitretin, acitretin alone, or UVB plus placebo. Results showed that patients receiving combination therapy with acitretin and UVB had more improvement than those who received monotherapy. In addition, patients treated with UVB plus acitretin required fewer treatments and a decreased cumulative dose of UVB than those patients receiving UVB monotherapy ($p < .05$) [65]. A recent retrospective study demonstrated that using the combination of low-dose acitretin (25 mg/day) and NB-UVB, at a 50% reduction in both starting doses and increments, allowed for clearing of psoriasis in the majority of study subjects with no increase in side effects associated with either retinoid or NB-UVB therapy [66]. Benefits of using acitretin in combination with phototherapy include lower ultraviolet doses and the possible suppression of cutaneous malignancy associated with PUVA [67]. Likewise, patients treated with a retinoid and topical anthralin have maintained remission for longer than those treated with monotherapy of either agent [59]. From these studies, there is evidence that patients with mild to moderate disease may benefit from maintenance therapy with topical agents or phototherapy with an oral retinoid available intermittently to treat relapses.

REFERENCES

1. Davis SA, Feldman SR. Combination therapy for psoriasis in the United States. *Journal of Drugs in Dermatology.* 2013;12(5):546–550.
2. Menter MA, See JA, Amend WJ, et al. Proceedings of the Psoriasis Combination and Rotation Therapy Conference. Deer Valley, Utah, Oct. 7–9, 1994. *Journal of the American Academy of Dermatology.* 1996;34(2 Pt 1):315–321.
3. Momtaz K, Parrish J. Combination of psoralens and ultraviolet A and ultraviolet B in the treatment of psoriasis vulgaris: a bilateral comparison study. *Journal of the American Academy of Dermatology.* 1984;10:481–486.
4. Calzavara-Pinton P. Narrowband UVB (311 nm) phototherapy and PUVA photochemotherapy: a combination. *Journal of the American Academy of Dermatology.* 1998;38:687–690.
5. Morison WL. Systemic and topical PUVA. *Treatment of Moderate to severe Psoriasis.* 2nd ed. New York: Marcel Dekker; 2003:91–114.
6. Grundmann-Kollmann M, Ludwig R, Zollner TM, et al. Narrowband UVB and cream psoralen-UVA combination therapy for plaque-type psoriasis. *Journal of the American Academy of Dermatology.* 2004;50(5):734–739.
7. Park YK, Kim HJ, Koh YJ. Combination of photochemotherapy (PUVA) and ultraviolet B (UVB) in the treatment of psoriasis vulgaris. *The Journal of Dermatology.* 1988;15(1):68–71.

8. Hecker D, Lebwohl M. Topical calcipotriene in combination with UVB phototherapy for psoriasis. *International Journal of Dermatology.* 1997;36(4):302–303.
9. Kragballe K. Combination of topical calcipotriol (MC903) and UVB radiation for psoriasis vulgaris. *Dermatologica.* 1990;181(3):211–214.
10. Kerscher M, Volkenandt M, Plewig G, Lehmann P. Combination phototherapy of psoriasis with calcipotriol and narrow-band UVB. *Lancet.* 1993;342(8876):923.
11. Molin L. Topical calcipotriol combined with phototherapy for psoriasis. The results of two randomized trials and a review of the literature. Calcipotriol-UVB Study Group. *Dermatology.* 1999;198(4):375–381.
12. Ramsay CA, Schwartz BE, Lowson D, Papp K, Bolduc A, Gilbert M. Calcipotriol cream combined with twice weekly broad-band UVB phototherapy: a safe, effective and UVB-sparing antipsoriatric combination treatment. The Canadian Calcipotriol and UVB Study Group. *Dermatology.* 2000;200(1):17–24.
13. Ring J, Kowalzick L, Christophers E, et al. Calcitriol 3 microg g-1 ointment in combination with ultraviolet B phototherapy for the treatment of plaque psoriasis: results of a comparative study. *The British Journal of Dermatology.* 2001;144(3):495–499.
14. Woo WK, McKenna KE. Combination TL01 ultraviolet B phototherapy and topical calcipotriol for psoriasis: a prospective randomized placebo-controlled clinical trial. *The British Journal of Dermatology.* 2003;149(1):146–150.
15. Frappaz ATJ. Calcipotriol in combination with PUVA: a randomized double blind placebo study in severe psoriasis. *European Journal of Dermatology.* 1993;3:351–354.
16. Speight EL, Farr PM. Calcipotriol improves the response of psoriasis to PUVA. *The British Journal of Dermatology.* 1994;130(1):79–82.
17. Torras H, Aliaga A, Lopez-Estebaranz JL, et al. A combination therapy of calcipotriol cream and PUVA reduces the UVA dose and improves the response of psoriasis vulgaris. *The Journal of Dermatological Treatment.* 2004;15(2):98–103.
18. Lebwohl M, Hecker D, Martinez J, Sapadin A, Patel B. Interactions between calcipotriene and ultraviolet light. *Journal of the American Academy of Dermatology.* 1997;37(1):93–95.
19. Lebwohl M, Menter A, Koo J, Feldman SR. Combination therapy to treat moderate to severe psoriasis. *Journal of the American Academy of Dermatology.* 2004;50(3):416–430.
20. Behrens S, Grundmann-Kollmann M, Schiener R, Peter RU, Kerscher M. Combination phototherapy of psoriasis with narrow-band UVB irradiation and topical tazarotene gel. *Journal of the American Academy of Dermatology.* 2000;42(3):493–495.
21. Koo JY, Lowe NJ, Lew-Kaya DA, et al. Tazarotene plus UVB phototherapy in the treatment of psoriasis. *Journal of the American Academy of Dermatology.* 2000;43(5 Pt 1):821–828.
22. Behrens S, Grundmann-Kollmann M, Peter RU, Kerscher M. Combination treatment of psoriasis with photochemotherapy and tazarotene gel, a receptor-selective topical retinoid. *The British Journal of Dermatology.* 1999;141(1):177.
23. Allergan, Inc. Tazorac prescribing information. Allergan, Inc., Irvine, CA; 2011.
24. Lebwohl M, Ali S. Treatment of psoriasis. Part 1. Topical therapy and phototherapy. *Journal of the American Academy of Dermatology.* 2001;45(4):487–498; quiz 499–502.
25. Hecker D, Worsley J, Yueh G, Kuroda K, Lebwohl M. Interactions between tazarotene and ultraviolet light. *Journal of the American Academy of Dermatology.* 1999;41(6):927–930.
26. Lebwohl M, Berman B, France DS. Addition of short-contact anthralin therapy to an ultraviolet B phototherapy regimen: assessment of efficacy. *Journal of the American Academy of Dermatology.* 1985;13(5 Pt 1):780–784.
27. Boer J, Smeenk G. Effect of short-contact anthralin therapy on ultraviolet B irradiation of psoriasis. *Journal of the American Academy of Dermatology.* 1986;15(2 Pt 1):198–204.
28. Swinehart JM, Lowe NJ. UVABA therapy for psoriasis. Efficacy with shortened treatment times with the combined use of coal tar, anthralin, and metal halide ultraviolet machines. *Journal of the American Academy of Dermatology.* 1991;24(4):594–597.
29. Hofmann UB, Eggert AA, Brocker EB, Goebeler M. Calcitriol vs. dithranol in combination with narrow-band ultraviolet B (311 nm) in psoriasis. *The British Journal of Dermatology.* 2003;148(4):779–783.
30. Lee E, Koo J. Modern modified 'ultra' Goeckerman therapy: a PASI assessment of a very effective therapy for psoriasis resistant to both prebiologic and biologic therapies. *The Journal of Dermatological Treatment.* 2005;16(2):102–107.

31. Bagel J. LCD plus NB-UVB reduces time to improvement of psoriasis vs. NB-UVB alone. *Journal of Drugs in Dermatology.* 2009;8(4):351–357.
32. Menkes A, Stern RS, Arndt KA. Psoriasis treatment with suberythemogenic ultraviolet B radiation and a coal tar extract. *Journal of the American Academy of Dermatology.* 1985;12(1 Pt 1):21–25.
33. Morison WL, Parrish JA, Fitzpatrick TB. Controlled study of PUVA and adjunctive topical therapy in the management of psoriasis. *The British Journal of Dermatology.* 1978;98(2):125–132.
34. Dover JSM, McEvoy MT, Rosen CF. Are topical steroids useful in phototherapy for psoriasis? *Journal of the American Academy of Dermatology.* 1989(20):748–754.
35. Meola T, Jr., Soter NA, Lim HW. Are topical corticosteroids useful adjunctive therapy for the treatment of psoriasis with ultraviolet radiation? A review of the literature. *Archives of Dermatology.* 1991;127(11):1708–1713.
36. Menter A, Gottlieb A, Feldman SR, et al. Guidelines of care for the management of psoriasis and psoriatic arthritis: section 1. Overview of psoriasis and guidelines of care for the treatment of psoriasis with biologics. *Journal of the American Academy of Dermatology.* 2008;58(5):826–850.
37. Krueger GGF, Feldman SR, Camisa C. Two considerations for patients with psoriasis and their clinicians: what defines mild, moderate, and severe psoriasis? What constitutes a clinically significant improvement when treating psoriasis? *Journal of the American Academy of Dermatology.* 2000;43(2 pt 1):281–285.
38. Choi J, Koo JY. Quality of life issues in psoriasis. *Journal of the American Academy of Dermatology.* 2003;49(2 Suppl):S57–61.
39. Mrowietz U. Advances in systemic therapy for psoriasis. *Clinical and Experimental Dermatology.* 2001;26(4):362–367.
40. Marchetti A, Feldman SR, Kimball AB, et al. Treatments for mild to moderate recalcitrant plaque psoriasis: expected clinical and economic outcomes for first-line and second-line care. *Dermatology Online Journal.* 2005;11(1):1.
41. Pearce DJ, Spencer L, Hu J, Balkrishnan R, Fleischer AB, Jr., Feldman SR. Class I topical corticosteroid use by psoriasis patients in an academic practice. *The Journal of Dermatological Treatment.* 2004;15(4):235–238.
42. Roenigk HH, Jr., Auerbach R, Maibach HI, Weinstein GD. Methotrexate in psoriasis: revised guidelines. *Journal of the American Academy of Dermatology.* 1988;19(1 Pt 1):145–156.
43. Roenigk HH, Jr., Auerbach R, Maibach H, Weinstein G, Lebwohl M. Methotrexate in psoriasis: consensus conference. *Journal of the American Academy of Dermatology.* 1998;38(3):478–485.
44. van de Kerkhof PC, Mali JW. Methotrexate maintenance following Ingram therapy in 'difficult' psoriasis. *The British Journal of Dermatology.* 1982;106(6):623–627.
45. Kumar B, Saraswat A, Kaur I. Short-term methotrexate therapy in psoriasis: a study of 197 patients. *International Journal of Dermatology.* 2002;41(7):444–448.
46. de Jong EM, Mork NJ, Seijger MM, et al. The combination of calcipotriol and methotrexate compared with methotrexate and vehicle in psoriasis: results of a multicentre placebo-controlled randomized trial. *The British Journal of Dermatology.* 2003;148(2):318–325.
47. Paul BS, Momtaz K, Stern RS, Arndt KA, Parrish JA. Combined methotrexate—ultraviolet B therapy in the treatment of psoriasis. *Journal of the American Academy of Dermatology.* 1982;7(6):758–762.
48. Morison WL, Momtaz K, Parrish JA, Fitzpatrick TB. Combined methotrexate-PUVA therapy in the treatment of psoriasis. *Journal of the American Academy of Dermatology.* 1982;6(1):46–51.
49. Lebwohl M, Ellis C, Gottlieb A, et al. Cyclosporine consensus conference: with emphasis on the treatment of psoriasis. *Journal of the American Academy of Dermatology.* 1998;39(3):464–475.
50. Berth-Jones J, Henderson CA, Munro CS, et al. Treatment of psoriasis with intermittent short course cyclosporin (Neoral). A multicentre study. *The British Journal of Dermatology.* 1997;136(4):527–530.
51. Ellis C, Madhu B. *Cyclosporine. Treatment of Moderate to Severe Psoriasis.* New York: Marcel Dekker; 2003.
52. Grossman RM, Thivolet J, Claudy A, et al. A novel therapeutic approach to psoriasis with combination calcipotriol ointment and very low-dose cyclosporine: results of a multicenter placebo-controlled study. *Journal of the American Academy of Dermatology.* 1994;31(1):68–74.
53. Griffiths CE, Powles AV, Baker BS, Fry L, Valdimarsson H. Combination of cyclosporine A and topical corticosteroid in the treatment of psoriasis. *Transplantation Proceedings.* 1988;20(3 Suppl 4):50–52.
54. Winterfield LS, Menter A, Gordon K, Gottlieb A. Psoriasis treatment: current and emerging directed therapies. *Annals of the Rheumatic Diseases.* 2005;64(Suppl 2):ii87–90; discussion ii91–82.

55. Wiegand UW, Chou RC. Pharmacokinetics of acitretin and etretinate. *Journal of the American Academy of Dermatology.* 1998;39(2 Pt 3):S25–33.
56. Larsen FG, Jakobsen P, Knudsen J, Weismann K, Kragballe K, Nielsen-Kudsk F. Conversion of acitretin to etretinate in psoriatic patients is influenced by ethanol. *The Journal of Investigative Dermatology.* 1993;100(5):623–627.
57. Linden KG, Weinstein GD. Psoriasis: current perspectives with an emphasis on treatment. *The American Journal of Medicine.* 1999;107(6):595–605.
58. van de Kerkhof P. The effect of addition of calcipotriol ointment (50 micrograms/g) to acitretin therapy in psoriasis. *The British Journal of Dermatology.* 1998;138(1):84–89.
59. Lowe NJ, Lazarus V, Matt L. Systemic retinoid therapy for psoriasis. *Journal of the American Academy of Dermatology.* 1988;19(1 Pt 2):186–191.
60. Rim JH, Park JY, Choe YB, Youn JI. The efficacy of calcipotriol + acitretin combination therapy for psoriasis: comparison with acitretin monotherapy. *American Journal of Clinical Dermatology.* 2003;4(7):507–510.
61. van der Rhee HJ, Tijssen JG, Herrmann WA, Waterman AH, Polano MK. Combined treatment of psoriasis with a new aromatic retinoid (Tigason) in low dosage orally and triamcinolone acetonide cream topically: a double-blind trial. *The British Journal of Dermatology.* 1980;102(2):203–212.
62. Christiansen JV, Holm P, Moller R, Reymann F, Schmidt H. Etretinate (Tigason) and betamethasone valerate (Celeston valerate) in the treatment of psoriasis. A double-blind, randomized, multicenter trial. *Dermatologica.* 1982;165(3):204–207.
63. Ruzicka T, Sommerburg C, Braun-Falco O, et al. Efficiency of acitretin in combination with UV-B in the treatment of severe psoriasis. *Archives of Dermatology.* 1990;126(4):482–486.
64. Tanew A, Guggenbichler A, Honigsmann H, Geiger JM, Fritsch P. Photochemotherapy for severe psoriasis without or in combination with acitretin: a randomized, double-blind comparison study. *Journal of the American Academy of Dermatology.* 1991;25(4):682–684.
65. Lowe NJ, Prystowsky JH, Bourget T, Edelstein J, Nychay S, Armstrong R. Acitretin plus UVB therapy for psoriasis. Comparisons with placebo plus UVB and acitretin alone. *Journal of the American Academy of Dermatology.* 1991;24(4):591–594.
66. Spuls PI, Rozenblit M, Lebwohl M. Retrospective study of the efficacy of narrowband UVB and acitretin. *The Journal of Dermatological Treatment.* 2003;14(Suppl 2):17–20.
67. Lebwohl M, Drake L, Menter A, et al. Consensus conference: acitretin in combination with UVB or PUVA in the treatment of psoriasis. *Journal of the American Academy of Dermatology.* 2001;45(4):544–553.

Chapter 13

Palmoplantar Psoriasis

Daniel C. Butler and April Armstrong

INTRODUCTION

Palmoplantar psoriasis is a clinical subtype of plaque psoriasis characterized by its predomination on the palms and soles. Although the palms and soles make up only 4% of a patient's body surface area, the condition is highly resistant to treatment, and its impact can result in severe disability. Patients may experience impaired ability to perform mundane tasks such as holding a pen or driving a car, or, more significantly, essential tasks such as feeding oneself or walking. The treatment of this condition presents unique challenges, but adequate management can help mitigate severe adverse effects on quality of life.

EPIDEMIOLOGY

The prevalence of palmoplantar psoriasis is reported in variable ranges, with the most recent literature revealing that 17.4% of psoriasis patients have palm and sole involvement [1]. The disease appears evenly in males and females, with the average age of onset estimated to be between 35 and 53 years [1,2]. The clinical variants of palmoplantar disease include, most commonly, hyperkeratotic type (50%), followed by pustular (16%), combined (12%), and indeterminate (20%) [3]. Further characterization found that 34% have severe disease, as indicated by quality-of-life measures, and 50% and 18% have moderate and mild severity, respectively [3].

PRESENTATION

The correct identification of the disease can prove difficult due to the variety of dermatologic diseases that present similarly on the palms and soles. Assessment should begin with a thorough discussion of personal history, family history, smoking history, and previous medication use, all of which can help differentiate psoriasis from other diseases. One study found that 33% of palmoplantar psoriasis patients have a positive family history of psoriasis, 30% have a positive history of psoriatic arthritis, and 31% have a positive history of smoking. A personal history of psoriasis is helpful diagnostically because 86.3% of palmoplantar patients have minimal or mild psoriasis elsewhere on the body [1,2,4].

On physical examination, palmoplantar psoriasis typically presents with erythematous, scaly plaques similar to those seen with plaque psoriasis. Patients often develop thickening of the involved skin (referred to as keratoderma) that can progress to form painful fissures. Lesions are generally well demarcated and rarely extend past the flexures of the wrist. The finger pads are frequently involved, but the lateral sides of each digit are usually unaffected. The presentation is usually symmetrical, although the disease may begin unilaterally and progress to involve both sides [1]. Nail involvement, particularly in the form of pitting, is also a guiding clinical clue in that 65% of palmoplantar psoriasis patients have nail findings [2].

There are other inflammatory skin diseases affecting the palms and soles that may be difficult to distinguish from palmoplantar psoriasis on clinical examination. Often, the most challenging distinction is between palmoplantar psoriasis and eczematous processes. Both clinical presentation and histopathology may share similar features. Clinically, eczema is generally poorly demarcated compared with psoriasis and is less likely to have characteristic nail findings. In a study of the atopic hand eruptions, hand eczema most commonly presented on the fingers and was less likely on the wrists. However, demographic comparison of palm and sole psoriasis and eczema patients showed no significant differences [5]. Histopathology may be the most reliable way to definitively distinguish between the two entities. However, biopsies in the palmoplantar region may impair activities that involve hands and feet in the short term. One study with pathologists blinded to clinical presentation identified multiple parakeratotic foci, placed vertically, alternating with orthohyperkeratosis as histologic findings that favor palmoplantar psoriasis [6]. Factors of a patient's history that may help distinguish eczema include a personal or family history of atopy.

Other diagnoses to consider include contact dermatitis, pityriasis rubra pilaris, acquired keratoderma, tinea manuum, or tinea pedis, as well as, in rare cases, tertiary syphilis and cutaneous T-cell lymphoma. Dermatophytosis is particularly important to note, because it can be easily assessed in the office with a potassium hydroxide preparation. In addition, nail findings can be difficult to distinguish between psoriasis and dermatophytes, but asymmetry and response to antifungal treatment are indicative of a fungal infection.

Palmoplantar pustulosis is a condition that has warranted significant discussion regarding its relatedness with palmoplantar psoriasis [7]. Palmoplantar pustulosis is identified by crops of sterile pustules presenting on the palms and soles that erupt intermittently over a chronic disease course spanning several years [8]. Historically, both diseases were considered variants of psoriasis on a spectrum of severity, where the pustular presentation represented more severe disease. However, in 2007, after several studies noted key differences between the patient populations, the International Psoriasis Council determined that palmoplantar pustulosis is a separate condition despite certain phenotypic similarities [4].

This classification continues to be challenged by recent literature that identifies clinical and epidemiologic similarities between the populations, including age of onset, disease duration, psoriasis family history, and smoking history. Perhaps most noteworthy is that 90% of those with palmoplantar pustulosis had evidence of plaque psoriasis in the palmoplantar region [3]. Conversely, females are more often affected and nail involvement is less common in palmoplantar pustulosis patients [2,9].

PATHOPHYSIOLOGY

The mechanisms underlying the development of palmoplantar psoriasis are not completely understood. The Koebnerization phenomenon is a well-known element of psoriasis, and it has been implicated in the development of hand and foot disease [1]. The hypothesis states that microtrauma or additional pressure to the skin causes Koebnerization in the area. One observation supporting this examined a group of patients with unilateral involvement and found that all had their dominant hand as the involved palm. Contact sensitivities may also play a role, because patients with palmoplantar involvement are more likely to have positive patch test results compared with those without palmoplantar involvement [10].

On a molecular level, there is ongoing research investigating the development of psoriasis variants. One study found elevated levels of interleukin-23 in patients with palmoplantar psoriasis, but no significant difference was noted compared with levels found in lesional plaque-type skin [11]. Although this does give a brief perspective into the pathophysiology and possible therapeutic options, questions remain regarding what contributes to the development of the different psoriasis subtypes.

Treatment Dosing and Regimen Information

Avoidance and Prevention Identification and avoidance of precipitating factors can be the initial intervention. Suggesting the avoidance of harsh cleaners, chemicals, and repeated drying can eliminate some of the common culprits. Clinicians can also counsel the patient that repeated microtrauma from repetitive hand or foot use can contribute to disease development. Some helpful strategies include the use of gloves during household tasks or different shoes for activities that require extended mobility.

Another preventative strategy is the regular use of moisturizers. Moisturizers help maintain the barrier function of the skin and reduce the potential for painful fissures. Ointments are more effective moisturizers than creams, but they can be functionally and cosmetically difficult to use due to their greasy nature, especially for patients with palm and sole involvement. Regular application of somewhat suboptimal emollients may be preferred to occasional application of a superior emollient. This can include the use of creams during the day to avoid lost productivity, and the use of ideal ointment-based emollients before bed or when patients are less active with their hands and feet.

Topical Corticosteroids When selecting a topical corticosteroid for palmoplantar patients, it is helpful to recognize the localized skin differences of the palms and soles, including increased thickness of the epidermis. Thus, these areas are less susceptible to the skin thinning effects of even the strongest topical steroids. Class I (superpotent) and class II (potent) agents can be used for greater lengths of time in these regions. In addition, because the palms and soles make up <4% of the total body surface area, adrenal suppression is highly unlikely, further supporting extended use beyond the recommended four-week maximum for superpotent agents.

Even with prolonged use of the strongest topical agents, palmoplantar disease is highly unresponsive to therapy. In a large retrospective analysis, most patients reported partial improvement, defined as <50% decrease in symptomatic severity or affected area, with twice-daily application of a superpotent agent for four weeks. One-quarter of patients reported more than a 75% decrease in severity and area involved using the same regimen, and close to 20% had no clinical response to the same four-week regimen [9]. The reason for this nonresponse, defined as no change in symptomatic severity or area of involvement, is likely to be multifactorial, with one factor being that the thickness of the regional skin minimizes penetration of the medication. Topical steroids, which have beneficial effects on the dermal immune process, cannot penetrate to their maximal therapeutic depth. In addition, scaling and hyperkeratosis create additional layers, inhibiting the response. One helpful strategy used in other forms of psoriasis is the addition of keratolytics [10,12]. Although literature specific to palmoplantar psoriasis is lacking, salicylic acid has proven effective at reducing thick scaling of the scalp when a 2% preparation is applied daily for three weeks mixed with a superpotent corticosteroid [13]. This treatment can benefit palmoplantar patients by reducing hyperkeratosis and desquamation, potentially improving penetration [14]. It is recommended that combination therapy with salicylic acid only be used temporarily as initial treatment, after which the steroid can be continued as monotherapy [15]. Calcipotriol, an alternative topical agent for psoriasis, is inactivated by salicylic acid, thus their concurrent use should be avoided [15].

Another way to increase penetration is occlusion with gloves or wraps. This process can enhance penetration up to 10 times the depth, subsequently increasing the potency of the medication [16]. However, the process of occlusion can be cumbersome on top of the regular application schedule. Because it requires coverage for hours at a time, occlusion may temporarily limit the function of hands and feet. For these reasons, occlusion is best done before bed or during hours of limited activity. Although longer occlusion is preferred, one to two hours can be sufficient to achieve a positive result.

In addition to limited penetration, another barrier to the success of topical agents is compliance. Compliance is a challenge for all patients using topical agents for chronic skin conditions, but it is even more difficult for palmoplantar patients, whose involved areas are essential for everyday functioning.

Other Topical Agents A variety of other topical medications have been used for palmoplantar psoriasis, but they too are limited by the same issues as topical corticosteroids and are shown to be less efficacious when used as monotherapy. One study showed 25% symptomatic improvement with calcipotriol applied twice daily to the palms and soles, whereas other literature reveals that up to 43% of patients had no symptomatic improvement [17,18]. The modest improvements when used as monotherapy likely necessitate supplementary intervention.

The literature shows that combination therapy with topical steroids is a more effective way to use other topical agents. The use of topical vitamin D derivatives with topical steroids did show additive benefits to monotherapy with corticosteroids, as did tazarotene with the same corticosteroids [9]. Even with the augmented effect, within a longitudinal study, most patients on combination topical therapy progressed to other options due to lack of efficacy [19]. The most effective combination supported in the literature is daily use of topical clobetasol with coal tar application at night. One study showed application of 0.05% clobetasol propionate cream twice daily with overnight application of 6% coal tar for 16 weeks proved to be faster, safer, and equal in efficacy to topical psoralen and ultraviolet A (PUVA) [20].

Phototherapy

Ultraviolet B Therapy In an open-label prospective study, 9 of 11 patients receiving narrowband ultraviolet B (UVB) three times a week for 12 weeks for topically resistant palmoplantar psoriasis showed >75% improvement in disease severity and area of involvement [21]. Another study showed similar results, with a 61% reduction in clinical severity; yet, this three times a week treatment for nine weeks was less effective than soak PUVA in a head-to-head comparison [22]. Narrowband UVB penetrates the thick stratum corneum less readily and may thus explain the discrepancy in efficacy [23].

PUVA Treatment Psoralen can be administered topically as a gel, lotion, or cream, but soaking the hands and feet in a bath of the dissolved medication is currently the preferred topical modality. The medication can also be ingested orally, but topical forms are generally preferred to avoid systemic photosensitizing effects. A comparison of the topical PUVA methods shows comparable efficacy across modalities [24]. For palmoplantar patients, oral PUVA is found to be most efficacious but involves more adverse effects, including nausea and dizziness [25]. The literature supports topical-soak PUVA as the most effective form of topical phototherapy [26–28]. The recommendation is to soak the hands and feet for 20 minutes in a psoralen concentration of 1.0 mg/L followed by exposure to 0.25–0.5 J/cm^2 UVA light three times per week. This treatment has been reported to result in nearly half of patients experiencing complete reduction in the severity of itching, erythema, scaling, and swelling [22,26].

Excimer Laser The 308-nm excimer laser is an effective option to treat both local and generalized psoriasis. Palmoplantar patients appear to be ideal candidates for the directed light therapy because it allows for localized, directed therapy to the palms and soles at higher therapeutic levels. Although the literature supports its successful use, the extent of success is variable, showing an average 52% symptomatic improvement with only 6.7% of patients achieving complete clearance [29,30].

Systemic Therapies

Retinoids Historically, etretinate, a chemical precursor of the more readily available acitretin, has shown efficacy as monotherapy for the treatment of palmoplantar psoriasis [31–33]. In recent decades, acitretin has taken preference over its precursor due to its shorter half-life. Retinoids are the most frequently used oral medication for palmoplantar patients, because they are effective against pustulation and hyperkeratosis [34]. The percentage of patients reporting complete symptomatic resolution is between 39% and 53% [34].

One reason retinoids are readily used in the population is their additive effect with phototherapy. Acitretin can be started in conjunction with phototherapy or as an adjunct to a subtherapeutic phototherapy regimen. Psoriasis Area Severity Index (PASI) scores show greater improvement in studies with narrowband UVB plus acitretin, as well as broadband UVB plus acitretin in comparison with phototherapy alone [35,36]. Moreover, the results of combination retinoids and PUVA therapy, also called re-PUVA (i.e., retinoid-PUVA), is even more pronounced. One study in palmoplantar patients showed that acitretin 25–75 mg daily combined with 0.6 mg/kg methoxypsoralen systemic PUVA three times per week resulted in greater clinical improvement than monotherapy with either agent [37–39].

When starting acitretin, 25 mg daily is found to be the optimal initial dose to maximize clinical improvement while minimizing side effects [40]. If greater efficacy is needed, dosage for patients can be increased by 10–25 mg every two to four weeks, as tolerated. It can take three to six months for the medication to show its full effect, and patients should be counseled regarding the delayed maximum result. When considering combination with light therapy, it is important to acknowledge that retinoids alter the skin's response to light by loosening cellular adhesion within the stratum corneum and by compromising barrier function [41,42]. It is recommended that before starting phototherapy, patients have a two-week "priming" period where acitretin is started and the patient adjusts to the subsequent skin alterations. If the patient is already on a phototherapeutic regimen, the dosimetry of phototherapy should be reduced by up to one-half to prevent phototoxicity. If no reaction is observed, the phototherapy dose can be titrated up to baseline [43]. The major concern with retinoids is their teratogenic potential; thus, the FDA contraindicates its use for women of childbearing age and advises women to avoid becoming pregnant for three years after taking the medication.

Methotrexate Methotrexate can also be effective for the treatment of palmoplantar psoriasis. One study showed that for patients on 20–30 mg methotrexate weekly for four months, there was >50% improvement in symptomatic severity and total area involvement in half of the patients, but other studies have failed to show that level of efficacy [9,19]. One potential benefit of methotrexate is that its maximal effect appears at least four weeks faster than that of acitretin [44]. However, the significant side effect profile, including cumulative liver toxicity, makes retinoids generally more preferable to methotrexate.

When initiating therapy with methotrexate, a laboratory workup including hepatitis screening, complete blood count (CBC), and liver function tests (LFTs) should be performed before administration of a 5 or 7.5 mg "test" dose. After this initial dose, the same labs should be checked a week later to assess for changes. Although the stated purpose of the test dose is to assess any idiosyncratic, acute bone marrow suppression effects from methotrexate, the test dose is not uniformly practiced by clinicians, and rigorous data are lacking regarding its utility. However, methotrexate use can result in acute and life-threatening bone marrow suppression. For palmoplantar psoriasis, after the initial testing dose, the usual starting dose is between 10 and 15 mg (4–6 tablets) once weekly [19]. Repeat labs should be completed every six weeks [45]. For a more complete discussion of methotrexate use, see Chapter 9 of *Moderate to Severe Psoriasis.*

Cyclosporine Cyclosporine is a highly effective treatment for the rapid remission of palmoplantar psoriasis. Rapid improvement can be seen within four weeks. The fast onset of action and therapeutic effects can be important in a population where severe disease can result in difficulties with walking or activities of daily living. The starting dose recommended is usually between 4 and 5 mg/kg/day [46]. This dose can be adjusted depending on the clinical response. Acceptable responses have been reported at doses of 2.5 mg/kg/day and even as low as 0.25 mg/kg/day [46,47]. If an inadequate response is observed, the dose can be gradually increased by 0.5 mg/kg/day at two- to four-week intervals, to a maximum of 5 mg/kg/day [45]. The literature shows that >90% of patients achieve at least 50% improvement in disease severity for patients taking low doses between 1.25 and 2.5 mg/kg over a three-month period [48].

Cyclosporine can be used as emergent short-term therapy while bridging to another medication or as a long-term solution. The maximum duration of treatment is controversial; the U.S. labeling recommends that treatment courses not exceed one year, although international standards suggest that two years of treatment are acceptable [45,46,49]. Studies show that effective maintenance doses range from 3.0 to 3.5 mg/kg/day, but lower doses are preferable to reduce the risk of systemic toxicity, including decreased renal function and hypertension. A screening laboratory workup before starting cyclosporine includes a CBC, blood urea nitrogen (BUN), creatinine, urinalysis, LFTs, lipid profile, magnesium, uric acid, and potassium as well as determination of hepatitis B and C, human immunodeficiency virus (HIV), and tuberculosis status [50]. Kidney function and blood pressure need to be monitored every other week for the first three months and then every four to six weeks thereafter, along with CBCs, LFTs, magnesium, uric acid, and potassium. For a more extensive discussion on the use of cyclosporine, see Chapter 10 of *Moderate to Severe Psoriasis*.

Tumor Necrosis Factor-α Inhibitors There are numerous studies supporting the safe and effective use of infliximab, etanercept, and adalimumab for palmoplantar psoriasis [51–56]. Infliximab groups were dosed at 5 mg/kg at weeks 0, 2, and 6 followed by every eight weeks, and severity was measured by improvements on the palms and soles only. Two-thirds of patients receiving infliximab experienced 50% improvement in symptoms, with 50.3% clearance of the mean surface area by week 14. In this same trial, one-third of all the patients experienced 75% symptomatic improvement as measured by a modified Palmoplantar Psoriasis Area Severity Index (m-PPPASI) [51]. One series noted a less substantial effect of infliximab on palmoplantar psoriasis compared with its effect on plaque psoriasis. In this comparison of groups dosed at 5 mg/kg at weeks 0, 2, 6, and every eight weeks thereafter, plaque-type patients experienced improvement as measured by a modified Psoriasis Area Severity Index (mPASI) of close to 90%, whereas palmoplantar disease severity improved by a mean of only 28% [52]. Although the reason for this phenomenon is not fully understood, it highlights the difficulty in treating palmoplantar psoriasis with the typical dosing used in plaque psoriasis.

In addition to infliximab, there are reports of successful treatment with etanercept, including in pediatric patients. These studies gave etanercept using standard dosing of 50 mg twice weekly for the first three months followed by once weekly for the duration of treatment. PASI-75 improvement was appreciated at week 24, and the medication was tolerated well without adverse effects [53–55].

Literature regarding adalimumab also addresses its successful use for palmoplantar psoriasis patients. Responses were seen with standard dosing of adalimumab, that is, one 80 mg injection followed by 40 mg injections every other week [56]. One double-blind study shows that nearly 75% of patients reported increased quality of life on the dermatology life quality index (DLQI), and 35% had complete symptomatic resolution with physician global assessment (PGA) scores of 0 [56]. Although adalimumab and the other anti-tumor necrosis factor (TNF) agents are successful in the treatment of palmoplantar psoriasis, there have not been any head-to-head studies comparing efficacy.

Even though improvements in disease severity and symptomatic relief are common for anti-TNF therapy, there are many reports of patients who develop palmoplantar psoriasis after initiating these medications. This response is seen in those receiving therapy for psoriasis as well as other conditions, and the unique presentation does not correspond to a particular anti-TNF agent or dosage [57]. More than 28 cases of this phenomenon have been reported, and the literature reports a variety of successful treatment options for the reaction, including discontinuation of the agent, switching to an alternative anti-TNF agent, or both [58]. Given the rare occurrence of this observation, anti-TNF agents remain safe and effective first-line options for patients with palmoplantar psoriasis.

Ustekinumab Ustekinumab has proven to be beneficial in the treatment of palmoplantar psoriasis. Although the literature is limited, patients appear to have a fast and robust improvement of symptomatic relief and clinical severity even after a single dose of this medication [59]. Studies followed standard dosing, giving patients 45 mg every third month for those who weigh <100 kg and 90 mg every third month for those who weigh >100 kg. In a study of 20 patients, complete clearance was seen in 35% of participants, with 60% of patients improving 1–2 points on their PGA scores. There was also a mean 56% improvement in DLQI scores. One interesting observation reveals a dose–response difference. It appears that those receiving 90 mg had more substantial improvement regarding both the percentage of patients who completely cleared and the percentage with those who improved their PGA scores [60].

INDIVIDUALIZING THERAPY FOR PALMOPLANTAR PSORIASIS

The approach to palmoplantar patients is unique in that it prioritizes symptomatic severity and quality-of-life impairment as they relate to a limited, local area. Treatment decisions should include an assessment of the individual's daily disease burden as well as the daily and long-term effects of the proposed therapy.

Topical steroids should be the initial therapy for mild to moderate disease, with preferential use of class I corticosteroids. Patients should be encouraged to apply agents twice daily; if patients can tolerate ointment-based topical formulations, ointment form is preferred over creams due to superior penetration of active ingredients. However, most patients prefer the cream formulation, and considerations must be made to balance compliance with medication efficacy. The addition of other topical agents, including calcipotriene or tazarotene, can augment the steroid's effect, but they should not be used as monotherapy unless the disease burden is minimal. Patients should be encouraged to use occlusion whenever possible at night, particularly if the therapeutic response is insufficient.

When mild to moderate disease continues to worsen despite an aggressive topical regimen, other options should be considered, including acitretin, PUVA, or narrowband UVB therapy.

If the patient is of childbearing age, light therapy should be preferred. For males and postmenopausal women, PUVA and UVB therapies are preferred over acitretin, but the logistics of three weekly treatments and potential light sensitivities can make acitretin the preferential option.

For moderate to severe disease, therapeutic options include biologic agents and a combination of acitretin with PUVA or UVB. This therapy is likely to have a more robust effect than either therapy used as monotherapy. Alternatively, for moderate to severe disease, patients can start with anti-TNF agents or ustekinumab. Etanercept and adalimumab are preferred to infliximab by patients due to ease of administration. The biologics are good alternatives for female patients who should avoid the use of acitretin or methotrexate.

In emergent or recalcitrant cases where patients are severely disabled or have failed to respond to other agents, cyclosporine is useful to control the symptoms quickly. Once the disease is under reasonable control, the dose of cyclosporine can be reduced, or clinicians can transition the patient to an alternative regimen of light therapy, acitretin, methotrexate, a biologic agent, or combination therapy. During all therapeutic options, patients should be counseled as to the benefits of continued topical corticosteroid application.

CONCLUSIONS

The palmoplantar psoriasis subtype population faces a variety of issues, including severe physical disability, challenging treatment regimens, and lack of inclusion in clinical trials due to limited body surface coverage [61]. The collective burden contributes to a frustrating disease course with limited research helping to explain unanswered questions. Nevertheless, progress has been made in understanding the palmoplantar subtype of psoriasis. Although these challenges are substantial, more research and better therapeutics will help strengthen the battle against this unique condition.

REFERENCES

1. Kumar B, Saraswat A, Kaur I. Palmoplantar lesions in psoriasis: a study of 3065 patients. *Acta Derm Venereol.* 2002;82(3):192–195.
2. Brunasso AM, Puntoni M, Aberer W, Delfino C, Fancelli L, Massone C. Clinical and epidemiological comparison of patients affected by palmoplantar plaque psoriasis and palmoplantar pustulosis: a case-series study. *Br J Dermatol.* 2013; 168(6):1243–1251.
3. Farley E, Masrour S, McKey J, Menter A. Palmoplantar psoriasis: a phenotypical and clinical review with introduction of a new quality-of-life assessment tool. *J Am Acad Dermatol.* 2009;60(6):1024–1031.
4. Griffiths CE, Christophers E, Barker JN, et al. A classification of psoriasis vulgaris according to phenotype. *Br J Dermatol.* 2007;156(2):258–262.
5. Diepgen TL, Andersen KE, Brandao FM, et al. Hand eczema classification: a cross-sectional, multicentre study of the aetiology and morphology of hand eczema. *Br J Dermatol.* 2009;160(2):353–358.
6. Aydin O, Engin B, Oguz O, Ilvan S, Demirkesen C. Non-pustular palmoplantar psoriasis: is histologic differentiation from eczematous dermatitis possible? *J Cutan Pathol.* 2008;35(2):169–173.
7. Ammoury A, El Sayed F, Dhaybi R, Bazex J. Palmoplantar pustulosis should not be considered as a variant of psoriasis. *J Eur Acad Dermatol Venereol.* 2008;22(3):392–393.
8. de Waal AC, van de Kerkhof PC. Pustulosis palmoplantaris is a disease distinct from psoriasis. *J Dermatolog Treat.* 2011;22(2):102–105.
9. Adisen E, Tekin O, Gulekon A, Gurer MA. A retrospective analysis of treatment responses of palmoplantar psoriasis in 114 patients. *J Eur Acad Dermatol Venereol.* 2009;23(7):814–819.

10. Caca-Biljanovska N, V'Lckova-Laskoska M, Balabanova-Stefanova M, Grivceva-Panovska V. Frequency of delayed-type hypersensitivity to contact allergens in palmo-plantar psoriasis. *Prilozi.* 2005;26(2):131–141.
11. Lillis JV, Guo CS, Lee JJ, Blauvelt A. Increased IL-23 expression in palmoplantar psoriasis and hyperkeratotic hand dermatitis. *Arch Dermatol.* 2010;146(8):910–919.
12. Chan CS, Van Voorhees AS, Lebwohl MG, et al. Treatment of severe scalp psoriasis: from the Medical Board of the National Psoriasis Foundation. *J Am Acad Dermatol.* 2009;60(6):962–971.
13. Elie R, Durocher LP, Kavalec EC. Effect of salicylic acid on the activity of betamethasone-17,21-dipropionate in the treatment of erythematous squamous dermatoses. *J Int Med Res.* 1983;11(2):108–112.
14. Coutanceau C, Carballido F, Le Maitre M. Clinical evaluation of the efficacy and the tolerance of a cream gel with 30% urea, 2% of salicylic acid, and 1% of lactic acid versus vehicle in subjects with localized hyperkeratosis. *J Am Acad Dermatol.* 2008;58(2):AB129.
15. Fluhr JW, Cavallotti C, Berardesca E. Emollients, moisturizers, and keratolytic agents in psoriasis. *Clin Dermatol.* 2008;26(4):380–386.
16. Volden G. Successful treatment of chronic skin diseases with clobetasol propionate and a hydrocolloid occlusive dressing. *Acta Derm Venereol.* 1992;72(1):69–71.
17. Duweb GA, Abuzariba O, Rahim M, al-Taweel M, al-Alem S, Abdulla SA. Occlusive versus nonocclusive calcipotriol ointment treatment for palmoplantar psoriasis. *Int J Tissue React.* 2001;23(2):59–62.
18. Thiers BH. The use of topical calcipotriene/calcipotriol in conditions other than plaque-type psoriasis. *J Am Acad Dermatol.* 1997;37(3 Pt 2):S69–71.
19. Spuls PI, Hadi S, Rivera L, Lebwohl M. Retrospective analysis of the treatment of psoriasis of the palms and soles. *J Dermatolog Treat.* 2003;14(Suppl 2):21–25.
20. Khandpur S, Sharma VK. Comparison of clobetasol propionate cream plus coal tar vs. topical psoralen and solar ultraviolet A therapy in palmoplantar psoriasis. *Clin Exp Dermatol.* 2011;36(6):613–616.
21. Nordal EJ, Christensen OB. Treatment of chronic hand dermatoses with UVB-TL01. *Acta Derm Venereol.* 2004;84(4):302–304.
22. Sezer E, Erbil AH, Kurumlu Z, Tastan HB, Etikan I. Comparison of the efficacy of local narrowband ultraviolet B (NB-UVB) phototherapy versus psoralen plus ultraviolet A (PUVA) paint for palmoplantar psoriasis. *J Dermatol.* 2007;34(7):435–440.
23. Berneburg M, Rocken M, Benedix F. Phototherapy with narrowband vs broadband UVB. *Acta Derm Venereol.* 2005;85(2):98–108.
24. Grundmann-Kollmann M, Behrens S, Peter RU, Kerscher M. Treatment of severe recalcitrant dermatoses of the palms and soles with PUVA-bath versus PUVA-cream therapy. *Photodermatol Photoimmunol Photomed.* 1999;15(2):87–89.
25. Hofer A, Fink-Puches R, Kerl H, Quehenberger F, Wolf P. Paired comparison of bathwater versus oral delivery of 8-methoxypsoralen in psoralen plus ultraviolet: a therapy for chronic palmoplantar psoriasis. *Photodermatol Photoimmunol Photomed.* 2006;22(1):1–5.
26. Schiener R, Gottlober P, Muller B, et al. PUVA-gel vs. PUVA-bath therapy for severe recalcitrant palmoplantar dermatoses. A randomized, single-blinded prospective study. *Photodermatol Photoimmunol Photomed.* 2005;21(2):62–67.
27. Layton AM, Sheehan-Dare R, Cunliffe WJ. A double-blind, placebo-controlled trial of topical PUVA in persistent palmoplantar pustulosis. *Br J Dermatol.* 1991;124(6):581–584.
28. Davis MD, McEvoy MT, el-Azhary RA. Topical psoralen-ultraviolet A therapy for palmoplantar dermatoses: experience with 35 consecutive patients. *Mayo Clin Proc.* 1998;73(5):407–411.
29. Goldberg DJ, Chwalek J, Hussain M. 308-nm Excimer laser treatment of palmoplantar psoriasis. *J Cosmet Laser Ther.* 2011;13(2):47–49.
30. Han L, Somani AK, Huang Q, et al. Evaluation of 308-nm monochromatic excimer light in the treatment of psoriasis vulgaris and palmoplantar psoriasis. *Photodermatol Photoimmunol Photomed.* 2008;24(5):231–236.
31. Thune P. Treatment of palmoplantar pustulosis with Tigason. *Dermatologica.* 1982;164(1):67–72.
32. White SI, Puttick L, Marks JM. Low-dose etretinate in the maintenance of remission of palmoplantar pustular psoriasis. *Br J Dermatol.* 1986;115(5):577–582.
33. White SI, Marks JM, Shuster S. Etretinate in pustular psoriasis of palms and soles. *Br J Dermatol.* 1985;113(5):581–585.

34. Marsland AM, Griffiths CE. Treatments for chronic palmoplantar pustular psoriasis. *Skin Therapy Lett.* 2001;6(12):3–5.
35. Ruzicka T, Sommerburg C, Braun-Falco O, et al. Efficiency of acitretin in combination with UV-B in the treatment of severe psoriasis. *Arch Dermatol.* 1990;126(4):482–486.
36. Spuls PI, Rozenblit M, Lebwohl M. Retrospective study of the efficacy of narrowband UVB and acitretin. *J Dermatolog Treat.* 2003;14(Suppl 2):17–20.
37. Rosen K, Mobacken H, Swanbeck G. PUVA, etretinate, and PUVA-etretinate therapy for pustulosis palmoplantaris. A placebo-controlled comparative trial. *Arch Dermatol.* 1987;123(7):885–889.
38. Lassus A, Lauharanta J, Eskelinen A. The effect of etretinate compared with different regimens of PUVA in the treatment of persistent palmoplantar pustulosis. *Br J Dermatol.* 1985;112(4):455–459.
39. Lawrence CM, Marks J, Parker S, Shuster S. A comparison of PUVA-etretinate and PUVA-placebo for palmoplantar pustular psoriasis. *Br J Dermatol.* 1984;110(2):221–226.
40. Ling MR. Acitretin: optimal dosing strategies. *J Am Acad Dermatol.* 1999;41(3 Pt 2):S13–17.
41. Yamauchi PS, Rizk D, Kormili T. Systemic retinoids. In: Weinstein GD, Gottlieb AB, ed. *Therapy of Moderate-to-Severe Psoriasis.* New York: Marcel Dekker; 2003:137–150.
42. Elias PM, Fritsch PO, Lampe M, et al. Retinoid effects on epidermal structure, differentiation, and permeability. *Lab Invest.* 1981;44(6):531–540.
43. Pang ML, Koo J, Yamauchi P, Lee CS. Systemic retinoids. In: Koo JYM, Lee CS, Lebwohl MG, Weinstein GD, Gottlieb AB, ed. *Moderate to Severe Psoriasis.* Vol 3. New York: Informa; 2009:159–172.
44. Janagond AB, Kanwar AJ, Handa S. Efficacy and safety of systemic methotrexate vs. acitretin in psoriasis patients with significant palmoplantar involvement: a prospective, randomized study. *J Eur Acad Dermatol Venereol.* 2012.
45. Menter A, Korman NJ, Elmets CA, et al. Guidelines of care for the management of psoriasis and psoriatic arthritis: section 4. Guidelines of care for the management and treatment of psoriasis with traditional systemic agents. *J Am Acad Dermatol.* 2009;61(3):451–485.
46. Griffiths CE, Katsambas A, Dijkmans BA, et al. Update on the use of ciclosporin in immune-mediated dermatoses. *Br J Dermatol.* 2006;155(Suppl 2):1–16.
47. Peter RU, Färber L, Wei J. Low-dose cyclosporin A in palmoplantar psoriasis: evaluation of efficacy and safety. *J Eur Acad Dermatol Venereol.* 1994;3(4):518–524.
48. Reitamo S, Erkko P, Remitz A, Lauerma AI, Montonen O, Harjula K. Cyclosporine in the treatment of palmoplantar pustulosis. A randomized, double-blind, placebo-controlled study. *Arch Dermatol.* 1993;129(10):1273–1279.
49. Lebwohl M, Ellis C, Gottlieb A, et al. Cyclosporine consensus conference: with emphasis on the treatment of psoriasis. *J Am Acad Dermatol.* 1998;39(3):464–475.
50. Amor KT, Ryan C, Menter A. The use of cyclosporine in dermatology: part I. *J Am Acad Dermatol.* 2010;63(6):925–946; quiz 947–928.
51. Bissonnette R, Poulin Y, Guenther L, Lynde CW, Bolduc C, Nigen S. Treatment of palmoplantar psoriasis with infliximab: a randomized, double-blind placebo-controlled study. *J Eur Acad Dermatol Venereol.* 2011;25(12):1402–1408.
52. Brunasso AM, Puntoni M, Delfino C, Massone C. Different response rates between palmoplantar involvement and diffuse plaque psoriasis in patients treated with infliximab. *Eur J Dermatol.* 2012;22(1):133–135.
53. Bissonnette R, Poulin Y, Bolduc C, et al. Etanercept in the treatment of palmoplantar pustulosis. *J Drugs Dermatol.* 2008;7(10):940–946.
54. Floristan U, Feltes R, Ramirez P, Alonso ML, De Lucas R. Recalcitrant palmoplantar pustular psoriasis treated with etanercept. *Pediatr Dermatol.* 2011;28(3):349–350.
55. Weinberg JM. Successful treatment of recalcitrant palmoplantar psoriasis with etanercept. *Cutis.* 2003;72(5):396–398.
56. Richetta AG, Mattozzi C, Giancristoforo S, et al. Safety and efficacy of adalimumab in the treatment of moderate to severe palmo-plantar psoriasis: an open label study. *Clin Ter.* 2012;163(2):e61–66.
57. Papadavid E, Gazi S, Dalamaga M, Stavrianeas N, Ntelis V. Palmoplantar and scalp psoriasis occurring during anti-tumour necrosis factor-alpha therapy: a case series of four patients and guidelines for management. *J Eur Acad Dermatol Venereol.* 2008;22(3):380–382.
58. Roux CH, Brocq O, Leccia N, et al. New-onset psoriatic palmoplantaris pustulosis following infliximab therapy: a class effect? *J Rheumatol.* 2007;34(2):434–437.

59. Morales-Munera C, Vilarrasa E, Puig L. Efficacy of ustekinumab in refractory palmoplantar pustular psoriasis. *Br J Dermatol.* 2013;168(4):820–824.
60. Au SC, Goldminz AM, Kim N, et al. Investigator-initiated, open-label trial of ustekinumab for the treatment of moderate to severe palmoplantar psoriasis. *J Dermatolog Treat.* 2012; 24(3):179–187.
61. Pettey AA, Balkrishnan R, Rapp SR, Fleischer AB, Feldman SR. Patients with palmoplantar psoriasis have more physical disability and discomfort than patients with other forms of psoriasis: implications for clinical practice. *J Am Acad Dermatol.* 2003;49(2):271–275.

Chapter 14

Scalp Psoriasis

Peter C. M. van de Kerkhof, Marloes M. Kleinpenning, and Rianne M. J. P. Gerritsen

INTRODUCTION

Psoriasis has the scalp as one of its predilection sites. Scalp psoriasis may seriously impair quality of life. In this chapter, we present the epidemiologic aspects, clinical morphology, and differential diagnosis of scalp psoriasis, followed by the classes of treatments.

EPIDEMIOLOGY

Involvement of the scalp is the most frequent manifestations of psoriasis. Indeed, 79% of Dutch patients with psoriasis indicated that the scalp was the most frequently affected area [1]. In many patients, psoriasis of the scalp is a major problem; in fact, 31% of patients with scalp psoriasis indicated that the condition is distressing [2].

In a questionnaire mailed to 6000 members of the Dutch Psoriasis Association, 57% of the respondents named scalp involvement as an important psychologic handicap [3]. In fact, scalp psoriasis had existed for more than five years in 81% of the respondents, and in 48%, psoriasis covered more than half of the scalp. Visibility of the lesions and itch were the most annoying symptoms in 34% and 26%, of respondents, respectively, with scalp psoriasis.

CLINICAL MORPHOLOGY

Classical scalp psoriasis manifests as sharply demarcated erythematous plaques with white-silvery scales. The scales extend as sleeves around the hair, a condition also described as "pseudo-teigne amiantacée." The lesions often expand onto the face, in particular in the hairline, but involvement of the retroauricular fold also is often seen. Figure 14.1 illustrates the classical manifestations of scalp psoriasis. Scalp psoriasis may itch in most patients, at least in some episodes.

It is the traditional view that scalp psoriasis is not characterized by hair loss or by atrophy of the skin. However, it has been shown that the number of telogen hairs in trichograms of plucks of hair is increased [4]. Scanning electron microscopy has revealed that hair of psoriatic patients shows cuticular breakage and an abraded cuticular surface [5]. Furthermore, it is borne out of clinical praxis that long-lasting psoriatic plaques may cause alopecia cicatricial [6–8].

Because scalp psoriasis may result in irreversible hair loss, it is important to convince the patient that active treatment is important not only for the immediate improvement of the condition but also for long-term personal appearance.

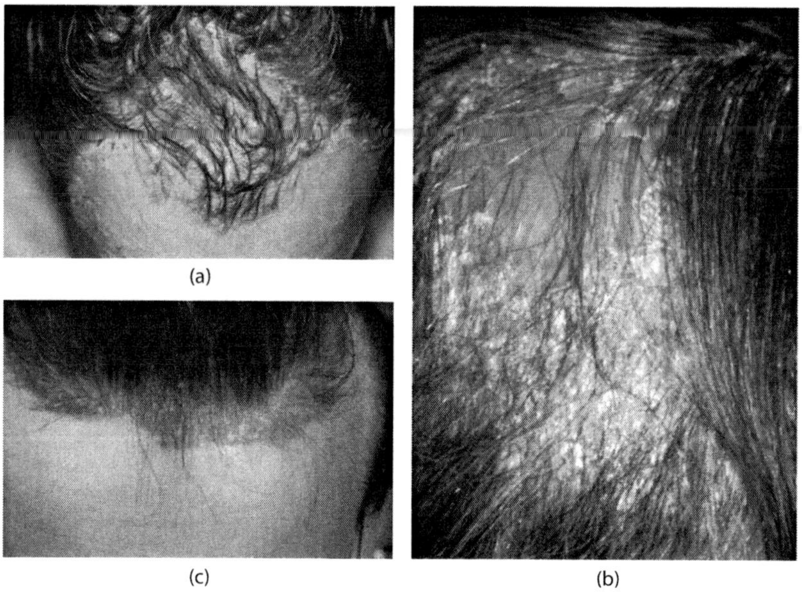

FIGURE 14.1 (See color insert.) Classical manifestations of scalp psoriasis. (a) Psoriasis of the scalp. (b) Scarring psoriatic alopecia. (c) Hairline psoriasis.

DIFFERENTIAL DIAGNOSIS

Scaling of the scalp may provide a challenge to the physician for adequate diagnosis and treatment. Classic psoriatic plaques elsewhere or classic manifestations of seborrheic dermatitis, lupus erythematosus, or lichen planopilaris may help the diagnosis. Therefore, inspection of the entire skin is important.

The scalp lesions of psoriasis may strongly resemble seborrheic dermatitis, another papulosquamous condition; however, seborrheic dermatitis has more yellow scales-crusts and preferential localization on upper trunk, face, and flexures. Fungal lesions also may strongly resemble scalp psoriasis. Broken hair, pustulation, and prominent atrophy may increase suspicion that a fungus is involved. Lichen planus is characterized by violaceous papules in follicular arrangement resulting in atrophy. Lupus erythematodes is also characterized by atrophy and follicular hyperkeratoses.

A group of 85 patients with scaling of the scalp (pityriasis amiantacea) were examined clinically, and they underwent histologic, bacteriologic, and mycological examinations [9]. Psoriasis was confirmed in only 35.3% of these cases. In 34.2% of the cases, the diagnosis was seborrheic dermatitis or atopic dermatitis. In 12.9% of the cases, a diagnosis of tinea capitis was confirmed by potassium hydroxide preparation, fungal culture, and periodic acid–Schiff staining. Overgrowth of *Staphylococcus* isolates was evident in 96.5% of the patients.

In another study, patients who had been diagnosed as having scalp psoriasis had colonization with *Malassezia* (*Pityrosporum*) species [10]. *Malassezia globosa*, *M. slooffiae*, and *M. restricta* were predominant species in 55%, 18%, and 10% of the patients, respectively. Therefore, in cases of pityriasis amiantacea, the differential diagnosis is broad, and in cases where the clinical picture is not conclusive, histologic examination and cultures may be indicated [11]. In psoriasis of the scalp, overgrowth of *Malassezia* species remains an important feature and may be of therapeutic relevance.

GENERAL THERAPEUTIC ASPECTS

A questionnaire mailed to patients of the Dutch Society for Psoriasis (n = 922 responders) [3] revealed that 99.6% of patients used a topical corticosteroid for scalp psoriasis. Shampoos were used by 51% of the patients and calcipotriol treatment by 28% of the patients responding to the questionnaire. The majority of these patients used the treatment for prolonged periods; 72% of them had indicated that they had used treatments for more than eight weeks. Of particular importance is the patients indicating the formulation that allows a cosmetically acceptable outcome. Although involvement of the scalp with psoriasis is frequent and the impairment of quality of life is important, few evidence-based studies on treatment of scalp psoriasis are available.

SHAMPOOS

Shampoos are used as a vehicle for active treatment principles. Although no double-blind studies are available on the efficacy of tar shampoos, the use of tar shampoo is a popular approach by patients suffering from scalp psoriasis.

Open studies indicated that shampoos containing 2%–10% coal tar may be effective in psoriasis [12,13]. Some reservation on the use of coal tar shampoos is justified because the secretion of 10-hydroxypyrene in urine is increased in patients using tar shampoo, indicating resorption of hydrocarbons through the skin [14].

Zinc pyrithione shampoos are well appreciated. But again, no double-blind studies are available to substantiate their efficacy. In open studies, scalp psoriasis proved to respond to zinc pyrithione–containing shampoos in concentrations between 1% and 2% [14–16].

More recently, clobetasol propionate shampoo 0.05% was reported to be a new option for the treatment of patients with moderate to severe scalp psoriasis [17]. In a multicenter, randomized, vehicle-controlled, double-masked, parallel-group study, clobetasol propionate shampoo was compared against the corresponding vehicle shampoo in patients with moderate to severe scalp psoriasis during a four-week treatment. A total of 143 patients were treated. Clobetasol shampoo was significantly more effective compared with the vehicle shampoo with the same safety profile. Clobetasol propionate 0.05% shampoo was compared with a 1% tar shampoo in 162 patients with scalp psoriasis. In this multicenter, randomized study, clobetasol propionate shampoo was more effective [18]. In another comparative study of 151 patients, clobetasol shampoo was more effective compared with 0.005% calcipotriol solution over a four-week period [19].

DESCALING OF THE SCALP

Debridement of the scalp by an automatized shampooing and debridement machine has been shown to empower markedly the response to antipsoriatic treatments [20].

Salicylic acid 5%–10% has been shown to have a marked keratolytic effect. Salicylic acid is formulated in an ointment that can be washed off easily. Application of salicylic acid ointments is done for a few days, before active treatment principles are used. An alternative for salicylic acid is urea that can be used in concentrations of up to 40% [21].

COAL TAR AND DITHRANOL

Coal tar may be indicated for itchy psoriasis. However, the unpleasant smell of coal tar is a limitation. Coal tar solution (5%–20%) can be formulated in a lotion or added to a topical corticosteroid preparation.

Dithranol is another time-honored therapy. Dithranol 0.1%–3% is manufactured in various formulations. The treatment is started at a low concentration and increased stepwise to provide a minimal degree of irritation. Dithranol treatment of the scalp may cause temporary discoloration of the hair. In an open study, dithranol in a cream formulation caused 58% reduction of the modified Psoriasis Area and Severity Index (PASI) score for the scalp during an eight-week treatment [22]. The application of dithranol in scalp psoriasis has been improved by manufacturing dithranol into detergents (Silix Waschöl N, Pacos GmbH, Halle, Germany). An emulsifying oil base (*Helianthus annulus*, octyl cocoate, polyethylene glycol [PEG]-40, sorbitan peroleate, PEG-40 hydrogenated castor oil, trideceth-9, propylparaben, butylated hydroxytoluene [BHT], ascorbyl palmitate, glyceryl stearate, glyceryl oleate, and citric acid) and crystalline monoglycerides (Micanol Bioglan, Giessen, Germany) have been shown to be suitable vehicles for dithranol treatment of scalp psoriasis [23].

IMIDAZOLE ANTIFUNGALS

Because scalp psoriasis is accompanied by an overgrowth of *Malassezia* species, an antifungal treatment seems to be a rational approach. The outcome of various studies on topical and systemic antifungal treatments is contradictory [24–27]. However, in treatment-resistant manifestations, a reduction of *Malassezia* overgrowth may be effective in improving the condition.

TOPICAL CORTICOSTEROIDS

Topical corticosteroids are frequently used in scalp psoriasis. From an epidemiologic survey we know that topical corticosteroids are used by the majority of patients for more than eight weeks [3].

In scalp psoriasis, the formulation is relevant, in particular, with respect to the cosmetic appearance. A cream or lotion is preferred over an ointment, although an ointment provides better bioavailability. More recently, a foam vehicle has become available. The advantage of the foam is that it spreads in the hair until it reaches the scalp, where it "melts." The total coverage area for 100 g of foam was comparable to the coverage area of 100 g of traditional vehicles [28]. In a comparative study against standard treatment (corticosteroid lotion or vitamin D_3 treatments), betamethasone-17-valerate in foam was more effective, resulting in clearing or nearly clearing in 88% of the patients [29]. In another study, it was shown that once-daily application of betamethasone-17-valerate in the foam vehicle was as effective as twice-daily application of the standard treatment [30]. The average sign scores (erythema plus induration plus scaling) reduced from 8.1 to 3.9 and from 7.7 to 3.0 during a four-week head-to-head study [31]. In a comparative study of clobetasol propionate foam 0.05% against clobetasol cream, the decrease of PASI during a two-week study was 41% versus 31%. Patients using foam had a significantly greater increase in quality-of-life parameters and had spent less time applying their medication [31]. The use of clobetasol propionate 0.05% shampoo (CPS) is an important innovation. CPS proved to be a good alternative to tar blend shampoo in the treatment of moderate to severe scalp psoriasis. In a comparative 24-week study against vehicle, the added value of clobetasol 0.05 shampoo was clearly shown. Health benefits were measured in disease-free days (DFDs). The economic analysis includes drug and physician costs. Depending on the country, the mean total number of DFDs per patient is 21%–42% higher with CPS compared with vehicle, and the mean total cost is 11%–31% lower. The mean costs per DFD are 30%–46% lower with CPS compared with the vehicle [32].

Side effects of topical corticosteroids on the scalp are limited. If the facial area is exposed to the steroids, perioral dermatitis may develop. It may be relevant, however, that topical corticosteroids may suppress hair growth [33] and that the skin of the scalp is by far more permeable to topical corticosteroids than skin in most other regions [34].

The efficacy and safety ratio of topical corticosteroids may be enhanced by applying corticosteroid preparations intermittently for two or three days per week. Furthermore, the addition of salicylic acid may increase the bioavailability of topical corticosteroids considerably, thereby enhancing efficacy. Plastic occlusion (e.g., a shower cap) may be helpful in enhancing the efficacy of corticosteroids. However, penetration may be enhanced considerably. Zinc pyrithione spray has been used in combination with a topical corticosteroid. In a double-blind study, the added value of zinc pyrithione could not be shown [35]. Combination treatments with vitamin D_3 analogs, the topical retinoid tazarotene [36], and ultraviolet B (UVB) phototherapy are important options for effective and safe control of scalp psoriasis.

VITAMIN D_3 ANALOGS

Calcipotriol, calcitriol, and tacalcitol are well-established, first-line treatments of psoriasis. Calcipotriol solution has become a mainstay in the topical treatment of scalp psoriasis. More recently, tacalcitol has become available in several countries.

In a four-week, double-blind comparative study, calcipotriol lotion proved to be effective, although less effective compared with betamethasone lotion [37]. In 73%–75% of the patients treated with betamethasone, a marked improvement or clearing was observed and in

57%–58% of the calcipotriol-treated patients, such an improvement was seen. The majority of the patients were treated for another six weeks with calcipotriol solution in an open-label phase that resulted in a marked improvement in 82.6% of the patients. In this respect, it should be noted that optimal efficacy with calcipotriol solution requires eight weeks, whereas a potent topical corticosteroid already results in maximum efficacy after two to three weeks. In another comparative study (open-label) during six weeks, both treatments were equally effective [38].

The combined use of calcipotriol ointment (80–100 g/week) and calcipotriol solution (30–50 mL/week) proved to be safe, without affecting the indices of calcium metabolism or bone turnover [39]. In 202 patients, the long-term efficacy and safety of twice-daily calcipotriol solution was studied. By week 28, the total sign score had reduced from 5.9 to 2.5. Facial irritation was observed in 91 of 276 events, and no significant changes of systemic calcium metabolism have been observed [40]. In a multicenter prospective observational cohort (<3396 patients) treated with calcipotriol solution twice daily over an eight-week period, the following observations were made [41]: (1) in the total cohort, the scalp severity index reduced from 18.4 to 5.6; (2) in 80% of patients, the improvement was rated as good to very good; and (3) in those patients who were treated only with calcipotriol solution without additional treatments, the scalp severity index decreased from 16.0 to 4.9 in the eight-week treatment.

More recently, tacalcitol in an emulsion has become available in various countries. Once-daily tacalcitol emulsion proved to be effective and safe in a double-blind, placebo-controlled study. After an eight-week treatment, the median sum score had decreased by 53% in the tacalcitol group, with 80% of the patients showing marked improvement to clearing [42]. Local adverse reactions were transient and uncommon, and systemic calcium metabolism was not affected.

Topical vitamin D_3 treatment can be combined with topical corticosteroids. An elegant, effective, and safe strategy is once-daily application of a topical corticosteroid during weekend days and once or twice daily a vitamin D_3 analog during weekdays [43]. A large program of phase II studies has been completed evaluating the efficacy and safety of a gel formulation containing calcipotriol and betamethasone dipropionate [44–48]. The fixed combination of calcipotriol and betamethasone as a suspension (also referred to as "gel" outside of the United States) has become a mainstay in the treatment of scalp psoriasis. This two-compound formulation had a faster improvement and more impressive efficacy compared with the monocomponent formulations The efficacy of the combination has been shown in large multicenter, double-blind, parallel-group studies. The proportion of patients with "absence of disease" or "very mild disease" at week 8 was significantly higher in the two-compound group (68.4%) than in the betamethasone dipropionate group (61.0%, $p = .0079$) or calcipotriol group (43.4%, $p < .0001$). The proportion of patients rating their scalp psoriasis as "clear" or "almost clear" was significantly higher for the two-compound scalp formulation (69.6%) than for betamethasone dipropionate (59.9%, $p = .0006$) or calcipotriol (44.7%, $p < .0001$). The incidence of lesional/perilesional adverse events was lower in the two-compound and betamethasone dipropionate groups than in the calcipotriol group [48].

PHOTOTHERAPY

Phototherapy, although effective in plaque psoriasis, has limited applications in scalp psoriasis because the hair prevents adequate UV exposure of the skin surface. The UVB/fiber optic comb has been shown in a pilot study in fewer than 14 patients to improve the treated sides well above that of the untreated sides [49]. The 308-nm excimer laser has also been investigated with respect to efficacy in the treatment of scalp psoriasis. In a study in fewer than 13 patients, excimer laser–treated sides improved well above that of untreated sides [50].

A challenging development is photodynamic therapy [51]. Application of aminolevulinic acid results in intracellular accumulation of protoporphyrin IX that can be activated by visible light to produce reactive oxygen species and free radicals. This process has an antipsoriatic potential. Visible light penetrates better through keratin structures compared with ultraviolet light and may well improve phototherapy of scalp psoriasis.

SYSTEMIC TREATMENTS

In general, scalp psoriasis can be managed by a topical treatment. If topical treatments are not effective and phototherapy does not provide an adequate solution, a systemic treatment may be indicated. Cyclosporin is a very effective antipsoriatic treatment that can be used up to one or two years for reason of cumulative toxicity. Methotrexate, fumarates, and acitretin may provide a satisfactorily long-term control.

TREATMENT STRATEGIES IN SCALP PSORIASIS

A spectrum of treatments is available for the management of scalp psoriasis. However, few double-blind, placebo-controlled studies and double-blind controlled studies against active comparators are available. Guidelines on the treatment of scalp psoriasis are largely based on the open studies described above and on expert opinions. In this section, we integrate the current knowledge into treatment recommendations for scalp psoriasis.

The first phase is active descaling. In mild scaling, regular shampooing is an option. Application of salicylic acid 5%–10% or urea up to 40% in a wash-off ointment may enhance descaling. An automatic shampooing machine may help at day care centers for efficient descaling.

The second phase is active clearing treatment. The first-line approach is a vitamin D_3 solution or emulsion once a day and a superpotent topical corticosteroid in a vehicle that is well accepted by the patient once a day. If this approach is not effective after eight weeks or not appreciated for reason of intolerance, a superpotent topical corticosteroid may be combined with UVB therapy. To optimize phototherapy of the scalp, a hair blower or a UVB fiber comb can be used. Another alternative for the second phase is dithranol and tar-based treatments at a day care center. If all these approaches are not effective, cultures for *Malassezia* species should be taken, and a systemic antifungal treatment can be started. If all these treatments are not effective, a systemic antipsoriatic treatment should be considered with methotrexate, fumarates, cyclosporine, or acitretin.

The third phase of treatment is stabilization with a vitamin D_3 analog on weekdays (once or twice daily) and a superpotent topical corticosteroid once daily during the weekend. If a vitamin D_3 analog is not tolerated, the patient may restrict to intermittent applications of the corticosteroid only.

The fourth phase is the maintenance phase. For this phase, a vitamin D_3 analog is the preferred treatment either once or twice daily. A tar shampoo may further support this phase.

CONCLUSIONS

Scalp psoriasis is a frequently occurring condition that may impair quality of life considerably. A spectrum of treatments (Table 14.1) for this condition is available, although few double-blind comparative studies support the efficacy of these treatments. Treatment phases comprise I, descaling; II, clearing; III, stabilization; and IV, maintenance.

TABLE 14.1 Actual Frequency of Use of Various Treatments in Scalp Psoriasis (n = 922 patients)

Treatment	No. of Patients
Corticosteroids	
Hydrocortisone cream	13
Clobetasone cream	14
Hydrocortisone butyrate cream	32
Hydrocortisone butyrate lotion	16
Hydrocortisone butyrate emulsion	18
Triamcinolone cream	28
Betamethasone valerate cream	65
Betamethasone valerate emulsion	19
Betamethasone valerate lotion	125
Clobetasol cream	106
Clobetasol lotion	101
Betamethasone dipropionate hydrogel	26
Betamethasone dipropionate cream	37
Betamethasone dipropionate lotion	72
Desoximetasone emulsion	292
Other treatments	
Calcipotriol ointment	258
Coal tar shampoo	474
UVB phototherapy	119
Salicylic acid	65
Other/unknown[a]	161

[a] Other/unknown implies a series of alternative treatment approaches.

REFERENCES

1. van de Kerkhof PCM, Steegers-Theunissen RPM, Kuipers MV. Evaluation of topical drug treatment in psoriasis. *Dermatology* 1998; 197: 31–36.
2. Poyner TF, Fell PJ. Frequency of patients with plaque psoriasis who had not consulted their doctor in the past year. *Br J Clin Res* 1995; 6: 201–207.
3. van de Kerkhof PCM, de Hoop D, de Korte J, et al. Scalp psoriasis, clinical presentations and therapeutic management. *Dermatology* 1998; 197: 326–334.
4. Schoorl WJ, Baar HJ, van de Kerkhof PCM. The hair root pattern in psoriasis of the scalp. *Acta Derm Venereol* 1992; 72: 141–142.
5. Plozzer C, Coletti C, Kokelj F, et al. Scanning electron microscopy study of hair shaft disorders in psoriasis. *Acta Derm Venereol Suppl* 2000: 9–11.
6. van de Kerkhof PCM, Chang A. Scarring alopecia and psoriasis. *Br J Dermatol* 1992; 126: 524–525.
7. Schuster S. Psoriatic alopecia. *Br J Dermatol* 1992; 87: 73–77.
8. Bardazzi F, Fanti PA, Orlandi C, et al. Psoriatic scarring alopecia: observations in four patients. *Int J Dermatol* 1999; 38: 765–768.
9. Abdel-Hamid IA, Agha SA, Moustafa YM, et al. Pityriasis amiantacea: a clinical and etiopathologic study of 85 patients. *Int J Dermatol* 2003; 42: 260–264.
10. Conti Diaz IA, Civila E, Veiga R. The importance of microscopic examination in the management of desquamative disease of the scalp. *Mycopathologica* 2002; 153: 71–75.
11. Prohic A. Identification of Malassezia species isolated from scalp skin of patients with psoriasis and healthy subjects. *Acta Dermatovenerol Croat* 2003; 11: 10–16.
12. Olansky S. Whole coal tar shampoo: a therapeutic hair repair system. *Cutis* 1980; 25: 99–104.
13. Lowe NJ, Breeding JH, Wortzmann MS. New coal tar extract and coal tar shampoos. *Arch Dermatol* 1982; 118: 487–489.
14. Jongeneelen FJ, Bos RP, Azion RBM. Biological monitoring of polycyclic aromatic hydrocarbons: metabolites in urine. *Scand J Work Environ Health* 1986; 12: 137–143.
15. Snijder FH, Beuhler EV, Winek CL. Safety evaluation of zinc-2-pyridinethiol 1-ozide in a shampoo formulation. *Toxicol Appl Pharmacol* 1965; 7: 425–437.
16. Orentreich N. A clinical evaluation of two shampoos in the treatment of psoriasis. *J Soc Cosmet Chem* 1972; 23: 189–194.
17. Jarrat M, Breneman D, Gottlieb AB, et al. Clobetasol propionate shampoo 0.05%: a new option to treat patients with moderate to severe scalp psoriasis. *J Drugs Dermatol* 2004; 3: 367–373.
18. Griffiths CEM, Finlay AY, Fleming CJ, et al. A randomized, investigator-masked clinical evaluation of the efficacy and safety of clobetasol propionate 0.05% shampoo and tar blend 1% shampoo in the treatment of moderate to severe scalp psoriasis. *J Dermatolog Treat* 2006; 17: 90–95.
19. Reygagne P, Mrowietz U, Decroix J, et al. Clobetasol propionate shampoo 0.05% and calcipotriol solution 0.005%: a randomized comparison of efficacy and safety in subjects with scalp psoriasis. *J Dermatol* 1999; 38: 628–632.
20. King L Jr, Webb B, Zanolli M. Experience in treating recalcitrant scalp psoriasis with automated shampooing and debridement. *J Am Acad Dermatol* 1999; 41: 638–651.
21. Shemer A, Nathansohn N, Kaplan B, et al. Treatment of scalp seborrheic dermatitis and psoriasis with an ointment of 40% urea and 1% bifonazole. *Int J Dermatol* 2000; 39: 532–534.
22. Prins M, Swinkels OQJ, Bertholet B, et al. Dithranol short contact treatment of scalp psoriasis. *J Dermatolog Treat* 1999; 10: 13–17.
23. Wulff-Woesten A, Ohlendorf D, Henz BM, et al. Dithranol in an emulsifying oil base (bio-wash-oil) for the treatment of psoriasis of the scalp. *Skin Pharmacol Physiol* 2004; 17: 91–97.
24. Farr PM, Krause LB, Marks JM, et al. Response of scalp psoriasis to oral ketoconazole. *Lancet* 1985; 8461(II): 921–922.
25. Faergemann J. Treatment of sebopsoriasis with itraconazole. *Mykosen* 1985; 28: 612–618.
26. Rosenberg EW, Belew PW, Skinner RB. Treatment of psoriasis with antimicrobial agents. *Semin Dermatol* 1985; 4: 307–311.
27. Jury CS, Hugh McL, Shankland GS, et al. A randomized, placebo-controlled trial of oral itraconazole in scalp psoriasis. *J Dermatolog Treat* 2000; 11: 85–89.
28. Feldman SR, Sangha N, Setaluri V. Topical corticosteroid in foam vehicle offers comparable covered compared with traditional vehicles. *J Am Acad Dermatol* 2000; 42: 1017–1020.

29. Andreassi L, Giannetti A, Milani M, et al. Efficacy of betamethasone valerate mousse in comparison with standard therapies on scalp psoriasis: an open, multicentre, randomized, controlled, cross-over study on 241 patients. *Br J Dermatol* 2003; 148: 134–138.
30. Feldman SR, Ravis SM, Fleischer AB, Jr, et al. Betamethasone valerate in foam vehicle is effective with both daily and twice a day dosing: a single blind, open label study of the treatment of scalp psoriasis. *J Cutan Med Surg* 2001; 5: 386–389.
31. Bergstrom KG, Arambula K, Kimball AB. Medication formulation affects quality of life: a randomized single-blind study of clobetasol propionate foam 0.05% comparison with a combined program of clobetasol cream 0.05% and solution 0.05% for the treatment of psoriasis. *Cutis* 2003; 72: 407–411.
32. Griffiths CE, Finlay AY, Fleming CJ, Barker JN, Mizzi F, Arsonnaud SJ. A randomized, investigator-masked clinical evaluation of the efficacy and safety of clobetasol propionate 0.05% shampoo and tar blend 1% shampoo in the treatment of moderate to severe scalp psoriasis. *Dermatolog Treat* 2006; 17(2): 90–95.
33. Robertson D, Maibach H. Topical corticosteroids. *Semin Dermatol* 1983; 2: 238–249.
34. Feldman RJ, Maibach HI. Penetration of 14-C hydrocortisone through normal skin, the effect of stripping and occlusion. *Arch Dermatol* 1965; 91: 661–666.
35. Housman TS, Keil KA, Mellen BG, et al. The use of 0.25% zinc pyrithione spray does not enhance the efficacy of clobetasol propionate 0.05% foam in the treatment of psoriasis. *J Am Acad Dermatol* 2003; 49: 79–82.
36. Gollnick HP, Finzi AF, Marks R, et al. Optimizing the use of tazarotene in clinical practice: consensus statement from the European advisory panel for tazarotene (Zorac™). *Dermatology* 1999; 199: 40–46.
37. Klaber MR, Hutchinson PE, Pedvis-Leftick A, et al. Comparative effects of calcipotriol solution 50 mg/mL in the treatment of scalp psoriasis. *Br J Dermatol* 1994; 131: 678–683.
38. Duweb GA, Abuzariba O, Rahim M, et al. Scalp psoriasis: topical calcipotriol 50 micrograms/g/mL solution vs. Betamethasone valerate 1% lotion. *Int J Clin Pharmacol Res* 2000; 20: 65–68.
39. van de Kerkhof PCM, Green C, Hamberg KJ, et al. Safety and efficacy of combined high-dose treatment with calcipotriol ointment and solution in patients with psoriasis. *Dermatology* 2002; 204: 214–221.
40. Barnes L, Altmeyer P, Forstrom L, et al. Long-term treatment of psoriasis with calcipotriol scalp solution and cream. *Eur J Dermatol* 2000; 10: 199–204.
41. Thaci D, Daiber W, Boehncke WH, et al. Calcipotriol solution for the treatment of scalp psoriasis: evaluation of efficacy, safety and acceptance in 3396 patients. *Dermatology* 2001; 203: 153–156.
42. Ruzicka T, Trompke C. Treatment of scalp psoriasis. An effective and safe tacalcitol emulsion. *Hautarzt* 2004; 55: 165–170.
43. Lebwohl M, Yoles A, Lombardi K, et al. Calcipotriene ointment and halobetasol ointment in the long-term of psoriasis: effects on the duration of improvement. *J Am Acad Dermatol* 1998; 39: 447–450.
44. Papp K, Berth-Jones J, Kragballe K, et al. Scalp psoriasis: a review of current topical treatment options. *J Eur Acad Dermatol Venereol* 2007; 21: 1151–1160.
45. Guenther LC. Treatments for scalp psoriasis with emphasis on calcipotriol plus betamethasone dipropionate gel (Xamiol). *Skin Therapy Lett* 2009; 14(4): 1–4.
46. Ortonne JP, Ganslandt C, Tan J, Nordin P, Kragballe K, Segaert S. Quality of life in patients with scalp psoriasis treated with calcipotriol/betamethasone dipropionate scalp formulation: a randomized controlled trial. *J Eur Acad Dermatol Venereol* 2009; 23(8): 919–926.
47. Kragballe K, Hoffmann V, Ortonne JP, Tan J, Nordin P, Segaert S. Efficacy and safety of calcipotriol plus betamethasone dipropionate scalp formulation compared with calcipotriol scalp solution in the treatment of scalp psoriasis: a randomized controlled trial. *Br J Dermatol* 2009; 161(1): 159–166.
48. van de Kerkhof PC, Hoffmann V, Anstey A, et al. A new scalp formulation of calcipotriol plus betamethasone dipropionate compared with each of its active ingredients in the same vehicle for the treatment of scalp psoriasis: a randomized, double-blind, controlled trial. *Br J Dermatol* 2009; 160(1): 170–176.
49. Taneja A, Racette A, Gourgouliatos Z, et al. Broad-band UVB fiber-optic comb for the treatment of scalp psoriasis: a pilot study. *Int J Dermatol* 2004; 43: 462–467.
50. Taylor CR, Racette AL. A 308 nm excimer laser for the treatment of scalp psoriasis. *Lasers Surg Med* 2004; 34: 136–140.
51. Gupta AK, Ryder JE. Photodynamic therapy and topical aminolevulinic acid: an overview. *Am J Clin Dermatol* 2003; 4: 699.

Chapter 15

Inverse Psoriasis

Lara Wine-Lee, Robert A. Lee, and Abby S. Van Voorhees

INTRODUCTION

Psoriasis is commonly described as a chronic relapsing disease characterized by erythematous well-circumscribed plaques with thick, silvery scale and a predilection for the extensor surfaces of the extremities, lower back, and umbilical area [1–3]. Yet, the morphology and presentation of cutaneous lesions can vary considerably and can be divided into subtypes, including chronic plaque psoriasis, guttate psoriasis, erythrodermic psoriasis, generalized pustular psoriasis, pustular palmar and plantar psoriasis, and inverse psoriasis [2]. Moreover, these subtypes are not mutually exclusive, with one type evolving into another over time. Inverse psoriasis is also known as flexural or intertriginous psoriasis because of its selective involvement of skin folds such as the axillae, groin, inframammary folds, navel, gluteal crease, and the palms, soles, and nails. Because of its particular location inverse psoriasis' impact is greater than the total body surface area and poses unique therapeutic challenges.

EPIDEMIOLOGY

In the United States, psoriasis affects approximately 2.2%–2.5% of the general population. Inverse psoriasis accounts for roughly 2%–6% of these cases [4,5]. The male-to-female ratio is approximately equal. The age of onset has a bimodal distribution, with the first peak at 22.5 years of age and second peak at 55 years of age [6].

Psoriasis appears to demonstrate a polygenic mode of inheritance. Approximately one-third of the patients with psoriasis also have a relative with the disease. Monozygotic twins exhibit a 65% rate of concordance, opposed to 30% for dizygotic twins. Certain major histocompatibility complex types (human leukocyte antigen [HLA]-Cw6, HLA-B57, HLA-DR7) [7,8] are associated with a higher incidence of psoriasis, with some corresponding to specific clinical patterns: pustular type (HLA-B27), guttate type (HLA-B13 and HLA-B17), and palmoplantar pustulosis (HLA-B8, HLABw35, HLA-Cw7, HLA-DR3) [9]. Linkage analysis and genome-wide association studies (GWASs) have identified >15 loci associated with psoriasis susceptibility. The identified genes fall within the broad categories of antigen presentation, skin barrier function, T-cell signaling, and the nuclear factor-κB (NF-κB) pathway [10]. No HLA type or specific loci have been associated with inverse psoriasis.

CLINICAL PRESENTATION

Inverse psoriasis often appears as glossy, sharply demarcated erythematous plaques with little to no scale (Figure 15.1a–d). Often, lesions are moist and can be fissured. Characteristic

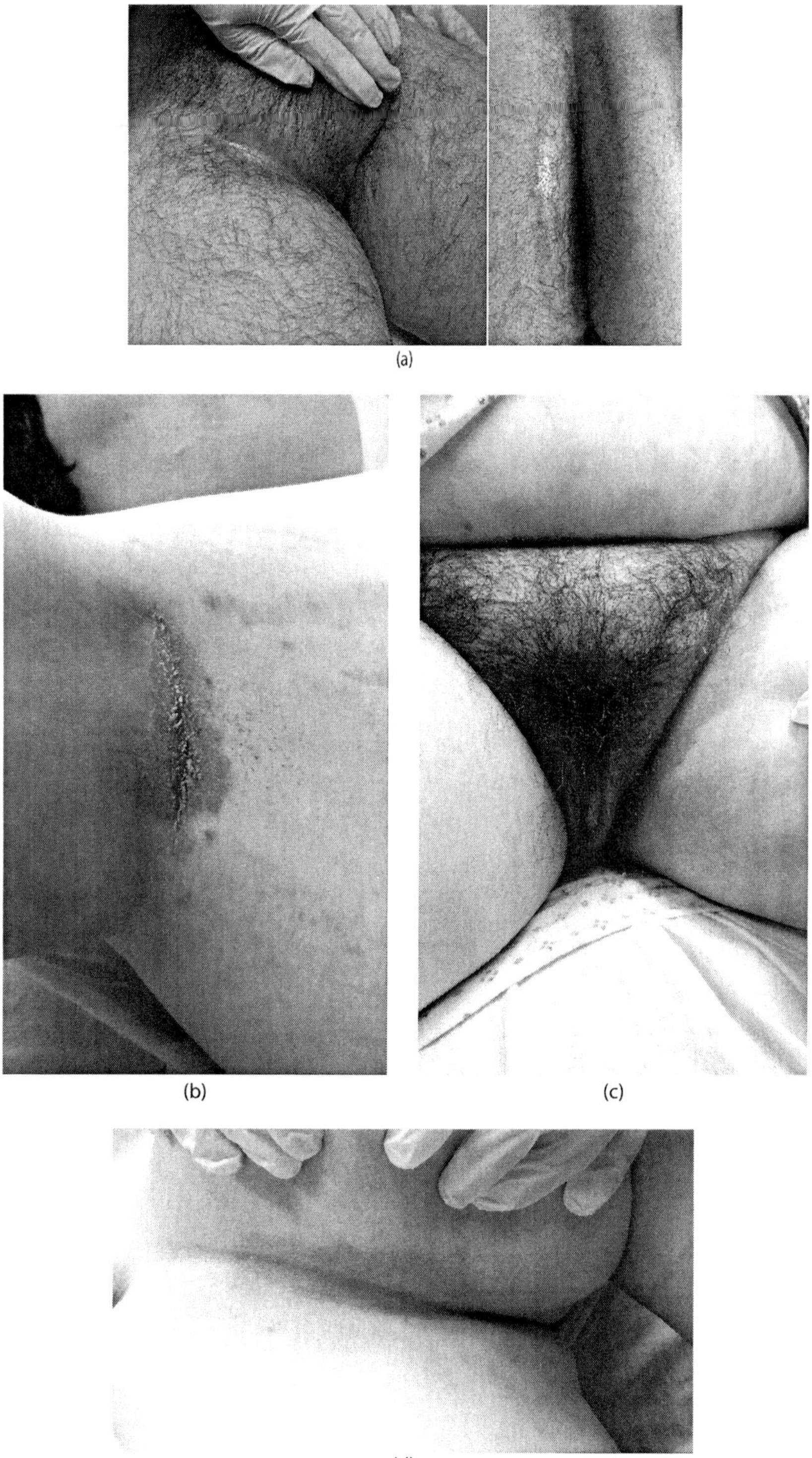

FIGURE 15.1 (See color insert.) Well-demarcated, red plaques in the inguinal crease and intergluteal cleft (a), axilla (b), inguinal crease (c) and inframammory fold (d) of patients with inverse psoriasis.

histopathology is identical for psoriasis vulgaris and inverse psoriasis and includes regular acanthosis, club-shaped dermal papillae, focally absent granular layer, focal parakeratosis, elongated and tortuous capillaries, and collections of neutrophils in the epidermis [11].

The effect of psoriasis on a patient is multidimensional, including the physical, social, and psychologic health of the person. Overall clinical severity of psoriasis, as assessed by the psoriasis area and severity index (PASI), and duration of psoriasis may not always be related directly to health-related quality-of-life measures [12]. Patients with psoriasis often ascribe a substantial negative effect on their quality of life [13]. The psychosocial effects of psoriasis on patients may be profound, resulting in considerable stigmatization, social isolation, and discrimination. Eighty-four percent of patients with psoriasis expressed difficulties in establishing social contacts and relationships and stated that this was the worst aspect of their psoriasis. Psoriasis patients also had reduction in physical and mental functioning comparable to that seen in cancer, arthritis, hypertension, heart disease, diabetes, and depression [14]. Although approximately 40% of patients report that psoriasis negatively affected their sexual activity and enjoyment, no study has been performed to specifically address the impact of inverse psoriasis [15]. For inverse psoriasis, the extent of skin involvement may not be a reliable guide to disability. By the same token, the presence of psoriasis on the face may contribute to depression. As a consequence, patients should be assessed using an approach that considers physical and psychologic measures [16].

ETIOLOGY

The pathogenesis of psoriasis is not well understood. The presence of numerous immune cells in psoriatic lesions implies an important role in disease progression and maintenance through secretion of various inflammatory cytokines. Also, hyperproliferation of keratinocytes is observed [3]. Often there is an inciting insult, such as infection, medication (Table 15.1) [16–18], or trauma (Koebner phenomenon). Friction, heat, and moisture in these areas are thought to induce psoriasis as a Koebner phenomenon. Although fungal infections have often been associated with inverse psoriasis, a recent study comparing untreated patients, topical steroid–treated patients, and control patients shows no evidence of *Candida* infection [19,20].

TABLE 15.1 Drugs That Exacerbate Psoriasis

Antimalarials
Lithium
β-Blockers
Nonsteroidal anti-inflammatory drugs
Trazodone
IFN-α
Terbinafine
Angiotensin-converting enzyme inhibitors
Gemfibrozil
Tetracycline
Penicillin

TABLE 15.2 Differential Diagnosis of Inverse Psoriasis

Intertrigo
Seborrheic dermatitis
Erythrasma
Cutaneous candidiasis
Contact dermatitis
Darier disease
Bowen disease
Extramammary Paget disease
Mycosis fungoides
Acrodermatitis enteropathica
Radiation dermatitis
Glucagonoma syndrome
Hailey–Hailey disease
Epidermolysis bullosa
Langerhans cell histiocytosis
Acanthosis nigricans
Axillary granular parakeratosis
Confluent and reticulated papillomatosis

DIFFERENTIAL DIAGNOSIS

Inverse psoriasis can be difficult to diagnose in the intertriginous areas because lesions often lack the characteristic silvery scale seen in plaque-type psoriasis (Table 15.2). The lesions are generally deep red, smooth, even glistening with a well-demarcated edge. Pustules or papules extending beyond the border suggest secondary *Candida* infection. Intertrigo, erythrasma, and seborrheic dermatitis may be indistinguishable in some cases.

MANAGEMENT

Topical Corticosteroids

Corticosteroids persist as the mainstay for topical treatment. Topical corticosteroids are categorized by the Stoughton–Cornell classification system based on the vasoconstriction of small blood vessels in the upper dermis. This system ranges from the superpotent class I steroids to the weaker class VII steroids. They are believed to reduce inflammation by reducing inflammatory cells and cytokines, including interleukin (IL)-1, IL-2, interferon (IFN)-γ, tumor necrosis factor (TNF)-α, and granulocyte macrophage–colony-stimulating factor (GM–CSF) [21–23].

Topical corticosteroids are first-line treatment for intertriginous psoriasis. An open-label study of 20 patients applying fluticasone propionate 0.005% (class III) twice a day for two weeks followed by twice-weekly application for 10 weeks demonstrated >75% clearance in 95% of facial and intertriginous lesions compared with 35% of nonfacial, nonintertriginous lesions [24]. There was no evidence of skin atrophy after 10 weeks. In recommendations published by the medical board of the National Psoriasis Foundation, a short (2 to 4 week) course of low to midpotency topical steroid is considered the most efficacious first-line therapy for intertriginous psoriasis [25]. Maintenance with low to potency topical steroids one or two times per week was also suggested [25].

Topical corticosteroids have side effects that limit their long-term use in the treatment of psoriasis. Common side effects can occur locally at the site of prolonged topical corticosteroid application, resulting in skin atrophy, irreversible striae, and telangiectasias. These findings are most often seen when high-potency corticosteroids are used on the face and intertriginous areas for prolonged periods. Intertriginous areas are even more sensitive to topical corticosteroids because of the thinness of the psoriasis lesions and likely occlusion in these areas. Long-term studies however are lacking for inverse psoriasis. Tachyphylaxis is also a common phenomenon with prolonged use [26]. Pulse therapy has been shown to prevent tachyphylaxis in psoriasis vulgaris but has not been studied for inverse psoriasis.

Topical Vitamin D Analogs

Topical vitamin D, available as calcipotriene or calcitriol, is commonly used for the treatment of psoriasis. Calcipotriene is a synthetic analog to the naturally occuring active for of Vitamin D3, (1,25-dihydroxyvitamin D_3). It binds to the vitamin D receptor found in keratinocytes, thereby halting proliferation and causing terminal differentiation. It also inhibits production of IL-2, IL-6, IFN-γ, and GM-CSF by T cells. Because it is not associated with skin atrophy, calcipotriene has potential advantages when used in intertriginous areas [27].

For psoriasis vulgaris, calcipotriene has been shown to be as effective as a class II corticosteroid. In a randomized, double-blind study with 114 subjects, mean scores of scaling and plaque elevation in calcipotriene-treated subjects were significantly lower by week 2 than in the fluocinonide-treated subjects and continued to be significantly lower through week 6 [28]. Calcipotriene can also be used in conjunction with topical corticosteroids to extend the duration of remissions while minimizing the adverse effects of chronic steroid use. In a randomized, double-blind study of 44 patients, 76% of patients using a combination of calcipotriene twice a day on weekdays and a class I corticosteroid twice a day on weekends were able to maintain remission at six months of treatment compared with 40% using a class I corticosteroid steroid twice a day on weekends and vehicle twice a day on weekdays [29]. There have been no randomized control studies studying the efficacy of calcipotriene for inverse psoriasis. In an open, uncontrolled trial, 10 or 12 patients with inverse psoriasis showed clinically significant improvement by six weeks of treatment [30]. Vitamin D analogs are recommended for chronic use in the treatment of intertriginous psoriasis [25].

However, calcipotriene can cause irritant contact dermatitis, particularly on the face and in intertriginous sites. Dilution of calcipotriene with petrolatum or the addition of a topical steroid may prevent the irritant contact dermatitis. Rarely, hypercalcemia can occur but is always associated with excess use over large surface area [31].

Topical Immunomodulators

Immunosuppression in the treatment of psoriasis can be achieved by inhibition of cytokine production, a process that is essential in the development of psoriasis [32]. Tacrolimus, a lipophilic agent produced by *Streptomyces tsukubaensis*, exhibits similar in vivo and in vitro biologic characteristics to cyclosporine A. Furthermore, it is more potent than cyclosporine A. Inhibition of calcineurin blocks the activity of nuclear factor of activated T cells (NF-AT) that, in turn, suppresses IL-2 production as well as T cell response. Both systemically and topically, tacrolimus inhibits T-cell infiltration and skin reddening, and levels of IL-2 receptors decrease during treatment. There is also inhibition of keratinocyte proliferation induced by epidermal growth factor (EGF), transforming growth factor (TGF)-α, or IL-6 through influence on the keratinocyte cell cycle at G0/G1 phases and dose-dependent inhibition of IL-8, which is elevated in psoriatic plaques.

Tacrolimus has a lower molecular weight and penetrates the skin better than cyclosporine. Therefore, it can be used topically. Adverse events include burning, heat sensation, itching, and erythema. In contrast to topical corticosteroids, there is no influence on collagen biosynthesis with resulting skin atrophy. Psoriatic plaques on the trunk and the extremities can be thick, and topical tacrolimus formulations are only minimally effective in treating these lesions [33]. However, several open-labeled trials indicating topical tacrolimus might be effective for intertriginous lesions [34,35]. A randomized, double-blind, vehicle-controlled study of inverse psoriasis with 167 patients using 0.1% tacrolimus showed 65.2% of the tacrolimus ointment group and 31.5% of the vehicle group were 90% clear by eight weeks [36]. None of the patients had skin atrophy, telangiectasias, or striae during the eight-week study. Recent studies have also confirmed its effectiveness in the pediatric setting [37,38]. Induction of lentigines in areas of prolonged tacrolimus use is reported [39,40].

Pimecrolimus also belongs to the macrolide group of immunomodulators. Compared with tacrolimus, it is 20 times more lipophilic and has a lower permeation potential through the skin. A 57-patient, randomized, double-blind, vehicle-controlled trial studying inverse psoriasis showed that 82% of the pimecrolimus group and 41% of the vehicle were 90% clear by eight weeks [41]. A direct comparison of topical 1% pimecrolimus, 0.005% calcipotriol, and 0.1% betamethasone demonstrated pimecrolimus to be the least effective of the three in treating inverse psoriasis but clearly superior to vehicle alone [42].

Risk of long-term use of topical tacrolimus and pimecrolimus remains inconclusive, and these agents should be used only as recommended [43–45]. Use of systemic tacrolimus has been shown to be associated with both lymphoid and nonlymphoid malignancies in the posttransplant setting [46,47]. Topical tacrolimus has been implicated in squamous cell carcinoma of the penis [48]. Oral pimecrolimus has been associated with development of lymphoma in monkey models [49]. In mouse models, topical tacrolimus has been shown to accelerate the development of squamous cell carcinomas [50]. In March 2005, the Food and Drug Administration (FDA) issued a public health advisory for topical pimecrolimus reporting 10 cases of cancer-related adverse events, including lymphoma, basal cell carcinoma, and squamous cell carcinoma [49]. At the same time, an advisory was also issued for topical tacrolimus, reporting 19 cases linking it with cancer-related adverse events, including lymphomas, squamous cell carcinoma, and malignant melanoma [49]. However, no long-term studies are yet available to evaluate the risk of topical formulations in humans. Therefore, prolonged use over large areas of the body should be done with caution.

Retinoids

Topical or oral retinoids have multiple effects on keratinocyte differentiation and proliferation and inflammatory processes that contribute to psoriasis. There are two classes of nuclear retinoid receptors that have been identified: the retinoic acid receptor (RAR) and retinoid X receptor (RXR) [51]. The function of these RARs and RXRs is not well understood in skin. In animal models, retinoids block induction of ornithine decarboxylase activity that is associated with cell proliferation and expression. In vitro skin models and cell cultures also demonstrate that retinoids suppresses epidermal hyperproliferation.

Acitretin is the active metabolite of etretinate, but it has a shorter half-life. It selectively binds RARs, albeit weakly. Re-esterification of acitretin into etretinate still limits use in women of childbearing potential. It is indicated in treating pustular and plaque psoriasis. Increased efficacy is seen when systemic retinoids are combined with phototherapy as well. There are no studies addressing the utility of acitretin in inverse psoriasis.

Tazarotene selectively binds to RARs. Generally, tazarotene is most effective for reducing plaque thickness. Because intertriginous psoriasis tends to have thin plaques and significant local irritation of tazarotene can be seen, it is not commonly used for intertriginous areas but may be effective on the face. There have been no randomized control studies studying the efficacy of tazarotene for inverse psoriasis. Common side effects from local application include irritation, pruritus, erythema, stinging, and desquamation [52]. Short contact with tazarotene minimizes the local irritation on the skin, which is especially applicable to intertriginous areas.

Light Therapy

Ultraviolet light causes DNA damage to cutaneous tissue and thereby can inhibit cell proliferation [2]. Specifically, it appears to target cutaneous immune cells and reduce the production of inflammatory cytokines important in psoriasis pathogenesis. It is widely used in the treatment of psoriasis vulgaris [22].

Broadband ultraviolet B (BB-UVB) and narrowband UVB (NB-UVB) can be used to treat plaque psoriasis. NB-UVB is generally more effective than BB-UVB in treating psoriasis but has the disadvantage of producing more severe and longer lasting burns than BB-UVB. The long-term effect of NB-UVB on carcinogenesis in plaque psoriasis remains unknown. Its overall safety is generally believed to be better than that of psoralen plus ultraviolet A (PUVA) [53]. Genitalia are often shielded due to the possible increased risk of carcinogenesis. Typical UVB light units are designed to treat large surface areas and generally do not reach intertriginous areas because of body habitus and positioning of the patient. A recent study using NB-UVB specifically for intertriginous areas in Asian patients demonstrated significant improvement in 41 of 48 patients. Side effects were limited to darkening of the skin and pruritus, side effects that resolved after stopping the treatments [54]. Smaller handheld units are promising alternatives to allow better targeting of occluded areas such as the axilla and inframammary folds. Specific studies addressing the efficacy and safety of BB-UVB and NB-UVB in inverse psoriasis have not been done.

PUVA is commonly used for widespread and resistant psoriasis. Psoralen, 8-methoxypsoralen, causes the formation of pyrimidine dimers that lead to cross-linkage of DNA strands and genomic instability and apoptosis. In a randomized trial involving 100 patients comparing NB-UVB with PUVA given twice weekly, 88% of patients were cleared with PUVA compared with 63% with NB-UVB [55]. Also PUVA-treated patients required significantly fewer treatments and had almost three times the remission rate at six months after treatment. The potential side effects of PUVA include an increased incidence of squamous cell carcinoma [56], basal cell carcinoma, and possibly malignant melanoma [57]. The genitalia are usually shielded during UVA exposure because of the risk of developing carcinoma in that region. PUVA is not commonly used for inverse psoriasis because of the tendency for intertriginous skin to burn, the risk of carcinogenesis, and the technical difficulty of delivering UV light to the intertriginous areas. No studies using PUVA specifically for inverse psoriasis have been performed.

Targeted ultraviolet light therapy allows for sparing of uninvolved skin and has recently been considered. In a preliminary case report, a single inverse psoriasis patient using the excimer laser (308 nm) obtained 90% improvement of her lesions after three weeks of treatment [58]. Excimer light therapy has also been reported to be effective in conjunction with topical tacrolimus [59]. Further studies are necessary to better demonstrate the efficacy and safety of this modality. The disadvantages of this approach include risk of burning, hyperpigmentation, and unknown risk of carcinogenesis.

Methotrexate

Methotrexate is a synthetic analog of folic acid and a competitive inhibitor of the enzyme dihydrofolate reductase [60]. The inhibition of thymidylate synthesis appears to be the most important effect exerted by methotrexate, resulting in inhibition of DNA synthesis and arrest of cell division in the S phase. T and B cells are preferentially targeted and thereby inhibit the elaboration of inflammatory cytokines. Methotrexate also suppresses epidermal cell division in psoriasis.

Methotrexate is indicated in patients with moderate to severe psoriasis and is indicated when other treatment modalities have failed [61,62]. It is most appropriately used for patients with plaque psoriasis with >10% body surface involvement; pustular psoriasis; erythrodermic psoriasis; psoriatic arthritis; and more localized, recalcitrant psoriasis. Because of its distribution, inverse psoriasis can be much more debilitating than that suggested by the total body surface area affected. In this case, intervention with methotrexate can be considered.

A randomized, single-blind, controlled trial comparing cyclosporine and methotrexate involving 88 patients with psoriasis vulgaris showed no significant difference in effectiveness or side effects between the two drugs. Sixty percent in the methotrexate group compared with 71% in the cyclosporine group achieved at least 75% clinical improvement over the 16 weeks of the study [63]. Also, the time needed to reach an almost complete remission and a partial remission did not differ significantly between the groups. No specific studies for the use of methotrexate in inverse psoriasis have been performed.

Methotrexate is contraindicated in patients who have renal impairment, persistent abnormalities in liver function enzymes, pregnancy, hepatitis, frequent alcohol use, and myelosuppression [64]. Common side effects associated with methotrexate include nausea and vomiting. Ulcerative stomatitis, pulmonary fibrosis, bone marrow suppression, and induction of lymphoma have also been described. The most serious long-term adverse effect associated with methotrexate is the induction of hepatotoxicity. The liver biopsy is the most definitive test for ascertaining whether fibrotic changes in the liver are present during methotrexate therapy.

Cyclosporine

Cyclosporine is an immunosuppressive agent derived from the fungus *Tolypocladium inflatum* Gams. Cyclosporine is used to prevent allograft rejection and is FDA approved for the treatment of psoriasis. Cyclosporine induces immunosuppression by inhibiting the first phase of T-cell activation. Cyclosporine binds to cyclophilins and then complexes to inhibit the enzyme calcineurin, a calcium-activated phosphatase. Calcineurin inhibition, in turn, results in the inhibition of the transcription factor NF-AT that is important for inflammatory cytokine expression [65].

Cyclosporine is indicated for the treatment of severe plaque psoriasis in patients who are not immunocompromised [66]. In addition, cyclosporine is effective in treating various forms of psoriasis that have been recalcitrant to other modalities. When used as monotherapy, cyclosporine can induce rapid clearance of plaques in a majority of patients with 60%–80% reduction at 8–12 weeks, respectively. Its use for inverse psoriasis has not been specifically studied [63,65].

Nephrotoxicity is the main adverse effect of cyclosporine therapy [64]. Acute renal toxicity is dose dependent and reversible upon lowering the dosage or discontinuation of the drug. Other common side effects include gastrointestinal symptoms such as nausea, vomiting, anorexia, and diarrhea. Hypertension, headache, myalgias, arthralgias, paresthesias, hyperesthesia, influenza-like symptoms, and fatigue are not uncommon. Dermatologic side effects include hypertrichosis and gingival hypertrophy. Cyclosporine has been associated with the induction of various lymphoproliferative disorders in transplant patients. In contrast, an increased incidence of nonmelanoma skin cancer has not been observed in psoriatic patients treated with cyclosporine, presumably because of much shorter courses of therapy with lower doses that have been used.

Biologic Agents

Psoriasis is thought to involve a complex pattern of overexpressed T-helper 1 (Th1) cytokines such as IL-2, IL-6, and IL-8 or IFN-γ and TNF-α [67]. In particular, TNF-α is involved in the activation of NF-κB, a transcription factor that regulates the expression of cytokines such as IL-6, IL-8, and colony stimulating factor (CSF). It also induces the expression of intercellular adhesion molecule (ICAM)-1 and vascular cell adhesion molecule type 1 (VCAM-1) on endothelial cells and keratinocytes, where both are involved in trafficking lymphocytes to inflammatory lesions. TNF-α also stimulates migration of Langerhans' cells to lymph nodes and enhances capability to present antigens to primed T cells. Several agents targeting specific steps in the immunopathogenesis of psoriasis are now available in clinical practice [68]. At present, there are no published data specifically addressing the effectiveness of the various biologics for the treatment of inverse psoriasis.

Etanercept is a recombinant soluble fusion protein consisting of two identical chains of the TNF-α receptor fused with the Fc portion of human IgG1. It is functioning as a competitive inhibitor for binding of TNF-α at its receptor. Inflammatory cytokines such as TNF have been implicated in the pathogenesis of psoriasis. In a randomized, double-blind study, 672 plaque psoriasis patients received either placebo or etanercept subcutaneously at 25 mg once weekly, 25 mg twice weekly, or 50 mg twice weekly. At 12 weeks, 14%, 34%, and 49% of patients, respectively, demonstrated a 75% reduction in severity compared with 4% of patients receiving placebo [69]. In another randomized, double-blind, placebo-controlled study, of the 148 plaque psoriasis patients receiving placebo or etanercept 25 mg, subcutaneously twice weekly, 30% of the etanercept-treated patients demonstrated 75% severity reduction compared with 1% of the patients in the placebo group at 12 weeks [70].

Infliximab is a humanized-mouse monoclonal chimeric antibody against the TNF-α molecules. Adalimumab is a humanized monoclonal antibody against the TNF-α molecules. Both bind to soluble and membrane-bound TNF, leading to cell lysis. In a randomized, double-blind study, 33 patients with plaque psoriasis received intravenous placebo, infliximab 5 mg/kg, at weeks 0, 2, and 6. At 10 weeks, 82% of patients in the infliximab 5 mg/kg group had a 75% improvement in the PASI scores compared with 18% of patients in the placebo group [71]. Long-term studies seemed to indicate that continuous therapy is superior to intermittent therapy with infliximab at 5 mg/kg given every 8 weeks, showing a PASI-75 of 78% at 26 weeks and a PASI-75 of 55% at 50 weeks [72]. Loss of long-term efficacy appears to correlate with a progressive reduction of serum infliximab concentrations to undetectable levels. This could be related to the dosing regimen as well as the development of neutralizing antibodies [73]. A large randomized control study of 1212 patients using adalimumab revealed 68% achieving a PASI-75 at week 12 compared with 5% of patients taking placebo. Loss of response was seen at much higher rate among responders who were reassigned to a placebo group compared to those who continued on the medications (5% vs. 28%) [74]. This strongly suggests that continued adalimumab therapy is required to maintain a response.

Ustekinumab is a human monoclonal antibody against IL-12 and IL-23. These proinflammatory cytokines have been shown to induce differentiation toward Th1 and Th17 cells that are important in the pathogenesis of psoriasis. In a randomized, placebo-controlled trial of 766 patients with moderate to severe psoriasis, those receiving 45 or 90 mg of ustekinumab at 12-week intervals showed PASI-75 of 67% and 66%, respectively [75]. Response was maintained for at least one year. In another randomized, placebo-controlled trial of 1230 patients, PASI 75 was achieved in 67% and 76% of patients receiving 45 mg and 90 mg, at 12-week intervals, respectively [76]. An increased response rate was achieved in partial responders by increasing 90 mg dosing to every eight weeks, but a similar trend was not seen with 45 mg dosing. Similar efficacy rates were demonstrated in a randomized trial showing better efficacy compared with etanercept 50 mg twice weekly, which showed a PASI-75 of 57% [77]. Ustekinumab has not been studied specifically in intertriginous psoriasis.

Other Treatments

Anthralin and tar can be moderately irritating and can stain skin and clothing. They are generally not well tolerated in intertriginous areas and are not widely used in the treatment of inverse psoriasis, having been replaced with better tolerated topical agents [22].

The role of microbial colonization of intertriginous psoriasis is still not fully elucidated. Although evidence of *Candida* species was not found in one series of patients, *Staphylococcus aureus* colonization was found but is not thought to contribute to the clinical presentation [19]. Nonetheless, the addition of a topical antifungal or antibacterial may be appropriate in cases of microbial colonization or overgrowth.

A single case series reported the use of botulinum toxin to treat inverse psoriasis. Thirteen of 15 patients appeared to respond favorably as early as two weeks after treatment, with a durable response through the 12-week follow-up period. No adverse reactions were reported. The mechanism is unclear, but it is thought to involve the decrease of sweating and thereby maceration in the area. The involvement of neuropeptides as mediators of inflammation may also play a role [78].

Dapsone is a sulfone antimicrobial initially used in the treatment of leprosy. Dapsone also has anti-inflammatory actions through its blockade of myeloperoxidase. It is not FDA labeled for treatment of psoriasis, but it has been successfully used for the treatment of pustular psoriasis in select patients. Systemic dapsone has been reported as being successful in the treatment of intertriginous psoriasis [79]. The most common serious adverse effects of dapsone include hemolysis and rarely hypersensitivity and agranulocytosis.

CONCLUSIONS

Inverse psoriasis is a common, chronic, relapsing, and potentially debilitating disease, the effect of which may be out of proportion with the total body surface area affected. Careful attention needs to be paid to the patient in assessing the true impact of the disease as well as designing an individualized treatment regimen that thoughtfully addresses the challenges of treating these patients. However, little research has focused directly on treatment of this often recalcitrant type of psoriasis. Investigation into effective treatments is also needed.

REFERENCES

1. Odom RB, James WD, Berger TG. *Andrews' Diseases of the Skin: Clinical Dermatology*, 9th ed. Philadelphia, PA: W. B. Saunders, 2000.
2. Fitzpatrick TB, Freedberg IM. *Fitzpatrick's Dermatology in General Medicine*, 6th ed. New York: McGraw-Hill, Medical Pub. Division, 2003.
3. van de Kerkhof PCM. *Textbook of Psoriasis*, 2nd ed. Malden, MA: Blackwell Science, 2003.

4. Koo J. Population-based epidemiologic study of psoriasis with emphasis on quality of life assessment. *Dermatol Clin* 1996; 14: 485–496.
5. Stern RS, Nijsten T, Feldman SR, et al. Psoriasis is common, carries a substantial burden even when not extensive, and is associated with widespread treatment dissatisfaction. *J Investig Dermatol Symp Proc* 2004; 9: 136–139.
6. Farber EM, Nall ML. The natural history of psoriasis in 5600 patients. *Dermatologica* 1974; 148: 1–18.
7. Watson W, Cann HM, Farber EM, et al. The genetics of psoriasis. *Arch Dermatol* 1972; 105: 197–207.
8. Tiilikainen A, Lassus A, Karvonen J, et al. Psoriasis and HLA-Cw6. *Br J Dermatol* 1980; 102: 179–184.
9. Zachariae H, Overgaard Petersen H, Kissmeyer Nielsen F, et al. HL-A antigens in pustular psoriasis. *Dermatologica* 1977; 154: 73–77.
10. Hébert HL, Ali FR, Bowes, et al. Genetic susceptibility to psoriasis and psoriatic arthritis: implications for therapy. *Br J Dermatol* 2012; 166: 474–482.
11. Lever WF, Elder DE. *Lever's Histopathology of the Skin*, 9th ed. Philadelphia, PA: Lippincott Williams, 2005.
12. Kirby B, Richards HL, Woo P, et al. Physical and psychologic measures are necessary to assess overall psoriasis severity. *J Am Acad Dermatol* 2001; 45: 72–76.
13. Fortune DG, Richards HL, Griffiths CE, et al. Psychological stress, distress and disability in patients with psoriasis: consensus and variation in the contribution of illness perceptions, coping and alexithymia. *Br J Clin Psychol* 2002; 41: 157–174.
14. Choi J, Koo JY. Quality of life issues in psoriasis. *J Am Acad Dermatol* 2003; 49: S57–S61.
15. Gupta MA, Gupta AK. Psoriasis and sex: a study of moderately to severely affected patients. *Int J Dermatol* 1997; 36: 259–262.
16. Yosipovitch G, Tang MB. Practical management of psoriasis in the elderly: epidemiology, clinical aspects, quality of life, patient education and treatment options. *Drugs Aging* 2002; 19: 847–863.
17. Pauluzzi P, Boccucci N. Inverse psoriasis induced by terbinafine. *Acta Derm Venereol* 1999; 79: 389.
18. Gilleaudeau P, Vallat VP, Carter DM, et al. Angiotensin-converting enzyme inhibitors as possible exacerbating drugs in psoriasis. *J Am Acad Dermatol* 1993; 28: 490–492.
19. Flytstrom I, Bergbrant IM, Brared J, et al. Microorganisms in intertriginous psoriasis: no evidence of Candida. *Acta Derm Venereol* 2003; 83: 121–123.
20. Leibovici V, Alkalay R, Hershko K, et al. Prevalence of Candida on the tongue and intertriginous areas of psoriatic and atopic dermatitis patients. *Mycoses* 2008; 51: 63–66.
21. Wolverton SE. *Comprehensive Dermatologic Drug Therapy*. Philadelphia, PA: Saunders, 2001.
22. Lebwohl M, Ali S. Treatment of psoriasis. Part 1. Topical therapy and phototherapy. *J Am Acad Dermatol* 2001; 45: 487–498; quiz 499–502.
23. Lebwohl M, Ting PT, Koo JY. Psoriasis treatment: traditional therapy. *Ann Rheum Dis* 2005; 64 (Suppl 2): ii83–ii86.
24. Lebwohl MG, Tan MH, Meador SL, et al. Limited application of fluticasone propionate ointment, 0.005% in patients with psoriasis of the face and intertriginous areas. *J Am Acad Dermatol* 2001; 44: 77–82.
25. Kalb RE, Bagel J, Korman NJ, et al. Treatment of intertriginous psoriasis: from the Medical Board of the National Psoriasis Foundation. *J Am Acad Dermatol* 2009; 60(1): 120–124.
26. du Vivier A, Stoughton RB. Tachyphylaxis to the action of topically applied corticosteroids. *Arch Dermatol* 1975; 111: 581–583.
27. Duweb GA, Eldebani S, Alhaddar J. Calcipotriol cream in the treatment of flexural psoriasis. *Int J Tissue React* 2003; 25: 127–130.
28. Bruce S, Epinette WW, Funicella T, et al. Comparative study of calcipotriene (MC 903) ointment and fluocinonide ointment in the treatment of psoriasis. *J Am Acad Dermatol* 1994; 31: 755–759.
29. Lebwohl M, Yoles A, Lombardi K, et al. Calcipotriene ointment and halobetasol ointment in the long-term treatment of psoriasis: effects on the duration of improvement. *J Am Acad Dermatol* 1998; 39: 447–450.
30. Kienbaum S, Lehmann P, Ruzicka T. Topical calcipotriol in the treatment of intertriginous psoriasis. *Br J Dermatol* 1996; 135: 647–650.
31. Russell S, Young MJ. Hypercalcaemia during treatment of psoriasis with calcipotriol. *Br J Dermatol* 1994; 130: 795–796.

32. Reynolds NJ, Al-Daraji WI. Calcineurin inhibitors and sirolimus: mechanisms of action and applications in dermatology. *Clin Exp Dermatol* 2002; 27: 555–561.
33. Zonneveld IM, Rubins A, Jablonska S, et al. Topical tacrolimus is not effective in chronic plaque psoriasis. A pilot study. *Arch Dermatol* 1998; 134: 1101–1102.
34. Freeman AK, Linowski GJ, Brady C, et al. Tacrolimus ointment for the treatment of psoriasis on the face and intertriginous areas. *J Am Acad Dermatol* 2003; 48: 564–568.
35. Martin Ezquerra G, Sanchez Regana M, Herrera Acosta E, et al. Topical tacrolimus for the treatment of psoriasis on the face, genitalia, intertriginous areas and corporal plaques. *J Drugs Dermatol* 2006; 5: 334–336.
36. Lebwohl M, Freeman AK, Chapman MS, et al. Tacrolimus ointment is effective for facial and intertriginous psoriasis. *J Am Acad Dermatol* 2004; 51: 723–730.
37. Brune A, Miller DW, Lin P, et al. Tacrolimus ointment is effective for psoriasis on the face and intertriginous areas in pediatric patients. *Pediatr Dermatol* 2007; 24: 76–80.
38. Steele JA, Choi C, Kwong PC. Topical tacrolimus in the treatment of inverse psoriasis in children. *J Am Acad Dermatol* 2005; 53: 713–716.
39. Castelo-Soccio L, Marcantonio DD, Shah P, et al. Induced lentiginosis with use of topical calcineurin inhibitors. *Arch Dermatol* 2012; 148: 766–768.
40. Hickey JR, Robson A, Barker JN, et al. Does topical tacrolimus induce lentigines in children with atopic dermatitis? A report of three cases. *Br J Dermatol* 2005; 152(1): 152–154.
41. Gribetz C, Ling M, Lebwohl M, et al. Pimecrolimus cream 1% in the treatment of intertriginous psoriasis: a double-blind, randomized study. *J Am Acad Dermatol* 2004; 51: 731–738.
42. Kreuter A, Sommer A, Hyun J, et al. 1% pimecrolimus, 0.005% calcipotriol, and 0.1% betamethasone in the treatment of intertriginous psoriasis: a double-blind, randomized controlled study. *Arch Dermatol* 2006; 142: 1138–1143.
43. Gupta AK, Adamiak A, Chow M. Tacrolimus: a review of its use for the management of dermatoses. *J Eur Acad Dermatol Venereol* 2002; 16: 100–114.
44. Gupta AK, Chow M. Pimecrolimus: a review. *J Eur Acad Dermatol Venereol* 2003; 17: 493–503.
45. Ashcroft DM, Dimmock P, Garside R, et al. Efficacy and tolerability of topical pimecrolimus and tacrolimus in the treatment of atopic dermatitis: meta-analysis of randomised controlled trials. *BMJ* 2005; 330: 516.
46. Siddiqui MA, Sullivan S, al-Mofadhi AM. Lymphomatoid papulosis and FK 506. *Int J Dermatol* 1997; 36: 202–205.
47. Jain AB, Yee LD, Nalesnik MA, et al. Comparative incidence of de novo nonlymphoid malignancies after liver transplantation under tacrolimus using surveillance epidemiologic end result data. *Transplantation* 1998; 66: 1193–1200.
48. Langeland T, Engh V. Topical use of tacrolimus and squamous cell carcinoma on the penis. *Br J Dermatol* 2005; 152: 183–185.
49. Administration UFaD. FDA Public Health Advisory: Elidel (pimecrolimus) cream and Protopic (tacrolimus) ointment; 2005.
50. Niwa Y, Terashima T, Sumi H. Topical application of the immunosuppressant tacrolimus accelerates carcinogenesis in mouse skin. *Br J Dermatol* 2003; 149: 960–967.
51. Duvic M, Nagpal S, Asano AT, et al. Molecular mechanisms of tazarotene action in psoriasis. *J Am Acad Dermatol* 1997; 37: S18–S24.
52. Yamauchi PS, Rizk D, Lowe NJ. Retinoid therapy for psoriasis. *Dermatol Clin* 2004; 22: 467–476, x.
53. Weischer M, Blum A, Eberhard F, et al. No evidence for increased skin cancer risk in psoriasis patients treated with broadband or narrowband UVB phototherapy: a first retrospective study. *Acta Derm Venereol* 2004; 84: 370–374.
54. Wang G, Li C, Gao T, et al. Clinical analysis of 48 cases of inverse psoriasis: a hospital based study. *Eur J Dermatol* 2005; 15: 176–178.
55. Gordon PM, Diffey BL, Matthews JN, et al. A randomized comparison of narrow-band TL-01 phototherapy and PUVA photochemotherapy for psoriasis. *J Am Acad Dermatol* 1999; 41: 728–732.
56. Stern RS, Lunder EJ. Risk of squamous cell carcinoma and methoxsalen (psoralen) and UV-A radiation (PUVA). A meta-analysis. *Arch Dermatol* 1998; 134: 1582–1585.
57. Stern RS, Nichols KT, Vakeva LH. Malignant melanoma in patients treated for psoriasis with methoxsalen (psoralen) and ultraviolet A radiation (PUVA). The PUVA Follow-Up Study. *N Engl J Med* 1997; 336: 1041–1045.

58. Mafong EA, Friedman PM, Kauvar AN, et al. Treatment of inverse psoriasis with the 308 nm excimer laser. *Dermatol Surg* 2002; 28: 530–532.
59. Carrascosa JM, Soria X, Domingo H, et al. Treatment of inverse psoriasis with excimer therapy and tacrolimus ointment. *Dermatol Surg* 2007; 33: 361–363.
60. Cronstein BN. The mechanism of action of methotrexate. *Rheum Dis Clin North Am* 1997; 23: 739–755.
61. Roenigk HH, Jr, Auerbach R, Maibach H, et al. Methotrexate in psoriasis: consensus conference. *J Am Acad Dermatol* 1998; 38: 478–485.
62. Naldi L, Griffiths CE. Traditional therapies in the management of moderate to severe chronic plaque psoriasis: an assessment of the benefits and risks. *Br J Dermatol* 2005; 152: 597–615.
63. Heydendael VM, Spuls PI, Opmeer BC, et al. Methotrexate versus cyclosporine in moderate-to-severe chronic plaque psoriasis. *N Engl J Med* 2003; 349: 658–665.
64. Lebwohl M, Ali S. Treatment of psoriasis. Part 2. Systemic therapies. *J Am Acad Dermatol* 2001; 45: 649–661; quiz 662–644.
65. Ho VC. The use of ciclosporin in psoriasis: a clinical review. *Br J Dermatol* 2004; 150(Suppl 67): 1–10.
66. Laburte C, Grossman R, Abi-Rached J, et al. Efficacy and safety of oral cyclosporin A (CyA; Sandimmun) for long-term treatment of chronic severe plaque psoriasis. *Br J Dermatol* 1994; 130: 366–375.
67. Krueger JG. The immunologic basis for the treatment of psoriasis with new biologic agents. *J Am Acad Dermatol* 2002; 46: 1–23; quiz 23–26.
68. Kipnis CD, Myers WA, Opeola M, et al. Biologic treatments for psoriasis. *J Am Acad Dermatol* 2005; 52: 671–682.
69. Leonardi CL, Powers JL, Matheson RT, et al. Etanercept as monotherapy in patients with psoriasis. *N Engl J Med* 2003; 349: 2014–2022.
70. Gottlieb AB, Matheson RT, Lowe N, et al. A randomized trial of etanercept as monotherapy for psoriasis. *Arch Dermatol* 2003; 139: 1627–1632; discussion 1632.
71. Chaudhari U, Romano P, Mulcahy LD, et al. Efficacy and safety of infliximab monotherapy for plaque-type psoriasis: a randomised trial. *Lancet* 2001; 357: 1842–1847.
72. Menter A, Feldman SR, Weinstein GD, et al. A randomized comparison of continuous vs. intermittent infliximab maintenance regimens over 1 year in the treatment of moderate to severe plaque psoriasis. *J Am Acad Dermatol* 2007; 56: 31.e1–15.
73. Reich K, Nestle FO, Papp K, et al. Infliximab induction and maintenance therapy for moderate-to-severe psoriasis: a phase III, multicentre, double-blind trial. *Lancet* 2005; 366: 1367–1374.
74. Menter A, Tyring SK, Gordon K, et al. Adalimumab therapy for moderate to severe psoriasis: a randomized, controlled phase III trial. *J Am Acad Dermatol* 2008; 58: 106–115.
75. Leonardi CL, Kimball AB, Papp KA, et al. Efficacy and safety of ustekinumab, a human interleukin-12/23 monoclonal antibody, in patients with psoriasis: 76-week results from a randomised, double-blind, placebo-controlled trial (PHOENIX 1). *Lancet* 2008; 371: 1665–1674.
76. Papp KA, Langley RG, Lebwohl M, et al. Efficacy and safety of ustekinumab, a human interleukin-12/23 monoclonal antibody, in patients with psoriasis: 52-week results from a randomised, double-blind, placebo-controlled trial (PHOENIX 2). *Lancet* 2008; 371: 1675–1684.
77. Griffiths CE, Strober BE, van de Kerkhof P, et al. Comparison of ustekinumab and etanercept for moderate to severe psoriasis. *N Engl J Med* 2010; 362: 118–128.
78. Zanchi M, Favot F, Bizzarini M, et al. Botulinum toxin type-A for the treatment of inverse psoriasis. *J Eur Acad Dermatol Venereol* 2008; 22: 431–436.
79. Guglielmetti A, Conlledo R, Bedoya J, et al. Inverse psoriasis involving genital skin folds: successful therapy with dapsone. *Dermatol Ther* 2012; 2: 15–23.

Chapter 16

Psoriasis of the Nails

Ashley A. Keyes, Richard K. Scher, Gabriele B. Poindexter, and Maithily A. Nendedkar-Thomas

INTRODUCTION

Nail psoriasis is a relatively common and often misdiagnosed disorder affecting millions of people worldwide. Current studies estimate that approximately 7.5 million people in the United States, or roughly 2.2% of the population, are affected [1]. Not everyone who develops psoriasis will have nail changes; in fact, no more than half of those patients who have cutaneous psoriasis will have associated nail findings [2]. There is a close association between nail disease and psoriatic arthritis, and reports suggest the development of psoriatic arthritis is nearly three times more likely in patients with nail dystrophy [3]. In addition, 63%–83% of patients who develop psoriatic arthritis will have nail changes as the first external indicator of joint disease [4]. Recognizing early clinical clues can prevent the development of debilitating and permanent joint destruction [4]. There are numerous types of psoriatic nail changes, some of which are more closely associated with arthropathy than others. Nail psoriasis without joint or skin involvement can also occur, presenting a diagnostic challenge.

The psychosocial impact and functional impairment of severe multinail psoriasis cannot be understated [5]. It is often a source of embarrassment for patients who try to disguise their fingernails with nail polish or hide their toenails under the safety of socks [6]. Psoriasis has also been found to be associated with an increased risk of cardiovascular disease, making the recognition of isolated nail psoriasis important for long-term risk stratification [7]. Although mild-to-severe psoriasis is associated with increased risk of myocardial infarction and stroke, severe psoriasis is associated with increased cardiovascular mortality [8].

This chapter discusses the various manifestations of nail psoriasis, its associations with systemic disease, mimicking conditions, and objective means of measuring nail changes. Furthermore, therapeutic options for this challenging disease are reviewed.

MANIFESTATIONS OF NAIL PSORIASIS

Psoriatic nail changes have various manifestations depending on the location of the disease within the nail unit (Figure 16.1) [9]. The largest portion of the nail unit is the nail plate, which is derived from the nail matrix and protected under the proximal nail fold. There are two portions of nail matrix, also known as the nail "growth center": distal and proximal. The distal matrix forms the ventral portion of the nail plate and the proximal matrix forms the dorsal part. In addition to the plate and matrix, the nail unit is composed of the nail bed

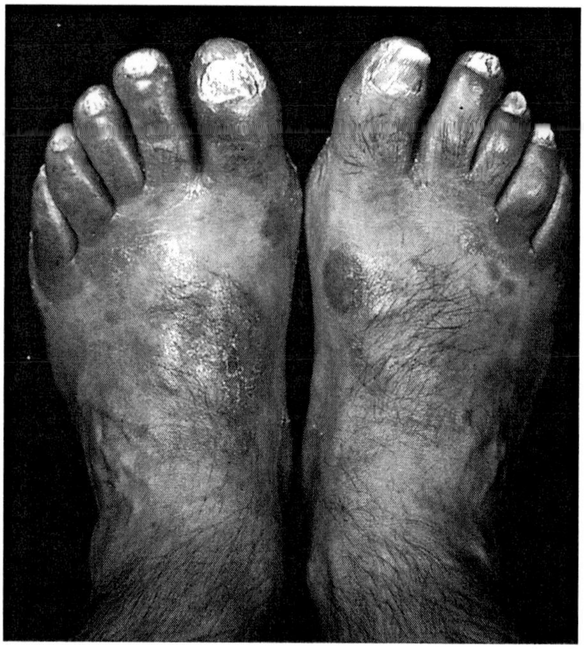

(a)

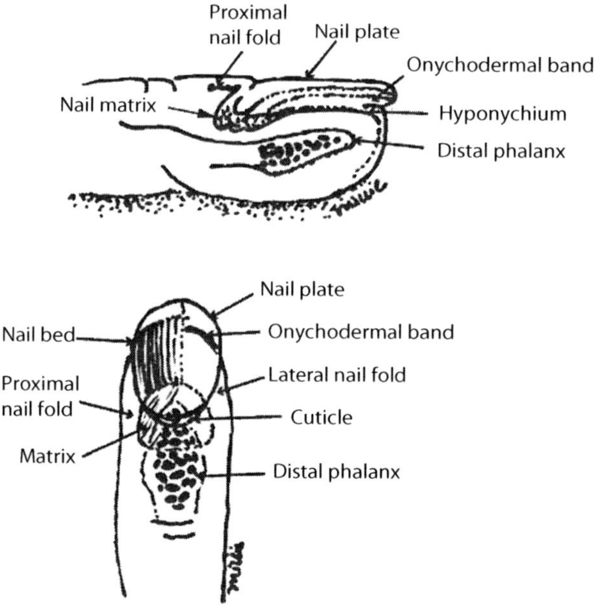

(b)

FIGURE 16.1 (See color insert.) (a) Plaque psoriasis with nail involvement. (b) The nail unit.

surrounded by the nail folds, which include the cuticle adjacent to the proximal nail fold. The most distal part of the nail unit is the hyponychium. The final component of the nail unit is the distal phalanx beneath the nail structures. Alterations in nail unit organization occur in a limited number of sites: nail matrix, nail bed, proximal nail fold, and hyponychium (Table 16.1) [2,10].

TABLE 16.1 Clinical Manifestation of Nail Psoriasis Based on Location of Psoriatic Change in the Nail Unit

Nail Unit Psoriasis Location					
Nail matrix, proximal involvement	**Nail bed, mid-distal matrix**	**Nail bed only**	**Nail bed and plate**	**Nail bed and hyponychium**	**Proximal nail fold**
Morphology due to pathologic change					
Pitting—deep, irregular indentations in the nail plate	Leukonychia	Oil spots	Onycholysis due to distal separation of the two structures progressing proximally	Subungual hyperkeratosis (when severe, this is the likely cause of onycholysis)	Chronic paronychia
Beau's lines	Red spots in the lunula	Hyperkeratosis			Splinter hemorrhages
Onychomadesis	Crumbling (all matrix)	Splinter hemorrhages			Classic silvery plaques
Trachyonychia					
Crumbling (due to total matrix involvement for a long duration)					

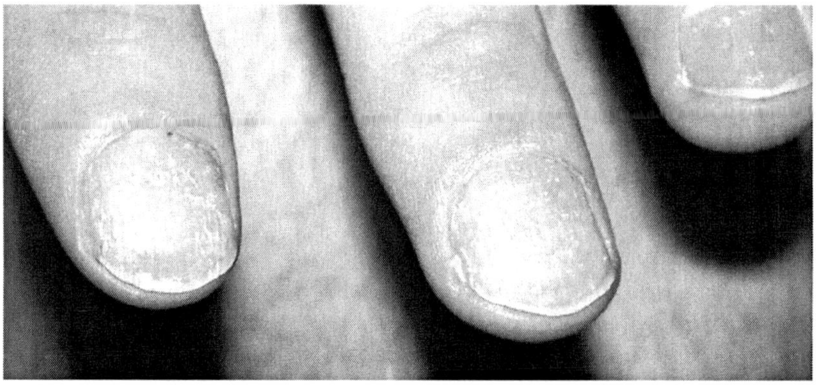

FIGURE 16.2 (See color insert.) Pitting in nail psoriasis.

Nail matrix involvement results in pitting and leukonychia (Figure 16.2). A phenomenon attributed to an abnormality in the maturation and keratinization of the proximal nail matrix, pitting is the most common nail lesion found in psoriasis [11,12]. The histopathology is the same as that of classic psoriasis but on a much smaller scale. The "pits" are produced by small foci of hyperproliferative, parakeratotic cells. As in classic psoriasis, the over exuberant cell turnover leads to a buildup of parakeratotic proximal matrix cells pressing against the dorsal nail plate [10]. Zaias' landmark study demonstrated that as the nail plate grows, the poorly adherent parakeratotic cells desquamate from the surface of the nail plate [10], leaving an indentation as clinical evidence of their former activity [13]. The nail pits' depth and shape depend upon the extent and duration the parakeratotic cells remain in place before becoming dislodged. This is a direct indicator of disease activity [2]. Although pitting may be seen in other disorders, the large size, irregular shape, and random distribution of the pits are the hallmark of fingernail psoriasis [10].

Interestingly, nail pitting is infrequently seen on toenails [14]. One possible mechanism to account for nail pitting in fingernails rather than toenails is the varying growth rates of fingernails versus toenails. In toenails, the growth rate is much slower; therefore, the parakeratotic focus and the nail plate may grow out toward the hyponychium together [2]. This process would explain for the lack of pitting and the marked increase in subungual hyperkeratosis as the key manifestation of toenail psoriasis. Subungual hyperkeratosis is analogous to plaque psoriasis on the skin and results from the deposition and collection of cells under the nail plate that have not undergone desquamation (Figure 16.1a) [15]. Like psoriasis elsewhere on the body, the hyponychial skin is subject to the Koebner phenomenon. Severe hyponychial involvement leading to subungual hyperkeratosis is more common in toenails because they are subject to more trauma than finger nails [10].

In addition to pitting, there are many other classic nail findings. Beau's lines are horizontal indentations in the nail plate due to temporary arrest of matrix growth during a period of inflammation [10]. Onychomadesis occurs when severe disease leads to separation of the nail plate from the proximal nail fold [10]. Proximal matrix disease manifests as roughened or "sandpaper" nails and is known as trachyonychia [16]. With severe trachyonychia and pitting, the patient develops crumbling. The whitish chalky plaque overlying the bed occurs when the entire matrix is involved for such a long duration that parakeratotic cells outnumber normal cells. As a result, no normal cell structure remains to which cells can adhere [10].

Red spots in the lunula are seen when the distal matrix is affected [2]. When the nail bed alone is affected, then "oil spots" [17], nail bed hyperkeratosis, and splinter hemorrhages [18] are common. Oil spots, also known as "salmon patches," refer to a yellow-orange discoloration due to psoriasis of the nail bed (Figure 16.3) [19]. Splinter hemorrhages are due to trauma and are analogous to the Auspitz sign associated with cutaneous psoriasis [10] (Figure 16.3a). Leukonychia is caused by midmatrix disease. The whitish areas are likely due to adherent foci of parakeratotic cells that cannot be dislodged. Onycholysis is a distinct phenomenon that results from separation of the nail bed from the plate (Figure 16.4). The separation begins distally and progresses proximally toward the matrix. The plate appears whitish rather than yellow due to trapped air beneath it. It is usually surrounded by a reddish hue [10] and is distinguished from true leukonychia by location. Leukonychia is usually seen on the proximal portion of the plate whereas onycholysis appears distally. Proximal nail fold plaques are marked by classic cutaneous psoriasis with silvery scales over a red base [2]. This may present as chronic paronychia [11].

Although there are numerous manifestations of nail psoriasis, very few are characteristic of psoriasis alone. The classic oil spot is the most diagnostic lesion [19], followed by fingernail pitting and subungual hyperkeratosis [13].

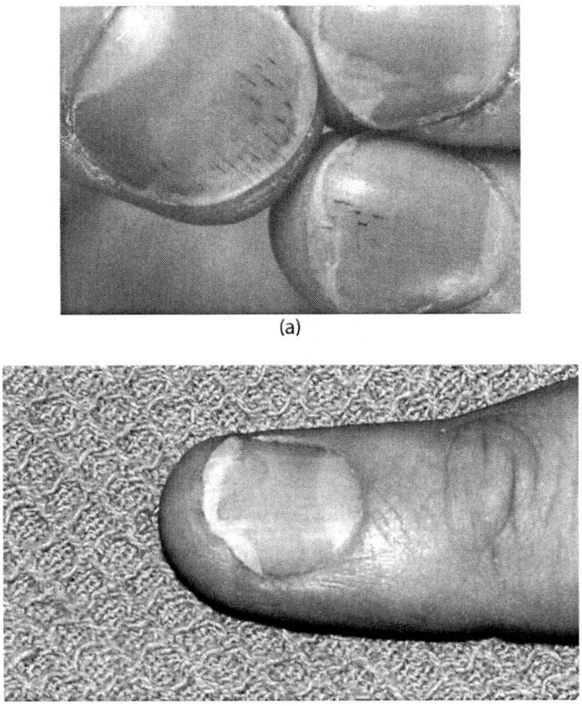

(a)

(b)

FIGURE 16.3 (See color insert.) (a) Splinter hemorrhages and oil spots in nail psoriasis. (b) Oil spot in nail psoriasis.

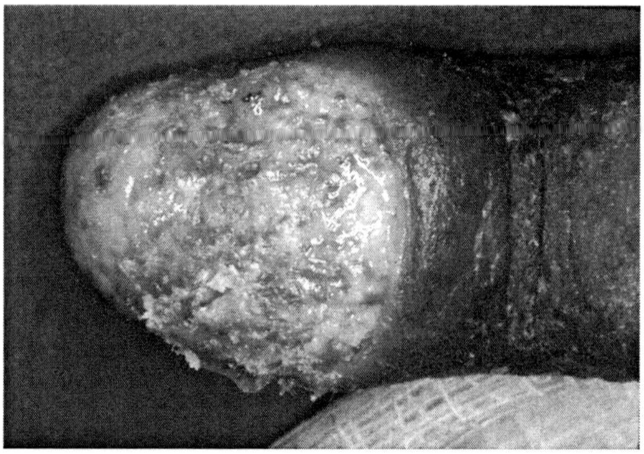

(a)

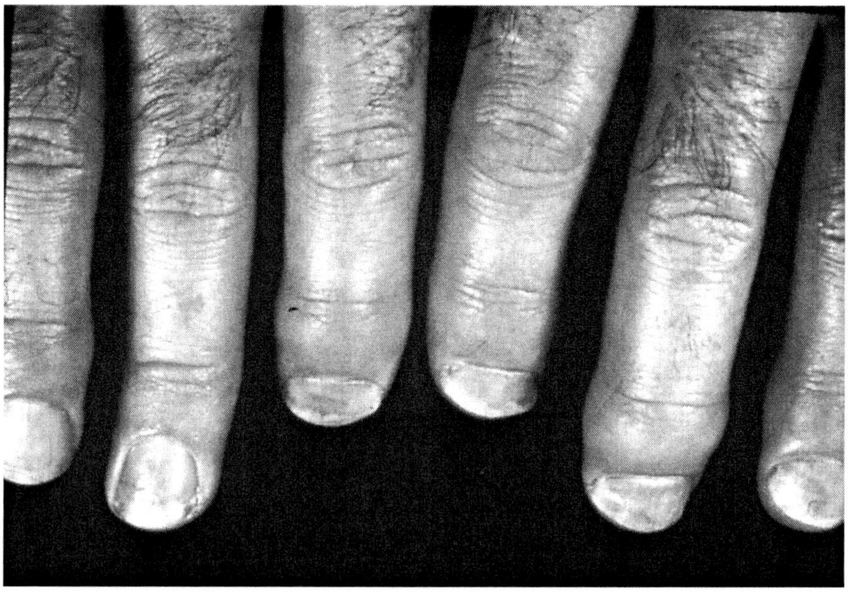

(b)

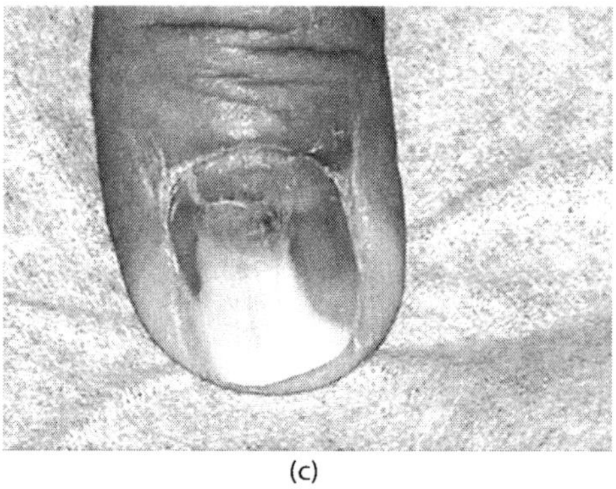

(c)

FIGURE 16.4 (See color insert.) (a) Severe pustular psoriasis (acrodermatitis continua of Hallopeau) in a patient with HIV. (b) Enthesitis in a patient with psoriatic arthritis. (c) Onycholysis in nail psoriasis.

Extensive onychodystrophy with painful pustules and loss of the nail plate is usually due to a more severe and distinct type of nail psoriasis known as acrodermatitis continua of Hallopeau [11]. Although most manifestations of nail psoriasis do not lead to scarring, pustular psoriasis is an exception (Figure 16.4a). Fortunately, this debilitating disorder is rare and often isolated to a single digit [14]. Despite several treatment options described in the literature, successful eradication of the disorder before anonychia and scarring is rare [20].

ASSOCIATION WITH PSORIATIC ARTHRITIS

Moll and Wright originally classified psoriatic arthritis into five types based on clinical features [21]. Type I refers to primarily distal interphalangeal (DIP) bone and joint erosion that radiographically presents as the classic "pencil in cup deformity." It affects approximately 5% of all patients. The rarest is type II, also known as arthritis mutilans, and presents as a severe mutilating arthritis that can have ocular involvement. Type III is a symmetric polyarthritis that affects the small joints of the hands and feet and the large joints of the legs, such as the hips and knees. Type IV is the most common type, affecting approximately 70% of those patients who present with psoriatic arthritis. Asymmetric oligoarthritis is the hallmark of this type of psoriatic arthritis. It affects the same joints as type III with variable DIP joint involvement. Type V is distinguished by axial disease that affects the spine and sacroiliac joints and usually presents with ankylosing spondylitis. Of all the psoriatic arthritis types, type V is least associated with nail disease. In addition to the five types of arthritis classically associated with psoriasis, pustulosis palmoplantaris with osteoarthritis sternoclavicularis and psoriatic onycho-pachydermo-periostitis is now linked to psoriatic arthritis [22].

The major distinguishing characteristic of the most common form of psoriatic arthritis, type IV, is that unlike rheumatoid arthritis, it usually presents with asymmetric joint disease. It is classified as a seronegative, inflammatory arthropathy, meaning rheumatoid factor is usually negative. Much like cutaneous psoriasis, it waxes and wanes unpredictably [23]. Symptoms include joint pain, stiffness, and enthesitis [24].

Enthesitis refers to inflammation of the tendons, ligaments, and joint capsule fibers at the site of bone insertion and may result in pain, reduction in mobility, and even joint destruction (Figure 16.4b) [25]. Recently, it has been shown that enthesopathy, detectable by ultrasonography, is common in psoriasis patients even without clinical signs of arthritis. Subclinical enthesopathy is associated with nail involvement, with more extensive nail involvement correlating with enthesopathy severity [25,26]. Many studies have established that patients with psoriatic DIP joint disease are likely to have associated psoriatic nail changes in the same digit [27,28]. Furthermore, even if arthritic changes are not clinically evident, radiographic changes may be seen in the DIP joint of the same fingertip with visible psoriatic nail disease [29]. More recently, studies show that the distal phalanx bone is the most affected by adjacent nail involvement, with worsening nail disease correlating with worsening bony destruction. It is theorized that DIP involvement may be the end result of this process [30,31].

Longitudinal evaluation of a small cohort of patients with psoriasis by ultrasound demonstrated that identification of patients with enthesopathy might be predictive of future development of psoriatic arthritis [32]. Another study sought to determine whether psoriatic nail alteration could be used as an independent predictor of psoriatic arthritis. Looking specifically at patients with the various types of psoriatic arthritis, 83% of patients had clinically evident nail disease [33]. As anticipated, those patients with DIP involvement had more severe nail damage. Likewise, the severity of nail psoriasis directly correlated with the severity of the enthesitis as well as skin psoriasis. The arthritis tended to be progressive and unremitting in these patients. However, dactylitis and axial disease were not associated with nail disease. In fact, the lesser the nail involvement, the more likely the patient was to have the human leukocyte antigen (HLA)-B27 genetic haplotype, which is associated with axial rather than DIP joint disease [33].

In addition, to severe nail involvement, one study found that scalp severity also correlates positively with the number of swollen joints, deformed joints, dactylitis, and DIP involvement. This correlation suggests that scalp involvement may also predict psoriatic joint involvement [4]. The association of scalp and nail disease with psoriatic arthritis highlights the importance of performing total body skin exams with complete review of symptoms to best identify patients who may benefit from early treatment.

ASSOCIATED GENETIC HAPLOTYPES

Although the exact pathogenesis of nail psoriasis remains unclear, certain key HLA subtypes are known to be associated with certain psoriatic phenotypes (Table 16.2) [34,35]. However, genetic factors alone cannot account for the occurrence of psoriasis. Environmental and immunologic factors most certainly play a role in its inception.

NAIL PSORIASIS: CHILDHOOD VERSUS ADULT ONSET

Characterizations of childhood psoriasis versus adult psoriasis are numerous and varied. Multiple epidemiologic studies report a mean age of onset of 8–11 years in pediatric patients, with a higher incidence of positive family history in pediatric-onset psoriasis versus adult-onset psoriasis of 68% versus 54%, respectively. Diagnosis before 13 years is more likely to be guttate or generalized pustular psoriasis with a more severe clinical course. There continues to be a discrepancy as to whether girls are more commonly affected than boys [36].

Most patients, regardless of sex, develop psoriasis after the age of 20 years as adults [37]. When a family history of psoriasis is found in association with juvenile-onset psoriasis, the disease

TABLE 16.2 Key Genetic Haplotypes Associated with Psoriatic Arthritis and Nail Disease

Major Histocompatibility Class I Type			
HLA B27 and HLA-Cw2	**HLA-Cw6**	**HLA-Cw6 negative**	**HLA-B13 and HLA-B57 (B17)**
Later onset; less nail disease; strong association with axial disease. If early onset, then linked to pediatric spondyloarthropathy, but still has a poor association with nail disease	Earlier onset; nail disease but less dystrophy than if Cw6 negative	Stronger association with dystrophic nails than if Cw6 positive	If more severe skin disease, then increased joint or nail disease

course is inevitably more severe [38], more strongly associated with psoriatic arthritis [39], and more likely to display nail changes [5]. Childhood onset of nail psoriasis is commonly precipitated by trauma or infectious disease [40,41]. Also, the later the onset of cutaneous psoriasis, the less often concomitant fingernail or toenail psoriasis occurs. This is especially true for toenail psoriasis [42]. Although rare, when a child presents with nail alteration as the sole manifestation of psoriasis, an evaluation for juvenile psoriatic arthritis should be considered [43].

DIAGNOSTIC CHALLENGE: ISOLATED NAIL PSORIASIS AND ITS IMPERSONATORS

Onychomycosis

The most common misdiagnosis for psoriatic nail disease is onychomycosis [2] due to the shared finding of subungual hyperkeratosis. Onychomycosis can also occur concomitantly in psoriatic nails. In a recent study conducted with 228 patients, 62% of patients had positive mycology results. These findings were consistent with some studies; however, overall they represent a higher incidence than the majority of previous reports [44]. Despite conflicting data, it is prudent to perform a potassium hydroxide (KOH) wet mount, culture, or nail clipping for a periodic acid–Schiff (PAS) stain to ensure there is no superimposed onychomycosis. Treatment of the overlying onychomycosis often reduces hyperkeratosis, allowing the more characteristic psoriatic changes to be revealed, as well as potential improvement in overall appearance. Onychomycosis is difficult to eradicate, especially if the superimposed infection is due to molds rather than dermatophytes [45].

Allergic Contact Dermatitis

Typically, most patients with ungual contact dermatitis also have skin involvement, helping to confirm the diagnosis. It is most commonly due to nail trauma [46] or nail cosmetics [47]. Like most diagnostic dilemmas, a thorough history and examination clarify the correct diagnosis.

Drug Reactions

Onycholysis is often seen in patients taking phototoxic drugs such as antibiotics [48]. However, drug-induced onycholysis may occur with no associated cutaneous photosensitivity, as in chemotherapy [49]. Beau's lines and onychomadesis are the most common abnormalities associated with drug reactions [50]. When they are also associated with onycholysis, the clinical picture can clearly mimic psoriasis [51]. A careful evaluation of the history of the lesions should identify the likely culprit. Psoriatic nail changes typically have a slower onset than those due to a drug reaction; the latter reactions are often be sudden and explosive.

Lichen Striatus

Lichen striatus is an interesting disorder that is also potentially confused with linear psoriasis. It is most commonly seen in children involving an isolated nail with characteristic findings of onychorrhexis and linear trachyonychia. Linear, lichenoid papules at the proximal nail fold and spontaneous regression within months clarify the diagnosis [52]. It does not present with pitting or onycholysis.

Parakeratosis Pustulosa

Parakeratosis pustulosa is a disorder that is seen exclusively in female children. It presents with isolated scaling and erythema in either the thumb or index finger; pitting is a common finding. Some believe this entity should not be considered a diagnosis but rather a symptom of nail apparatus inflammatory disease such as psoriasis, as well as contact dermatitis or atopic dermatitis. Although many patients will experience spontaneous resolution, the development of psoriasis is possible and therefore warrants anticipatory guidance for the patient's parents [52].

Squamous Cell Carcinoma

Although rare, squamous cell carcinoma (SCC) arising in a psoriatic nail has been reported [53]. Interestingly, this patient had an exophytic verrucous plaque arising from a psoriatic thumbnail that became progressively larger. Pain prompted the patient to seek medical attention. Due to substantial progression, the terminal phalanx required amputation. Histologic examination of the amputated digit revealed well-differentiated SCC with erosion through the dermis and into the bone. The important feature of this case is that there was a delay in diagnosis because both the patient and the physician assumed the excess hyperkeratosis was due to worsening psoriasis.

DIAGNOSTIC PROCEDURE: THE NAIL BIOPSY

Numerous excellent textbooks [2,54,55] describe the appropriate method for punch biopsy of the nail bed versus the nail matrix [56]. It is a simple, straightforward procedure that is safely and routinely performed in the office setting. With challenging cases, the biopsy can be invaluable in ascertaining the cause of the nail abnormality, distinguishing between neoplasms, infection, and inflammatory conditions. On occasions, both the nail bed and the matrix require biopsy simultaneously. In this case, a longitudinal biopsy may be appropriate [57].

MEASUREMENT OF SEVERITY: THE NAIL PSORIASIS SEVERITY INDEX

An objective scale is needed to measure disease severity. The Psoriasis Area and Severity Index (PASI) is used primarily for cutaneous psoriasis but does not adequately measure nail disease activity. Therefore, the Nail Psoriasis Severity Index (NAPSI) was developed by Rich and Scher to objectively quantify the severity of nail disease in a reproducible manner [58]. It was also designed to assess efficacy of drug therapy for different manifestations of nail psoriasis (e.g., pitting vs. subungual hyperkeratosis). Using the NAPSI, the nail is divided into four quadrants, each of which is graded based on the presence or absence of nail matrix or nail bed disease. The highest score possible for each fingernail is 8, for a total of 80. If toenails are included, the maximum total number increases to 160 (Tables 16.3 and 16.4). The sum of the scores is calculated and used to judge the severity of nail psoriasis. Not included in this grading system are proximal nail fold psoriasis, pustular psoriasis, and psoriatic arthritis. Other methods have also been proposed, but the NAPSI has been found to be consistent, reproducible, and simple to use; thousands of patients have been evaluated in clinical trials [59–61].

TABLE 16.3 NAPSI Scoring System

NAPSI Scoring System[a]	Nail Matrix[b]	Nail Bed[c]	Total Score[d]
0	None	None	0
1	Present in 1 quadrant	Present in 1 quadrant	Possible points: 1 or 2 Enter score:
2	Present in 2 quadrants	Present in 2 quadrants	Possible points: 2 or 4 Enter score:
3	Present in 3 quadrants	Present in 3 quadrants	Possible points: 3 or 6 Enter score:
4	Present in 4 quadrants	Present in 4 quadrants	Possible points: 4 or 8 Enter score:

[a] For each nail, score the points as shown in the column.
[b] Evidence of any (1) pitting, (2) leukonychia, (3) red spots in the lunula, or (4) crumbling.
[c] Evidence of any (1) onycholysis, (2) splinter hemorrhages, (3) subungual hyperkeratosis, or (4) oil spots/salmon patches.
[d] There is a minimum of 0 and a maximum of 8 points awarded for each nail: 4 possible points for evidence of matrix disease and 4 possible points for evidence of nail bed disease.

TABLE 16.4 NAPSI Scoring Table

Nail Scoring Table—Compile the Score for Each Nail			
Nail 1	Nail 2	Nail 3	Nail 4
Nail 5	Nail 6	Nail 7	Nail 8
Nail 9	Nail 10		
Final score total:			

Note: Minimum score is 0 and maximum score is 80.

Another measurement of psoriatic nail disease severity is the modified NAPSI (mNAPSI) that was developed by rheumatologists with particular focus on patients with psoriatic arthritis. Based on the original NAPSI, the assessment of nails by quadrants was eliminated and the severity of the most common nail findings, such as nail pitting, onycholysis, and nail crumbling, is graded on a scale of 0–3 [61]. Other features, such as splinter hemorrhages, leukonychia, red spots in the lunula, oil spots, and hyperkeratosis, are graded based on presence or absence exclusively. Due to its complexity, the mNAPSI has been used much less frequently.

TREATMENT OPTIONS AND SIDE EFFECTS

There are a variety of treatments for nail psoriasis. This condition tends to be chronic and persistent, and with slow nail growth, many months of treatment are required to appreciate results. Topical medications are theoretically ideal because they have the advantage of direct application to the affected area without the risk of systemic side effects, drug interactions, or the pain of intralesional injections. Nevertheless, the low permeability of the nail plate is a challenge in topical drug therapy [62]. Currently, the drugs used for psoriatic nail disease are usually classified as follows: steroids, biologic agents, retinoids, and other miscellaneous therapies, such as chemotherapy or phototherapy. Each therapeutic class is now discussed in detail (Table 16.5).

TABLE 16.5 Therapeutic Options for Nail Psoriasis

Topical	Corticosteroids
	Calcipotriol
	Tazarotene
	5-Fluorouracil
	Cyclosporine
	Anthralin
Intralesional	Corticosteroids
Oral	Acitretin and isotretinoin
	Cyclosporine
	Sulfasalazine
Subcutaneous or intravenous	Etanercept, infliximab, adalimumab
	Alefacept
	Efalizumab
Radiation	PUVA
Combinations	Topical corticosteroid and topical calcipotriol
	Topical corticosteroid and topical salicylic acid
	Oral cyclosporine and topical corticosteroid

Steroids and Steroid-Like Drugs

The high-potency topical steroids are likely the most used form of therapy for nail psoriasis. Typically, a high-potency corticosteroid ointment such as clobetasol is applied to both the nail plate and proximal nail fold nightly [63]. A lacquer formulation is also available. A small, prospective, randomized control trial showed statistically significant improvement, as measured by NAPSI and mNAPSI, with 8% nail lacquer clobetasol compared with 0.05% and 1% nail lacquer clobetasol [64]. Although topical corticosteroids are relatively inexpensive, readily available, and easy to apply without concern for systemic side effects or pain, both steroid atrophy of the nail fold and tachyphylaxis can occur with prolonged use. There have been a few reports of a "disappearing digit" after extreme prolonged use as well [65]. Penetration of the topical corticosteroid alone is a problem and seems to result in marginal efficacy. When combined with salicylic acid ointment, efficacy of topical corticosteroids increases with reduction of hyperkeratosis and nail thickness [66]. Clobetasol nail lacquer in combination with a vitamin D_3 analog has been studied as well [67]. The most effective corticosteroid vehicle for nail matrix psoriasis appears to be the triamcinolone acetonide (TAC) (2.5–10 mg/mL) injection administered into the proximal and/or lateral nail fold every month for six months. Some dermatologists prefer using a ring block for anesthesia before the injection [68]. In our experience, dilution of the TAC with 1% lidocaine and application of anesthetic refrigerant spray before rapid injection minimizes patient discomfort and increases tolerability. One report found that 0.4 mL of 10 mg/mL TAC injected intralesionally into the nail bed and nail matrix worked best for subungual hyperkeratosis, ridging, and thickening, whereas only moderate results were obtained for pitting and onycholysis [68]. Other studies have found good results with injection only into the proximal nail fold [69,70]. The major complications from this therapy are pain, hemorrhage under the nail plate [2], and steroid-induced atrophy or hypopigmentation of the skin and subcutaneous tissues [71]. Careful injection at the inflammatory psoriatic site with small amounts at a concentration of 2.5 mg/mL steroid does not cause major atrophy or telangiectasias. As an added positive side effect, some patients report that associated painful DIP joint arthritis seems to diminish with repeated injections.

Calcipotriene is a vitamin D_3 analog that binds to a similar steroid receptor in the skin. The ointment form has been studied in comparison with class 1 topical steroids combined with salicylic acid for use in the treatment of nail psoriasis, and both were equally effective in decreasing hyperkeratosis [66]. Calcipotriene may be most effective in treating subungual hyperkeratosis, onycholysis, and discoloration [72]. The ideal use of calcipotriene appears to be in combination with other oral agents, such as cyclosporine [73] or even topical steroids [74]. With this medication, there are no injections, no risk of atrophy, tachyphylaxis or hemorrhage, and patients experience minimal side effects.

Biologic Agents

There are several biologic agents available to manage cutaneous psoriasis. Although many studies focus on plaque-type psoriasis and psoriatic arthritis with varying degrees of success [75–77], very little reproducible evidence exists with regard to biologic agents and nail psoriasis. These medications target either tumor necrosis factor (TNF)-α or T cells. TNF-α is a cytokine required for cell-mediated inflammation [78]. The key cell in the inflammatory milieu is the activated T-cell [79]. The rationale for use of biologics is that they are designed to diminish TNF-α or inhibit T-cell activity and decrease the inflammatory, destructive component of psoriasis, resulting in clinical improvement in the disease condition. These medications can be loosely grouped as TNF-α inhibitors (e.g., etanercept, adalimumab, and infliximab) and T-cell modulators (efalizumab).

Etanercept is a TNF-α receptor antibody fusion protein that competitively binds free TNF-α and is administered subcutaneously one to two times a week [80]. Infliximab is a chimeric mouse/human monoclonal antibody against TNF-α. It also binds to TNF-α and blocks its function. It is administered intravenously once every two months [81]. The human monoclonal antibody adalimumab is an antibody against TNF-α and is administered subcutaneously every two weeks [78]. Although adalimumab and infliximab are structurally distinct from etanercept with a discrete mechanism of action, the end result is similar. All three drugs bind TNF-α, blocking its ability to bind to its receptor and thereby reducing localized inflammation [78].

These three biologic agents are all Food and Drug Administration (FDA) approved for the treatment of psoriasis and pregnancy category B. Only one randomized controlled trial for adalimumab has provided data specifically on nail psoriasis, showing 50% improvement in NAPSI compared with 8% in the placebo group [82]. Other trials have similarly shown significant reduction in the NAPSI in patients with both cutaneous psoriasis and psoriatic arthritis [82]. Data on the efficacy of etanercept is similarly limited. The CRYSTEL trial compared two different dosing regimens for the treatment of psoriasis and showed an overall improvement in nail symptoms of >50%; the results were not stratified by treatment group [83]. There is one case of rapid improvement and cure of nail psoriasis with etanercept [84]. Infliximab has been studied in more detail for psoriasis. A double-blind, placebo-controlled study of infliximab found marked and sustained nail improvement in onycholysis, splinter hemorrhages, oil drop discoloration, and hyperkeratosis. Clearance of psoriasis in the target nail was achieved in about 50% patients by week 50 [85]. A recent small, open, prospective trial compared all three agents for the treatment of nail psoriasis. Evaluation with NAPSI at weeks 0, 14, and 24 showed significant improvement overall, with higher efficacy in the infliximab group at week 14 [86].

Although the TNF-α inhibitors have shown success in treating psoriasis and nail psoriasis, these treatments are considered second line after failure or intolerance to at least two conventional therapies, and the cost is prohibitive for many patients. In addition, any active chronic infection such as tuberculosis or hepatitis B is a contraindication to therapy [87]. The possibility of increasing the risk of lymphoma is also debated in the literature [87]. Relative contraindications to therapy include heart failure, prior malignancies, and family or personal history of systemic lupus or multiple sclerosis [87]. Recently, there have been reports of a paradoxical phenomenon occurring with all three of these mediations—the induction of psoriasis—including nail psoriasis by TNF-α inhibitors [88].

A newer class of biologic therapy is the human monoclonal antibody to interleukin (IL)-12 and IL-23, ustekinumab. This antibody binds to the p40 subunit, a subunit that is shared by both IL-12 and IL-23 and is overexpressed in psoriatic lesions. The function of these two cytokines is then neutralized. Although ABT-874 is no longer available in the United States, ustekinumab has received FDA approval for the treatment of psoriasis. Case reports and data have shown improvement in nail-related symptoms; however, randomized controlled trials are still lacking [89–91].

Efalizumab is a humanized monoclonal antibody against the CD11 portion of the LFA-1 molecule on T cells. It prevents binding to intercellular adhesion molecule (ICAM) on the antigen-presenting cell and prevents T-cells from migrating to the skin [92]. Because it does not actually destroy the activated pathogenic T cells, the psoriasis can actually worsen upon cessation of the drug due to a sudden influx of T cells into the skin. Efalizumab was FDA approved for the treatment of psoriasis; however, it was withdrawn from the market in 2009 due to increased risk of developing progressive multifocal leukoencephalopathy [93].

Retinoids

Tazarotene 0.1% gel is a topical retinoid whose active metabolite tazarotenic acid binds with high affinity to the gamma subunit of the retinoic acid receptors (RARs) in the skin and nails. RAR-γ is the predominate type of RAR in the epidermis [94]. Topical tazarotene impairs keratinocyte proliferation and inflammation, one of the mechanisms of onycholysis. One study by Scher et al. [95] demonstrated that tazarotene under occlusion appears to reduce onycholysis and also improves the appearance of pitting. A subsequent study confirmed this finding [96]. A double-blind comparison trial of tazarotene cream 0.1% versus clobetasol cream 0.05% found marked improvement in both groups in pitting, hyperkeratosis, onycholysis, and salmon patches, with regression after therapy cessation [97]. All studies found the drug to be well tolerated; repeated use caused minimal irritation.

Acitretin and isotretinoin are systemic retinoids that are more effective when combined with phototherapy, either UVB or PUVA [98,99]. Acitretin is the treatment of choice for pustular psoriasis but is less effective against plaque psoriasis [100]. There is one report of near total clearance of severe nail psoriasis with acitretin [101]. Another report compared low-dose, short-term cyclosporine with etretinate and found significant alleviation of nail involvement in both the groups [102]. A small open study evaluating acitretin in patients with isolated nail psoriasis showed 41% improvement in the NAPSI and 50% improvement in the mNAPSI, results comparable to other systemic treatments [103]. Although these are impressive results, oral retinoids are not the best choice for isolated nail psoriasis given the systemic side effects of hyperlipidemia and hyperostosis, and the localized side effects of xerosis and periungual pyogenic granulomas [104]. One major limitation of both topical and systemic retinoids is that they are pregnancy category X.

Oral or Topical Chemotherapy and Keratolytic Agents

Cyclosporine is well established as an effective oral immunosuppressive agent for the treatment of generalized psoriasis as well as nail psoriasis [102,105]. Although highly effective, the systemic side effects make cyclosporine imperfect for long-term therapy or for isolated nail disease. Side effects include hypertension, renal insufficiency, increased risk of skin cancers, and elevated lipids. It is also pregnancy category C. It is rarely used topically because it is a relatively large, highly lipophilic molecule that is unable to permeate the nail plate. Unlike the skin and gastrointestinal (GI) tract that have lipid-permeable membranes, the nail plate is a concentrated hydrogel [105]. Therefore, small hydrophilic molecules preferentially diffuse through the structure to the nail bed. Gels (e.g., tazarotene 0.1% gel rather than cream) or other water-based preparations are necessary when choosing a topical agent for nail psoriasis.

Numerous case series have shown that daily topical 1%–5% 5-fluorouracil is effective for the treatment of psoriatic nails, with improved pitting, subungual hyperkeratosis, onycholysis, and oil spots [106,107]. Fluorouracil is a chemotherapeutic agent that inhibits the enzyme thymidylate synthetase, leading to a decrease in cellular proliferation. Using the low-dose formulation of the drug in a delayed nail penetration vehicle such as urea or propylene glycol enhances penetration [108]. Like most agents that interfere with DNA synthesis, it is pregnancy category X. Most studies have shown localized irritation with occlusive dressings as the most serious adverse effect. However, there is one report of transient rhabdomyolysis occurring after the use of topical 5-fluorouracil [109].

There are no reports of isolated nail psoriasis treated with methotrexate. Like fluorouracil, it inhibits DNA synthesis, but the exact mechanism for blocking inflammation is still unknown. Because methotrexate is an immunosuppressive agent like cyclosporine, it is difficult to justify use of this agent for isolated nail psoriasis, except if there is severe impairment of digit function. Methotrexate is pregnancy category X.

Sulfasalazine is a sulfonamide pregnancy category B used to treat psoriatic arthritis. There is one case report of improvement in nail psoriasis with its use [110]. However, in this report, the patient had previously been treated with acitretin for 12 months. Like most oral medications, the benefit of the drug for isolated nail psoriasis must outweigh the potential side effects.

Topical anthralin is not usually a first-line medication due to the risk of long-term pigmentation of the nail plate. It has been used with moderate success for refractory nail psoriasis, with improvement in onycholysis, pachyonychia, and pitting [111]. In this study, anthralin was carefully washed away after 30 minutes of contact, followed by application of 10% triethanolamine to prevent pigmentation.

Phototherapy

Topical psoralen and ultraviolet A (PUVA) has been reported to be effective for all the different manifestations of nail psoriasis except pitting [112], presumably due to the inability of the light to penetrate the proximal nail fold skin sufficiently to affect matrix normalization. The major drawback of this therapy is the risk of severe PUVA burns with overexposure. Although there are no studies evaluating the efficacy of narrowband ultraviolet B (UVB) in the treatment of nail psoriasis, one study evaluated the usefulness of 308-nm excimer light and found no benefit [113]. Pulsed dye laser (595 nm) with once-monthly treatments has been well tolerated and demonstrates reduction in the NAPSI [114].

CONCLUSIONS

Compared with classic cutaneous psoriasis, nail psoriasis is a poorly studied entity for many reasons. For example, nail psoriasis is commonly misdiagnosed or diagnosis is delayed because it mimics other disorders. Even if a proper diagnosis is made, nail psoriasis remains difficult to treat. Traditional systemic therapies show inconsistent benefit for nail psoriasis. The most promising of all therapies are the newer biologic agents, such as infliximab. Undoubtedly, a definitive treatment is yet to be developed. Meanwhile, for isolated nail psoriasis, the best treatment remains intralesional corticosteroids.

REFERENCES

1. Kupetsky EA, Keller M. Psoriasis vulgaris: an evidence-based guide for primary care. *J Am Board Fam Med* 2013; 26(6):787–801.
2. Rich P, Scher R. *Nail Manifestations in Cutaneous Disease. An Atlas of Diseases of the Nail.* Parthenon Publishing Group, Inc; 2003. pp. 51–54.
3. Wilson FC, Icen M, Crowson CS, et al. Incidence and clinical predictors of psoriatic arthritis in patients with psoriasis: a population-based study. *Arthritis Rheum* 2009; 61(2): 233–239.
4. Elkayam O, Ophir J, Yaron M, et al. Psoriatic arthritis: interrelationships between skin and joint manifestations related to onset, course and distribution. *Clin Rheumatol* 2000; 19(4): 301–305.
5. de Jong EM, Seegers BA, Gulinck MK, et al. Psoriasis of the nails associated with disability in a large number of patients: results of a recent interview with 1728 patients. *Dermatology* 1996; 193(4): 300–303.
6. Fortune DG, Richards HL, Main CJ, et al. What patients with psoriasis believe about their condition. *J Am Acad Dermatol* 1998; 39(2 Pt 1): 196–201.
7. Neimann AL, Shin DB, Wang X, et al. Prevalence of cardiovascular risk factors in patients with psoriasis. *J Am Acad Dermatol* 2006; 55(5): 829–835.

8. Armstrong EJ, Harskamp CT, Armstrong AW. Psoriasis and major adverse cardiovascular events: a systematic review and meta-analysis of observational studies. *J Am Heart Assoc* 2013; 2(2): e000062.
9. Del-Rosso J, Basuk P, Scher R. Dermatological diseases. In: Scher RK, Daniel C, eds. *Nails: Therapy, Diagnosis, Surgery*. 3rd edn. Oxford, UK: Elsevier Saunders; 2005.
10. Zaias N. Psoriasis of the nail. A clinical-pathologic study. *Arch Dermatol* 1969; 99(5): 567–579.
11. Tosti A, Piraccini BM. Biology of nails and nail disorders. In: Wolff K, Goldsmith L, Katz S, et al., eds. *Fitzpatrick's Dermatology in General Medicine*. 7th edn. New York, NY: McGraw Hill; 2008. pp. 778–793.
12. Tham SN, Lim JJ, Tay SH, et al. Clinical observations on nail changes in psoriasis. *Ann Acad Med Singapore* 1988; 17(4): 482–485.
13. Kaur I, Saraswat A, Kumar B. Nail changes in psoriasis: a study of 167 patients. *Int J Dermatol* 2001; 40(9): 601–603.
14. Tosti A, Piraccini B. Dermatological diseases that affect the nail. In: Hordinsky M, Sawaya M, Scher R, eds. *Atlas of Hair and Nails*. Philadelphia, PA: Churchill Livingstone; 2000. pp. 47–49.
15. Jiaravuthisan MM, Sasseville D, Vender RB, et al. Psoriasis of the nail: anatomy, pathology, clinical presentation, and a review of the literature on therapy. *J Am Acad Dermatol* 2007; 57(1): 1–27.
16. Scheinfeld NS. Trachyonychia: a case report and review of manifestations, associations, and treatments. *Cutis* 2003; 71(4): 299–302.
17. Rich P. Nail disorders. Diagnosis and treatment of infectious, inflammatory, and neoplastic nail conditions. *Med Clin North Am* 1998; 82(5): 1171–1183, vii.
18. Saladi RN, Persaud AN, Rudikoff D, et al. Idiopathic splinter hemorrhages. *J Am Acad Dermatol* 2004; 50(2): 289–292.
19. Kouskoukis CE, Scher RK, Ackerman AB. The "oil drop" sign of psoriatic nails. A clinical finding specific for psoriasis. *Am J Dermatopathol* 1983; 5(3): 259–262.
20. Yerushalmi J, Grunwald MH, Hallel-Halevy D, et al. Chronic pustular eruption of the thumbs. Diagnosis: Acrodermatitis Continua of Hallopeau (ACH). *Arch Dermatol* 2000; 136(7): 925–930.
21. Moll JM, Wright V. Psoriatic arthritis. *Semin Arthritis Rheum* 1973; 3(1): 55–78.
22. Ruzicka T. Psoriatic arthritis. New types, new treatments. *Arch Dermatol* 1996; 132(2): 215–219.
23. Winchester R. Psoriatic arthritis. In: Wolff K, Goldsmith L, Katz S, et al., eds. *Fitzpatrick's Dermatology in General Medicine*. 7th edn. New York, NY: McGraw Hill; 2008. pp. 194–207.
24. Mease P, Goffe BS. Diagnosis and treatment of psoriatic arthritis. *J Am Acad Dermatol* 2005; 52(1): 1–19.
25. Ash ZR, Tinazzi I, Gallego CC, et al. Psoriasis patients with nail disease have a greater magnitude of underlying systemic subclinical enthesopathy than those with normal nails. *Ann Rheum Dis* 2012; 71(4): 553–536.
26. Sakkas LI, Alexiou I, Simopoulou T, et al. Enthesitis in psoriatic arthritis. *Semin Arthritis Rheum* 2013; pii: S0049-0172(13)00060-7.
27. Jones SM, Armas JB, Cohen MG, et al. Psoriatic arthritis: outcome of disease subsets and relationship of joint disease to nail and skin disease. *Br J Rheumatol* 1994; 33(9): 834–839.
28. Cohen MR, Reda DJ, Clegg DO. Baseline relationships between psoriasis and psoriatic arthritis: analysis of 221 patients with active psoriatic arthritis. Department of Veterans Affairs Cooperative Study Group on Seronegative Spondyloarthropathies. *J Rheumatol* 1999; 26(8): 1752–1756.
29. Scarpa R, Manguso F, Oriente A, et al. Is the involvement of the distal interphalangeal joint in psoriatic patients related to nail psoriasis? *Clin Rheumatol* 2004; 23(1): 27–30.
30. Scarpa R, Soscia E, Peluso R, et al. Nail and distal interphalangeal joint in psoriatic arthritis. *J Rheumatol* 2006; 33(7): 1315–1319.
31. Serarslan G, Guler H, Karazincir S. The relationship between nail- and distal phalangeal bone involvement severity in patients with psoriasis. *Clin Rheumatol* 2007; 26(8): 1245–1247.
32. Tinazzi I, McGonagle D, Biasi D, et al. Preliminary evidence that subclinical enthesopathy may predict psoriatic arthritis in patients with psoriasis. *J Rheumatol* 2011; 38(12): 2691–2692.
33. Williamson L, Dalbeth N, Dockerty JL, et al. Extended report: nail disease in psoriatic arthritis—clinically important, potentially treatable and often overlooked. *Rheumatology (Oxford)* 2004; 43(6): 790–794.
34. Gudjonsson JE, Karason A, Antonsdottir AA, et al. HLA-Cw6-positive and HLA- Cw6-negative patients with psoriasis vulgaris have distinct clinical features. *J Invest Dermatol* 2002; 118(2): 362–365.
35. Henseler T. The genetics of psoriasis. *J Am Acad Dermatol* 1997; 37(2 Pt 3): S1–S11.

36. Shah KN. Diagnosis and treatment of pediatric psoriasis: current and future. *Am J Clin Dermatol* 2013; 14(3): 195–213.
37. Farber EM, Nall ML. The natural history of psoriasis in 5600 patients. *Dermatologica* 1974; 148(1): 1–18.
38. Melski JW, Stern RS. The separation of susceptibility to psoriasis from age at onset. *J Invest Dermatol* 1981; 77(6): 474–477.
39. Henseler T, Christophers E. Psoriasis of early and late onset: characterization of two types of psoriasis vulgaris. *J Am Acad Dermatol* 1985; 13(3): 450–456.
40. Nyfors A, Lemholt K. Psoriasis in children. A short review and a survey of 245 cases. *Br J Dermatol* 1975; 92(4): 437–442.
41. Farber EM, Carlsen RA. Psoriasis in childhood. *Calif Med* 1966; 105(6): 415–420.
42. Stuart P, Malick F, Nair RP, et al. Analysis of phenotypic variation in psoriasis as a function of age at onset and family history. *Arch Dermatol Res* 2002; 294(5): 207–213.
43. Duran-McKinster C, Ortiz-Solis D, Granados J, et al. Juvenile psoriatic arthritis with nail psoriasis in the absence of cutaneous lesions. *Int J Dermatol* 2000; 39(1): 32–35.
44. Zisova L, Valtchev V, Sotiriou E, et al. Onychomycosis in patients with psoriasis—a multicentre study. *Mycoses* 2012; 55(2): 143–147.
45. Staberg B, Gammeltoft M, Onsberg P. Onychomycosis in patients with psoriasis. *Acta Derm Venereol* 1983; 63(5): 436–438.
46. Wilkinson DS. Dermatitis from repeated trauma to the skin. *Am J Ind Med* 1985; 8(4–5): 307–317.
47. Hemmer W, Focke M, Wantke F, et al. Allergic contact dermatitis to artificial fingernails prepared from UV light-cured acrylates. *J Am Acad Dermatol* 1996; 35(3 Pt 1): 377–380.
48. Gould JW, Mercurio MG, Elmets CA. Cutaneous photosensitivity diseases induced by exogenous agents. *J Am Acad Dermatol* 1995; 33(4): 551–573; quiz 574–576.
49. Gilbar P, Hain A, Peereboom VM. Nail toxicity induced by cancer chemotherapy. *J Oncol Pharm Pract* 2009; 15(3): 143–155.
50. Piraccini BM, Iorizzo M, Tosti A. Drug-induced nail abnormalities. *Am J Clin Dermatol* 2003; 4(1): 31–37.
51. Robbins TO, Kouskoukis CE, Ackerman AB. Onycholysis in psoriatic nails. *Am J Dermatopathol* 1983; 5(1): 39–41.
52. Richert B, André J. Nail disorders in children: diagnosis and management. *Am J Clin Dermatol* 2011; 12(2): 101–112.
53. Dobson CM, Azurdia RM, King CM. Squamous cell carcinoma arising in a psoriatic nail bed: case report with discussion of diagnostic difficulties and therapeutic options. *Br J Dermatol* 2002; 147(1): 144–149.
54. Baran R, Dawber R, Deberker D, et al. *Diseases of the Nails and their Management*. 3rd edn. New York, NY: Blackwell Science; 2001.
55. Scher R, Daniel C. *Nails: Therapy, Diagnosis, Surgery*. 3rd edn. New York, NY: Elsevier Saunders; 2005.
56. Krull E, Zook E, Baran B, et al. *Nail Surgery; A Text and Atlas*. New York, NY: Lippincott Williams & Wilkins; 2000.
57. Grover C, Khandpur S, Reddy BS, et al. Longitudinal nail biopsy: utility in 20-nail dystrophy. *Dermatol Surg* 2003; 29(11): 1125–1129.
58. Rich P, Scher RK. Nail Psoriasis Severity Index: a useful tool for evaluation of nail psoriasis. *J Am Acad Dermatol* 2003; 49(2): 206–212.
59. Kacar N, Ergin S, Erdogan BS. The comparison of Nail Psoriasis Severity Index with a less time-consuming qualitative system. *J Eur Acad Dermatol Venereol* 2008; 22(2): 219–222.
60. Baran RL. A Nail Psoriasis Severity Index. *Br J Dermatol* 2004; 150(3): 568–569.
61. Cassell SE, Bieber JD, Rich P, et al. The modified Nail Psoriasis Severity Index: validation of an instrument to assess psoriatic nail involvement in patients with psoriatic arthritis. *J Rheumatol* 2007; 34(1): 123–129.
62. Murdan S. 1st meeting on topical drug delivery to the nail. *Expert Opin Drug Deliv* 2007; 4(4): 453–455.
63. de Berker D. Management of nail psoriasis. *Clin Exp Dermatol* 2000; 25(5): 357–362.
64. Nakamura RC, Abreu Ld, Duque-Estrada B, et al. Comparison of nail lacquer clobetasol efficacy at 0.05%, 1% and 8% in nail psoriasis treatment: prospective, controlled and randomized pilot study. *An Bras Dermatol* 2012; 87(2): 203–211.
65. Wolf R, Tur E, Brenner S. Corticosteroid-induced 'disappearing digit'. *J Am Acad Dermatol* 1990; 23(4 Pt 1): 755–756.

66. Tosti A, Piraccini BM, Cameli N, et al. Calcipotriol ointment in nail psoriasis: a controlled double-blind comparison with betamethasone dipropionate and salicylic acid. *Br J Dermatol* 1998; 139(4): 655–659.
67. Sanchez Regana M, Marquez Balbas G, Umbert Millet P. Nail psoriasis: a combined treatment with 8% clobetasol nail lacquer and tacalcitol ointment. *J Eur Acad Dermatol Venereol* 2008; 22(8): 963–969.
68. de Berker DA, Lawrence CM. A simplified protocol of steroid injection for psoriatic nail dystrophy. *Br J Dermatol* 1998; 138(1): 90–95.
69. Grover C, Bansal S, Nanda S, et al. Efficacy of triamcinolone acetonide in various acquired nail dystrophies. *J Dermatol* 2005; 32(12): 963–968.
70. Khoo BP, Giam YC. A pilot study on the role of intralesional triamcinolone acetonide in the treatment of pitted nails in children. *Singapore Med J* 2000; 41(2): 66–68.
71. Deffer TA, Goette DK. Distal phalangeal atrophy secondary to topical steroid therapy. *Arch Dermatol* 1987; 123(5): 571–572.
72. Zakeri M, Valikhani M, Mortazavi H, et al. Topical calcipotriol therapy in nail psoriasis: a study of 24 cases. *Dermatol Online J* 2005; 11(3): 5.
73. Feliciani C, Zampetti A, Forleo P, et al. Nail psoriasis: combined therapy with systemic cyclosporin and topical calcipotriol. *J Cutan Med Surg* 2004; 8(2): 122–125.
74. Rigopoulos D, Ioannides D, Prastitis N, et al. Nail psoriasis: a combined treatment using calcipotriol cream and clobetasol propionate cream. *Acta Derm Venereol* 2002; 82(2): 140.
75. Goedkoop AY, de Rie MA, Picavet DI, et al. Alefacept therapy reduces the effector T- cell population in lesional psoriatic epidermis. *Arch Dermatol Res* 2004; 295(11): 465–473.
76. Weinberg JM. An overview of infliximab, etanercept, efalizumab, and alefacept as biologic therapy for psoriasis. *Clin Ther* 2003; 25(10): 2487–2505.
77. Weinberg JM, Saini R, Tutrone WD. Biologic therapy for psoriasis—the first wave: infliximab, etanercept, efalizumab, and alefacept. *J Drugs Dermatol* 2002; 1(3): 303–310.
78. Saripalli YV, Gaspari AA. Focus on: biologics that affect therapeutic agents in dermatology. *J Drugs Dermatol* 2005; 4(2): 233–245.
79. Mehlis SL, Gordon KB. The immunology of psoriasis and biologic immunotherapy. *J Am Acad Dermatol* 2003; 49(2 Suppl): S44–S50.
80. Goffe B, Cather JC. Etanercept: an overview. *J Am Acad Dermatol* 2003; 49(2 Suppl): S105–S111.
81. Gottlieb AB. Infliximab for psoriasis. *J Am Acad Dermatol* 2003; 49(2 Suppl): S112–S117.
82. Jemec GB, Ibler KS. Treatment of nail psoriasis with TNF-α or IL12/23 inhibitors. *J Drugs Dermatol* 2012; 11(8): 939–942.
83. Luger TA, Barker J, Lambert J, et al. Sustained improvement in joint pain and nail symptoms with etanercept therapy in patients with moderate to severe psoriasis. *J Eur Acad Dermatol Venereol* 2009; 23(8): 896–904.
84. Rallis E, Stavropoulou E, Rigopoulos D, et al. Rapid response of nail psoriasis to etanercept. *J Rheumatol* 2008; 35(3): 544–545.
85. Rich P, Griffiths CE, Reich K, et al. Baseline nail disease in patients with moderate to severe psoriasis and response to treatment with infliximab during 1 year. *J Am Acad Dermatol* 2008; 58(2): 224–231.
86. Saraceno R, Pietroleonardo L, Mazzotta A, et al. TNF-α antagonists and nail psoriasis: an open, 24-week, prospective cohort study in adult patients with psoriasis. *Expert Opin Biol Ther.* 2013; 13(4):469–473.
87. Menter A, Gottlieb A, Feldman SR, et al. Guidelines of care for the management of psoriasis and psoriatic arthritis: section 1. Overview of psoriasis and guidelines of care for the treatment of psoriasis with biologics. *J Am Acad Dermatol* 2008; 58(5): 826–850.
88. Wollina U, Hansel G, Koch A, et al. Tumor necrosis factor-alpha inhibitor-induced psoriasis or psoriasiform exanthemata: first 120 cases from the literature including a series of six new patients. *Am J Clin Dermatol* 2008; 9(1): 1–14.
89. Rallis E, Kintzoglou S, Verros C. Ustekinumab for rapid treatment of nail psoriasis. *Arch Dermatol* 2010; 146(11): 1315–1316.
90. Rigopoulos D, Gregoriou S, Makris M, et al. Efficacy of ustekinumab in nail psoriasis and improvement in nail-associated quality of life in a population treated with ustekinumab for cutaneous psoriasis: an open prospective unblended study. *Dermatology* 2011; 223(4): 325–329.
91. Patsatsi A, Kyriakou A, Sotiriadis D. Ustekinumab in nail psoriasis: an open-labeled, uncontrolled, nonrandomized study. *J Dermatol Treat* 2013; 24(2): 96–100.

92. Leonardi CL. Efalizumab: an overview. *J Am Acad Dermatol* 2003; 49(2 Suppl): S98–S104.
93. Ladizinski B, Heller MM, Bhutani T, et al. Progressive multifocal leukoencephalopathy and reversible progressive leukoencephalopathy syndrome in dermatologic therapy. *J Drugs Dermatol* 2013; 12(2): e20–24.
94. Van Laborde S, Scher RK. Developments in the treatment of nail psoriasis, melanonychia striata, and onychomycosis. A review of the literature. *Dermatol Clin* 2000; 18(1): 37–46.
95. Scher RK, Stiller M, Zhu YI. Tazarotene 0.1% gel in the treatment of fingernail psoriasis: a double-blind, randomized, vehicle-controlled study. *Cutis* 2001; 68(5): 355–358.
96. Bianchi L, Soda R, Diluvio L, et al. Tazarotene 0.1% gel for psoriasis of the fingernails and toenails: an open, prospective study. *Br J Dermatol* 2003; 149(1): 207–209.
97. Rigopoulos D, Gregoriou S, Katsambas A. Treatment of psoriatic nails with tazarotene cream 0.1% vs. clobetasol propionate 0.05% cream: a double-blind study. *Acta Derm Venereol* 2007; 87(2): 167–168.
98. Roenigk RK, Gibstine C, Roenigk HH, Jr. Oral isotretinoin followed by psoralens and ultraviolet A or ultraviolet B for psoriasis. *J Am Acad Dermatol* 1985; 13(1): 153–155.
99. Lebwohl M. Acitretin in combination with UVB or PUVA. *J Am Acad Dermatol* 1999; 41(3 Pt 2): S22–S24.
100. Moy RL, Kingston TP, Lowe NJ. Isotretinoin vs. etretinate therapy in generalized pustular and chronic psoriasis. *Arch Dermatol* 1985; 121(10): 1297–1301.
101. Brazzelli V, Martinoli S, Prestinari F, et al. An impressive therapeutic result of nail psoriasis to acitretin. *J Eur Acad Dermatol Venereol* 2004; 18(2): 229–230.
102. Mahrle G, Schulze HJ, Farber L, et al. Low-dose short-term cyclosporine versus etretinate in psoriasis: improvement of skin, nail, and joint involvement. *J Am Acad Dermatol* 1995; 32(1): 78–88.
103. Tosti A, Ricotti C, Romanelli P, et al. Evaluation of the efficacy of acitretin therapy for nail psoriasis. *Arch Dermatol* 2009; 145(3): 269–271.
104. Lebwohl M, Ali S. Treatment of psoriasis. Part 2. Systemic therapies. *J Am Acad Dermatol* 2001; 45(5): 649–661; quiz 62–64.
105. Murdan S. Drug delivery to the nail following topical application. *Int J Pharm* 2002; 236(1–2): 1–26.
106. Schissel DJ, Elston DM. Topical 5-fluorouracil treatment for psoriatic trachyonychia. *Cutis* 1998; 62(1): 27–28.
107. Fredriksson T. Psoriatic nails and 5-fluorouracil. *J Am Acad Dermatol* 1982; 6(1): 117.
108. de Jong EM, Menke HE, van Praag MC, et al. Dystrophic psoriatic fingernails treated with 1% 5-fluorouracil in a nail penetration-enhancing vehicle: a double-blind study. *Dermatology* 1999; 199(4): 313–318.
109. Schmied E, Levy PM. Transient rhabdomyolysis connected with topical use of 5-fluorouracil in a patient with psoriasis of the nails. *Dermatologica* 1986; 173(5): 257–258.
110. Gerster JC, Hohl D. Nail lesions in psoriatic arthritis: recovery with sulfasalazine treatment. *Ann Rheum Dis* 2002; 61(3): 277.
111. Yamamoto T, Katayama I, Nishioka K. Topical anthralin therapy for refractory nail psoriasis. *J Dermatol* 1998; 25(4): 231–233.
112. Marx JL, Scher RK. Response of psoriatic nails to oral photochemotherapy. *Arch Dermatol* 1980; 116(9): 1023–1024.
113. Aubin F, Vigan M, Puzenat E, et al. Evaluation of a novel 308-nm monochromatic excimer light delivery system in dermatology: a pilot study in different chronic localized dermatoses. *Br J Dermatol* 2005; 152(1): 99–103.
114. Treewittayapoom C, Singvahanont P, Chanprapaph K, et al. The effect of different pulse durations in the treatment of nail psoriasis with 595-nm pulsed dye laser: a randomized, double-blind, intrapatient left-to-right study. *J Am Acad Dermatol* 2012; 66(5): 807–812.

Chapter 17

Dietary Therapy for Psoriasis: Protein-Restricted Diets

Whitney A. Fisk, Ethan C. Levin, Judith Hong, and John Y. M. Koo

INTRODUCTION

One of the most frequent questions posed by patients with psoriasis is what role, if any, diet plays in psoriasis and whether there are specific dietary recommendations that can enhance psoriasis treatment or improve psoriasis as an alternative to traditional medication. There are no consensus recommendations regarding dietary therapy nor have there been any large controlled studies. Some patients report that weight-reducing diets [1] and gluten-free diets have been helpful [2,3]. This chapter focuses on the role of protein restriction in dietary therapy for psoriasis.

EPIDEMIOLOGIC RESEARCH

Epidemiologic data from the past half-century suggest that there might be an association between dietary protein intake and psoriasis. Per capita meat consumption has steadily risen since the 1960s in the United States [4], and the annual incidence of psoriasis has nearly doubled in this time [5,6]. This association is confounded by a concurrent increase in obesity, which can make psoriasis worse and harder to treat.

However, in Japan, obesity rates have only slightly increased over the same period, whereas both meat consumption and psoriasis rates have increased more dramatically. Since the 1960s, the Japanese diet has become increasingly "westernized," and per capita meat consumption has risen considerably [7–9]. Similarly, during this period, the incidence of psoriasis has increased—the prevalence was estimated to be <1% in the 1960s [7] and is now almost 5% [10]. Importantly, the rates of obesity (defined as body mass index [BMI] >30) have not precipitously risen in Japan [11] since the 1960s. According to the National Obesity Society, in 2005, 34.3% of the adult U.S. population was obese compared with only 3.9% of the adult Japanese population. These data are consistent with the hypothesis that meat consumption may contribute to or exacerbate psoriasis. However, there are other factors that may influence the prevalence of psoriasis, including other dietary habits (e.g., ethanol consumption) or better detection of the disease.

CLINICAL RESEARCH

In the 1960s, researchers reported significant improvement in psoriatic plaques when patients were placed on low-protein diets and low-tryptophan diets [12–17]. For example, one case series reported that several patients with generalized psoriasis nearly cleared after several weeks on a low-tryptophan diet [17]. Tryptophan is one of 20 amino acids that can compose protein. Low-protein diets and amino acid–restricted diets lost favor in the late 1960s after further studies failed to find a therapeutic benefit in psoriasis patients [15]. However, there were critical flaws in study methodology. In fact, one study reported using turkey as a primary component of a low-tryptophan diet [16]. It is now known that turkey is a tryptophan-rich food.

More recent clinical studies suggest that protein-restricted diets may improve psoriasis (Table 17.1). Five dietary plans are included in these studies: a vegetarian diet (n = 1) [18], a low-energy diet (n = 1) [19], a low-protein diet (n = 4) [20–23], and a taurine-restricted diet (n = 1) [24]. In six of seven studies, the study investigators concluded that improvement in psoriasis was at least due in part to a low-protein diet. Only one study restricted intake of a specific amino acid. This study reported improvement in psoriasis in those patients on a taurine-deficient diet who were limited to <40 g of total protein/day [24]. Taurine is frequently referred to as an amino acid, even though it is actually a derivative of the amino acid cysteine [25].

Several interesting observations can be made in reviewing the available clinical data. The quantity and source of protein may both affect control of psoriasis. Nonanimal sources of protein did not inhibit therapeutic effects. Red meat was more likely to precipitate symptoms than poultry or fish [21,22]. The success of the diets appeared to be independent of total calorie restriction and weight loss. None of the studies reported significant weight loss associated with improvement of psoriasis, including a study that specifically restricted total calories [19]. These results must be interpreted cautiously as many of the reviewed studies included multiple interventions or allowed participants to use other antipsoriasis therapies.

BASIC SCIENCE RESEARCH

Possible mechanisms through which protein restriction may improve psoriasis have been investigated in nonclinical studies. Decades ago, low-protein diets were hypothesized to improve psoriasis by depriving keratinocytes of amino acids. Recent research suggests several alternative explanations. Low-protein diets are associated with suppression of systemic inflammation, angiogenesis, and oxidative stress [1,26]. Each of these factors might contribute to improvement of psoriasis. Furthermore, restricting the availability of a single amino acid induces a physiologic state of altered gene expression called the "amino acid starvation response" or "amino acid response" (AAR) that suppresses specific inflammatory cascades [27,28].

TOTAL PROTEIN RESTRICTION AND ANIMAL PROTEIN RESTRICTION

Restricting total protein intake may improve psoriasis by suppressing systemic inflammation and inhibiting angiogenesis, thereby creating an environment in which psoriasis is less easily triggered and is more responsive to therapy.

TABLE 17.1 Summary of Dietary Clinical Studies

Publication; Study Design	No. of Patients; Disease Severity	Intervention(s)	Results	Limitations
Brown 2004; Prospective Case Series	5; Baseline PASI: 2.3–37.0	Low-protein diet without red meat	PASI-50 reached after 6 months, average improvement, 18.2–8.7	Dietary compliance self-reported and differed between subjects Use of topical medications permitted
Festugato 2011; uncontrolled clinical trial	43; not reported	Low-protein diet with limited red meat	88% of participants improved in redness, scaling, time between outbreaks, and quality of life after 2-year study	Dietary compliance not described; use of topical medications and PUVA permitted
Rucevic 2003; uncontrolled clinical trial	82; hospitalized patients with >30% BSA involvement	(1) 40 g protein/day without animal protein (2) 90 g protein/day (control)	After 4 weeks, psoriasis significantly improved in treatment group (p value not reported)	Subjects not randomly assigned; nonstandard method of assessing psoriasis (assessed with 3-point scale)
Lithel 1983; uncontrolled clinical trial	20; hospitalized patients with psoriasis ($n = 10$), rosacea, or atopic eczema	Low-energy diet followed by a vegan/low-protein diet (9% calories from protein, no animal protein)	Psoriasis patients improved during 3-week vegan diet but did not improve during 2-week fasting period	Baseline psoriasis severity not reported objectively with PASI or BSA
Zackheim 1969; Prospective Case Series	13; hospitalized patients with baseline BSA <50% ($n = 3$), ≥50% ($n = 10$)	(1) Low-protein diet (4–11 g/day) (2) High-protein diet (up to 162 g/day)	Patients improved on all diets, and low-protein diet did not appear superior to high-protein diet (p value not reported)	Results may not be generalizable to patients with less severe disease
Roe 1965; uncontrolled clinical trial	15; baseline BSA <5% ($n = 8$), >5% ($n = 7$)	Low taurine[a] diet (i.e., limited animal protein)	After 2 months, nine patients reported clearing and six patients reported disease improvement	Dietary compliance self-reported; concurrent therapy and other confounding variables such as weight loss were not reported

[a] Taurine is a derivative of the amino acid cysteine that is found in most animal meat.
BSA, body surface area.

Suppression of inflammation

Consumption of animal protein is associated with increased serum concentrations of several proinflammatory agents (e.g., interleukin-6 and tumor necrosis factor) and markers of inflammation (e.g., C-reactive protein [26,29]. The fatty acid profile of poultry and red meat, characterized by a high ratio of omega-6 to omega-3 fatty acids, may contribute to this proinflammatory effect [30,31]. Epidemiologic research correlates long-term diets high in red meat with increased markers of oxidative stress, independent of weight, BMI, or waist circumference [32]. Thus, increased systemic inflammation caused by high-protein meals may contribute to psoriatic disease.

One potential proinflammatory compound in red meat is a monosaccharide known as Neu5Gc. Neu5Gc accumulates in tissues after excess consumption of meat and dairy and is thought to be immunogenic [33,34]. When meat is consumed regularly, it may lead to low levels of chronic inflammation that may increase the risk for autoimmune disease and cancer [33,34]. Psoriasis patients are at increased baseline risk for some malignancies, including nonmelanoma skin cancers, lymphoma, and esophageal cancer, and this risk increases with more severe disease [35]. Thus, by reducing meat intake, psoriasis patients may decrease systemic inflammation, improve psoriasis, and possibly decrease cancer risk. However, the role of Neu5Gc in psoriasis has not been specifically examined.

Suppression of angiogenesis

In addition to its proinflammatory effects, excess consumption of animal protein may enhance angiogenesis, a pathologic component of both psoriasis and cancer [36]. Increased angiogenesis in psoriatic plaques is needed for keratinocyte hyperproliferation and recruitment of lymphocytes, neutrophils, and dendritic cells. The angiogenic mediators insulin-like growth factor 1 (IGF-1) [37, 38–40] and vascular endothelial growth factor (VEGF) [40] are shown to increase after high-protein meals. IGF-1 facilitates angiogenesis in several ways, including increasing the sensitivity of endothelial cells to VEGF [39,40]. Animal proteins have a unique ability to raise serum IGF-1 levels through upregulated hepatic synthesis and enhanced glucose-dependent insulin secretion [41]. Epidemiologic studies show an association between animal protein consumption and increased IGF-1 levels [42–44].

Interestingly, dietary factors, when consumed in normal amounts, can markedly affect pathologic angiogenesis [45]. Anti-angiogenic foods, such as cruciferous vegetables, are associated with decreased cancer risk [45]. Cruciferous vegetables contain phytochemicals that have anti-angiogenic properties, including inhibiting endothelial cell proliferation. Importantly, dietary factors have not been shown to suppress angiogenesis required for normal tissue metabolism [45].

Therapies that suppress angiogenesis may also improve psoriasis [46,47]. Psoriasis symptoms have been reported to clear completely in cancer patients treated with bevacizumab and improve significantly with sunitinib and sorafenib; all of these drugs are VEGF antagonists used for cancer chemotherapy [46,47]. Several other therapies are being investigated, including VEGF receptor mimics and a topical tyrosine kinase inhibitor with anti-angiogenesis action [47].

AMINO ACID RESTRICTION

Amino acid–restricted diets are a type of low-protein diet that limits intake of a specific amino acid. Dietary proteins are composed of varying proportions of 20 amino acids [48]. Protein from animal meat is considered complete or high-quality protein because it contains significant amounts of all 20 amino acids. Protein supplied by vegetables, grain, nuts, and legumes may be deficient in one or more amino acids. These foods also contain a significantly smaller proportion of calories from protein compared with animal protein. For example, rice contains minimal concentrations of lysine, and legumes provide limited quantities of methionine [48]. Diets limited in any amino acid would require elimination of meat and dairy.

Despite the minimal clinical evidence evaluating the benefits of amino acid–restricted diets, two recent developments support their potential role in treating psoriasis: (1) the discovery of the T-helper (Th)17 cell [49] and (2) the anti-inflammatory effect of limiting amino acid availability [27,28].

When specific amino acids are unavailable or scarce, the body enters a protective mode of decreased gene expression called AAR [27,28]. AAR includes decreased expression of cytokines that are characteristic of inflammatory pathways [50]. Th17 differentiation is suppressed, and regulatory T-cell function that protects against autoimmune disease is enhanced [51,52]. Psoriasis patients are shown to have functionally deficient regulatory T cells that likely contribute to disease progression [53]. Thus, dietary restriction of amino acids may be one method of normalizing function of regulatory T cells. Other immune cells, including Th1 and Th2 cells, are not affected by the amino acid response, suggesting that vital immune functions are preserved in this state [50]. The AAR has been demonstrated by limiting several different amino acids, including tryptophan, methionine, and leucine [54].

Given that the AAR appears to specifically affect the Th17 pathway, triggering this response with a pharmacologic agent could be therapeutic for psoriasis patients. A molecule called halofuginone has been developed that induces a state of altered gene expression characteristic of amino acid depletion [53,54]. In animal models, this molecule improves autoimmune disease [50], but it has not yet been studied in human subjects.

CLINICAL APPLICATION

Low-protein diets, especially those limited in animal protein and red meat, may be beneficial for some psoriasis patients. Evidence from nonclinical studies suggests that diets deficient in one or more amino acids may be especially therapeutic due to induction of the AAR. Such a diet would permit most fruits and vegetables, some legumes and grains, and exclude all animal protein and dairy.

Future studies are needed before amino acid–restricted diets can be recommended. However, these diets may be particularly suitable for patients who do not respond to conventional therapies. It is known that previously failed therapies can become effective when used with or after an immunomodulating medication. For patients who do not respond to therapy, amino acid restriction may sufficiently weaken proinflammatory stimuli to allow conventional therapies to take effect. Later, dietary restriction may be replaced by more conventional therapy.

Dietary modification should be monitored closely in psoriasis patients because metabolic syndrome and other comorbidities are common in this population. Low-protein diets can be high in refined carbohydrates that would be inappropriate for diabetic patients. Involvement of a nutritionist can ensure that patients are consuming a healthy and balanced low-protein diet.

CONCLUSIONS

Decreased total protein intake may suppress systemic inflammation, oxidative stress, and angiogenesis, all of which contribute to disease severity. Amino acid restriction may specifically inhibit Th17 cells, cells that are critically involved in driving psoriatic inflammation. Clinical studies assessing the role of low-protein diets in psoriasis are limited, and further research is needed to demonstrate which dietary modification strategies are reliably therapeutic in psoriasis patients.

REFERENCES

1. Wolters M. Diet and psoriasis: experimental data and clinical evidence. *Br J Dermatol* 2005;153:706–14.
2. Michaelsson G, Ahs S, Hammarstrom I, Lundin IP, Hagforsen E. Gluten-free diet in psoriasis patients with antibodies to gliadin results in decreased expression of tissue transglutaminase and fewer Ki67+ cells in the dermis. *Acta Derm Venereol Suppl* 2003;83:425–9.
3. Michaelsson G, Gerden B, Hagforsen E, Nilsson B, Pihl-Lundin I, Kraaz W, et al. Psoriasis patients with antibodies to gliadin can be improved by a gluten-free diet. *Br J Dermatol* 2000;142:44–51.
4. Daniel CR, Cross AJ, Koebnick C, Sinha R. Trends in meat consumption in the USA. *Public Health Nutr* 2011;14:575–83.
5. Icen M, Crowson CS, McEvoy MT, Dann FJ, Gabriel SE, Maradit Kremers H. Trends in incidence of adult-onset psoriasis over three decades: a population-based study. *J Am Acad Dermatol* 2009;60:394–401.
6. Cordain L, Eaton SB, Sebastian A, Mann N, Lindeberg S, Watkins BA, et al. Origins and evolution of the Western diet: health implications for the 21st century. *Am J Clin Nutr* 2005;81:341–54.
7. Aoki T, Yoshikawa K. Psoriasis in Japan. *Arch Dermatol* 1971;104:328–9.
8. Kromhout D, Keys A, Aravanis C, Buzina R, Fidanza F, Giampaoli S, et al. Food consumption patterns in the 1960s in seven countries. *Am J Clin Nutr* 1989;49:889–94.
9. Akter S, Nanri A, Pham NM, Kurotani K, Mizoue T. Dietary patterns and metabolic syndrome in a Japanese working population. *Nutr Metabol* 2013;10:30.
10. Furue M, Yamazaki S, Jimbow K, Tsuchida T, Amagai M, Tanaka T, et al. Prevalence of dermatological disorders in Japan: a nationwide, cross-sectional, seasonal, multicenter, hospital-based study. *J Dermatol* 2011;38:310–20.
11. Obesity: preventing and managing the global epidemic. Report of a WHO consultation. *World Health Organ Techl Rep Ser* 2000;894:i–xii, 1–253.
12. Caplan RM. The low-tryptophan diet in psoriasis. *J Am Med Assoc* 1969;207:758.
13. Carruthers R. Low tryptophan diet in the treatment of psoriasis. *Med J Aust* 1968;1:493–5.
14. Ellis JP, Sanderson KV, Savin JA. The turkey diet in psoriasis. *Lancet* 1968;1:1429–30.
15. Petrozzi JW, Rosenbloom J. Low-tryptophan diet in treatment of psoriasis. *J Am Med Assoc* 1968;205:345–6.
16. Spiera H, Lefkovits AM. Turkey, tryptophan, and psoriasis. *Lancet* 1967;2:1418.
17. Spiera H, Lefkovits AM. Remission of psoriasis with low dietary tryptophan. *Lancet* 1967;2:137–9.

18. Lithell H, Bruce A, Gustafsson IB, Hoglund NJ, Karlstrom B, Ljunghall K, et al. A fasting and vegetarian diet treatment trial on chronic inflammatory disorders. *Acta Derm Venereol Suppl* 1983;63:397–403.
19. Rucevic I, Perl A, Barisic-Drusko V, Adam-Perl M. The role of the low energy diet in psoriasis vulgaris treatment. *Coll Antropol* 2003;27 (Suppl 1):41–8.
20. Zackheim HS, Farber EM. Low-protein diet and psoriasis. A hospital study. *Arch Dermatol* 1969;99:580–6.
21. Lerner MR, Lerner AB. Psoriasis and protein intake. *Arch Dermatol* 1964;90:217–25.
22. Brown AC, Hairfield M, Richards DG, McMillin DL, Mein EA, Nelson CD. Medical nutrition therapy as a potential complementary treatment for psoriasis – five case reports. *Altern Med Rev: J Clin Therapeut* 2004;9:297–307.
23. Festugato M. Pilot study on which foods should be avoided by patients with psoriasis. *An Bras Dermatol* 2011;86:1103–8.
24. Roe DA. Nutrient requirements in psoriasis. *NY State J Med* 1965;65:1319–26.
25. Yamori Y, Taguchi T, Hamada A, Kunimasa K, Mori H, Mori M. Taurine in health and diseases: consistent evidence from experimental and epidemiological studies. *Br J Biomed Sci* 2010;17 (Suppl 1):S6.
26. Montonen J, Boeing H, Fritsche A, Schleicher E, Joost HG, Schulze MB, et al. Consumption of red meat and whole-grain bread in relation to biomarkers of obesity, inflammation, glucose metabolism and oxidative stress. *Eur J Nutr* 2013;52:337–45.
27. Chu TL, Guan Q, Nguan CY, Du C. Halofuginone suppresses T cell proliferation by blocking proline uptake and inducing cell apoptosis. *Int Immunopharm* 2013;16:414–23.
28. Tsalikis J, Croitoru DO, Philpott DJ, Girardin SE. Nutrient sensing and metabolic stress pathways in innate immunity. *Cell Microbiol* 2013;15(10):1632–41.
29. Barbaresko J, Koch M, Schulze MB, Nothlings U. Dietary pattern analysis and biomarkers of low-grade inflammation: a systematic literature review. *Nutr Rev* 2013;71:511–27.
30. Calder PC. n-3 polyunsaturated fatty acids, inflammation, and inflammatory diseases. *Am J Clin Nutr* 2006;83:1505S–19S.
31. Calder PC. Polyunsaturated fatty acids, inflammatory processes and inflammatory bowel diseases. *Mol Nutr Food Res* 2008;52:885–97.
32. Meyer KA, Sijtsma FP, Nettleton JA, Steffen LM, Van Horn L, Shikany JM, et al. Dietary patterns are associated with plasma F(2)-isoprostanes in an observational cohort study of adults. *Free Radic Biol Med* 2013;57:201–9.
33. Hedlund M, Padler-Karavani V, Varki NM, Varki A. Evidence for a human-specific mechanism for diet and antibody-mediated inflammation in carcinoma progression. *Proc Natl Acad Sci USA* 2008;105:18936–41.
34. Padler-Karavani V, Yu H, Cao H, Chokhawala H, Karp F, Varki N, et al. Diversity in specificity, abundance, and composition of anti-Neu5Gc antibodies in normal humans: potential implications for disease. *Glycobiology* 2008;18:818–30.
35. Beyaert R, Beaugerie L, Van Assche G, Brochez L, Renauld JC, Viguier M et al. Cancer risk in immune-mediated inflammatory diseases: IMID and Cancer Risk. *Molecular cancer* 2013;12:98.
36. Heidenreich R, Rocken M, Ghoreschi K. Angiogenesis drives psoriasis pathogenesis. *Int J Exp Pathol* 2009;90:232–48.
37. Smith WJ, Underwood LE, Clemmons DR. Effects of caloric or protein restriction on insulin-like growth factor-I (IGF-I) and IGF-binding proteins in children and adults. *J Clin Endocrinol Metabol* 1995;80:443–9.
38. Crowe FL, Key TJ, Allen NE, Appleby PN, Roddam A, Overvad K, et al. The association between diet and serum concentrations of IGF-I, IGFBP-1, IGFBP-2, and IGFBP-3 in the European Prospective Investigation into Cancer and Nutrition. *Cancer Epidemiol Biomarkers Prev* 2009;18:1333–40.
39. Dunn SE. Insulin-like growth factor I stimulates angiogenesis and the production of vascular endothelial growth factor. *Growth Horm IGF Res* 2000;10 (Suppl A):S41–2.
40. Kwon YW, Kwon KS, Moon HE, Park JA, Choi KS, Kim YS, et al. Insulin-like growth factor-II regulates the expression of vascular endothelial growth factor by the human keratinocyte cell line HaCaT. *J Investig Dermatol* 2004;123:152–8.
41. McCarty MF. A wholly nutritional 'multifocal angiostatic therapy' for control of disseminated cancer. *Med Hypotheses* 2003;61:1–15.

42. Young NJ, Metcalfe C, Gunnell D, Rowlands MA, Lane JA, Gilbert R, et al. A cross-sectional analysis of the association between diet and insulin-like growth factor (IGF)-I, IGF-II, IGF-binding protein (IGFBP)-2, and IGFBP-3 in men in the United Kingdom. *Canc Causes Contr* 2012;23:907–17.
43. Vrieling A, Voskuil DW, Bueno de Mesquita HB, Kaaks R, van Noord PA, Keinan-Boker L, et al. Dietary determinants of circulating insulin-like growth factor (IGF)-I and IGF binding proteins 1, -2 and -3 in women in the Netherlands. *Canc Causes Contr* 2004;15:787–96.
44. Lemozy S, Pucilowska JB, Underwood LE. Reduction of insulin-like growth factor-I (IGF-I) in protein-restricted rats is associated with differential regulation of IGF-binding protein messenger ribonucleic acids in liver and kidney, and peptides in liver and serum. *Endocrinology* 1994;135:617–23.
45. Li WW, Li VW, Hutnik M, Chiou AS. Tumor angiogenesis as a target for dietary cancer prevention. *J Oncol* 2012;2012:879623.
46. Akman A, Yilmaz E, Mutlu H, Ozdogan M. Complete remission of psoriasis following bevacizumab therapy for colon cancer. *Clin Exp Dermatol* 2009;34:e202–4.
47. Crawshaw AA, Griffiths CE, Young HS. Investigational VEGF antagonists for psoriasis. *Expet Opin Investig Drugs* 2012;21:33–43.
48. Elango R, Ball RO, Pencharz PB. Amino acid requirements in humans: with a special emphasis on the metabolic availability of amino acids. *Amino Acids* 2009;37:19–27.
49. Nwe SM, Champlain AH, Gordon KB. Rationale and early clinical data on IL-17 blockade in psoriasis. *Expet Rev Clin Immunol* 2013;9:677–82.
50. Sundrud MS, Koralov SB, Feuerer M, Calado DP, Kozhaya AE, Rhule-Smith A, et al. Halofuginone inhibits TH17 cell differentiation by activating the amino acid starvation response. *Science* 2009;324:1334–8.
51. Cobbold SP, Adams E, Farquhar CA, Nolan KF, Howie D, Lui KO, et al. Infectious tolerance via the consumption of essential amino acids and mTOR signaling. *Proc Natl Acad Sci USA* 2009;106:12055–60.
52. Waldmann H, Cobbold S. Regulatory T cells: context matters. *Immunity* 2009;30:613–5.
53. Soler DC, Sugiyama H, Young AB, Massari JV, McCormick TS, Cooper KD. Psoriasis patients exhibit impairment of the high potency CCR5 T regulatory cell subset. *Clin Immunol* 2013;149:111–8
54. Gallinetti J, Harputlugil E, Mitchell JR. Amino acid sensing in dietary-restriction-mediated longevity: roles of signal-transducing kinases GCN2 and TOR. *Biochem J* 2013;449:1–10.

INDEX